CHILDREN with TOURETTE SYNDROME

A Parents' Guide

Edited by Tracy Lynne Marsh

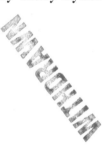

Woodbine House ∷ 2007

Published in the United States of America by Woodbine House, Inc., 6510 Bells Mill Rd.,
Bethesda, MD 20817. 800-843-7323. www.woodbinehouse.com

Cover art by Nancy Bea Miller (www.nancybeamiller.com)

Photographs on pages 128, 248, 292, 295, and 309 are courtesy of JuliAnne Jonker,
Jonker Portrait Gallery.

Photographs on pages 16, 64, 116, 168, 170, 182, 262, 281, and 304 are courtesy of
Mike Gandrud.

Library of Congress Cataloging-in-Publication Data

Children with Tourette syndrome : a parents' guide / edited by Tracy Haerle. -- 2nd ed.
   p. cm.
 Includes bibliographical references and index.
 ISBN-13: 978-1-890627-36-2 (pbk.)
 1. Tourette syndrome in children--Popular works. I. Haerle, Tracy.
 RJ496.T68C45 2007
 618.92'83--dc22

                                     2006032676

Published in the United States of America

10 9 8 7 6 5 4 3 2

This book is dedicated to my children,

Katie and Jeff.

*Without them I would have never
had the passion to put together this book
or the wisdom and understanding I have gained
by raising a child with Tourette Syndrome.*

TABLE

OF

CONTENTS

ACKNOWLEDGEMENTS

Many people were more than generous with their time, their expertise, and their support in the development of this book. I was so impressed with and appreciative of the generosity of our chapter authors in the first edition of this book. Now, after fifteen years, I was again pleasantly surprised that the chapter authors were ready to do it again! I want to thank every one of these chapter authors for making time in their busy schedules to revise their original chapters:

Larry Burd	Jim Eisenreich
Patricia Furer	Carl R. Hansen
Robin Jewers	Marilynn Kaplan
Sonja D. Kerr	Rosanne B. Papadopoulos
William V. Rubin	Gary Shady
Rox Wand	

We have added some new chapter authors. Dr. Jacob Kerbeshian is a board certified child and adolescent psychiatrist who is Clinical Professor of Neuroscience at the University of North Dakota School of Medicine and Health Sciences. He also practices medicine at the Altru Health System in Grand Forks, ND. He has updated our chapter on "Medical Treatments and Healthcare Professionals." I am so thankful that he was available and so willing to get the word out on TS treatments.

Another new chapter author is John Piacentini, Ph.D. He has written a new chapter on the newer area of treatment for tic disorders called "Behavior Therapies for Tourette Syndrome." This is thought-provoking new information and presented in a way that is very easy to understand.

Thanks go to Lisa Barrett Mann, who worked closely with me in editing chapters. Lisa's personal fingerprint is evident throughout the book. I so much appreciated her personal knowledge of the issues, and am also grateful to her son with TS and Asperger syndrome, who is surely responsible for giving her such a passion for all she knows on the subject. The revisions couldn't have been done without her.

I also want to thank Susan Stokes for her continued hard work through all the years and to the rest of the Woodbine House staff for all the things they do behind the scenes.

After years of being out of Tourette syndrome advocacy, I am very thankful to my friends in the TS community for opening up and helping me get back in the swing of things. Leslie Packer, Ph.D., has been a friend of mine throughout the years, and all the support and advice she offered as I started the revision was amazing. As busy as she is, she found time to help me solicit parent statements for the book, and she "advertised" the book revision on her very successful website on TS (which is listed in our Resource Guide at the back of this book). My friends at the Minnesota Tourette Syndrome Association were also very helpful in finding parent statements and were supportive of this work.

I would also like to recognize Mike Gandrud, whom I first met when he was a boy attending Minnesota Tourette Syndrome Family Camp. Mike was always very active in camp, eventually becoming a counselor, and always taking pictures. Thanks to Mike for many of the pictures in this edition. Thanks also to Julieann Jonker, from Jonker Portrait Gallery, for contributing many great photos. She is not only a world renowned photographer, but also my sister and the parent of a son with TS. In addition, thanks to all the parents of children with TS and adults with TS who shared pictures of themselves and their families.

Finally, I would like to thank my family for being so open and willing to share our family life with others. It goes without saying that if it weren't for them, I would never have been inspired to join in the crusade for better information, support, and services for people with Tourette syndrome, and this book would never have been written.

FOREWORD

Jim Eisenreich

Back in 1984, my dream of playing professional baseball almost came to an end. Only two years into my career with the Minnesota Twins, the motor and vocal tics I'd had since I was six became so pronounced that I sometimes had to leave the field in the middle of an inning. I was bounced from one doctor to another and was treated for problems that I didn't have. It was a nightmare.

Fortunately, I eventually received the correct diagnosis—Tourette syndrome—and proper treatment allowed me to once again lead a normal life.

I completed my baseball career in 1998 with the Los Angeles Dodgers. That added up to nearly fourteen years in the major leagues with five different teams—the Twins, Royals, Phillies, Marlins, and Dodgers—including two trips to the World Series, and a bunch of wonderful experiences. The 1997 Marlins gave me my World Series Championship.

I'm now retired from baseball. My wife, Leann, and I have four children and are busy raising them and running them to their various activities.

I still travel and speak to many children and families who are getting diagnosed with Tourette for the first time, and I check in with others I first met years ago. And the news is good: children are being diagnosed earlier, and there are more effective treatments becoming available every day.

I feel we have come a long way in our effort to create awareness for those who didn't understand Tourette syndrome. We still want to go further down the road, but a lot of people who come in contact with our kids—doctors, teachers, counselors, politicians, and most importantly, our families and friends—have really accepted us for who we are, and not what problem we have.

Research seems to be right on the doorstep of finding a cure. Wouldn't that be wonderful?

Until the happy day when a cure is found, enjoy this second edition of *Children with Tourette Syndrome: A Parents' Guide.* When you have Tourette syndrome, one of the most important things you can do is educate yourself and others about the disorder. This book provides a great deal of useful information and does so in understandable terms. It also depicts the very broad range of Tourette syndrome, from almost unnoticeable symptoms to those that are quite visible and severe. Share it with people who may not know yet what Tourette is (or what it's not).

We have come a long way. Let's keep going.

INTRODUCTION

Tracy Marsh

The first time I heard the words "Tourette Syndrome" was the day my seven-year-old son was diagnosed by a pediatric neurologist in 1987. We had been searching for answers to our son's puzzling behavior since he was a toddler.

At that time, information on Tourette Syndrome (TS) or any neurobiological disorder was hard to come by. I began searching through medical research articles and the few scholarly texts available to me (remember, this was before most families had Internet access). Also, I became involved with the Tourette Syndrome Association, attended a support group, and started helping other families navigate the maze of issues that we had experienced. I found myself writing articles for teachers and parents, translating the scholarly material into layman's language to help caretakers of children with TS better understand the disorder. As I learned about how misunderstood children with Tourette syndrome were, it became my passion to increase public awareness about the condition and to make this world a better place for children and adults with TS. This led me to put together the first edition of **Children with Tourette Syndrome**—the first book especially for parents of children with TS to bring together a variety of experts on school, medical, family, and legal issues with the goal of helping families anticipate, prevent, and deal with common problems.

It has been fifteen years since the first edition of this book was published. There is now much more information available on Tourette syndrome and other neurobiological disorders of childhood! It is exciting to search the Internet and see the many websites and online articles that provide information and support to all members of the family and all age groups. Still, with all the information available, it can be overwhelming to know what to trust, especially when you need some basic information and fast. Anyone can say anything on the Internet, so where do you go and whom do you trust? Clearly, parents still need a trustworthy source of basic information that will give them the background knowledge they need to evaluate the conflicting advice they may encounter. We hope that this revised edition of **Children with Tourette Syndrome** will be that trustworthy source for you, and that it will make your introduction into the world of TS less stressful for your family than it was for mine.

Our aim with this book is to provide basic facts about how TS can affect all areas of a child's life, to help prepare your family for the challenges ahead. One important point I need to make very clear: no two children with TS have exactly the same symptoms. The majority of people with TS have mild tics that may worsen through the adolescent years and then diminish to the point where they no longer interfere or cause any concern. Other people have more moderate to severe tics that may persist throughout life. Besides the great variety in tic severity is the added dimension of "associated disorders" that often accompany TS. As you are reading this book, please do not worry that your child will develop problems that are not already present. Although we need to cover all levels of severity of symptoms in the book, that does not mean that your child will have all of these symptoms or any at all. If your child does have some of these symptoms, hopefully the information we provide will help guide your family to some good treatments.

Chapters cover medical, educational, legal, family life, daily care, newer behavior training methods, and emotional issues as they apply to children from first diagnosis through adolescence. We also provide a look at what can be expected in the future. You will notice that I've used the personal pronouns "he" and "she" alternately by chapter. Although more boys than girls have Tourette syndrome, I didn't want to imply that all children with TS are boys, and it can be cumbersome to constantly use "he or she" to refer to a child.

New to this revised edition is a chapter on habit reversal training, a behavioral method of treatment that is being used more frequently to help children and adults control their tics. The medical chapter covers all the newer medicines now available, with in-depth explanations of what symptoms they address. The legal chapter covers the latest updates to important laws that apply to children with TS and other disabilities, especially in education law. One exciting new law change is something that myself and a few other parents of children with TS started advocating for in the late 1980s. Children with TS were not being served properly in the public school systems because they were not being properly labeled for special education services. All too frequently, children with TS were being labeled as having EBD (Emotional Behavior Disorder), which did not meet the needs of students who had a neurological impairment. We talked to the state department of education and we went to senators from the education committee in our state (Minnesota), advocating for children with TS to be classified under OHI (Other Health Impaired) instead. People looked at us like we were "crazy housewives." Even other school advocates disagreed with us. It is so exciting to see these changes in the law finally implemented, and at the federal level! It really taught me the value of fighting for what you believe is right, even when no one will listen to you.

We also have added many new Parent Statements to this revised edition. (Parent Statements are quotations at the ends of the chapters in which parents share their feelings, thoughts, and experiences. Parent statements contain nuggets of practical advice and can help you realize you are not in this alone.) Some of the new Parent Statements reflect the fact that many older children with TS are doing much better than they were fifteen years ago. With more knowledge about TS in the schools and the general public, children with TS are increasingly being accepted and allowed the freedom and support to achieve their personal goals. I have also included a glossary at the back of the book to help you decipher medical and educational jargon you may come across.

Just as we stated in the first edition of **Children with Tourette Syndrome,** we do not intend this book to be the final authority on TS. There is ongoing research (much of it funded by the Tourette Syndrome Association) into causes and treatments such as better medications, and ultimately to find a cure for TS. Please use the Book List at the end of the book for suggestions on other publications with valuable information. Also, you should contact the National Tourette Syndrome Association to keep updated on newly discovered information. See the Resource Guide at the end of the book for information on how to contact the Tourette Syndrome Association, and many other helpful organizations and websites.

Studies show that the severity of a child's Tourette syndrome is not what determines how successful he is in life. More important are high self-esteem and the acquisition of skills that enable him to cope with TS in a society that does not always fully understand neurological disorders. My dream is that this book will help families get started in that all-important task of preparing their child with TS for adult life. My ultimate goal is that all children who have Tourette syndrome will be accurately diagnosed and treated, and that they will be given every opportunity to reach their highest potential.

1

WHAT IS TOURETTE SYNDROME?

Carl R. Hansen, Jr., M.D.

▪▪ Introduction

Tourette syndrome (TS) is a baffling disorder.

In many people, Tourette syndrome (also known as Tourette's disorder) is so mild that it is never diagnosed. A child can go through life with a few tics and twitches, and his family and friends think nothing of it. In fact, this is the typical case of TS. On the other hand, for some, TS causes such disabling verbal outbursts, involuntary movements, and associated disorders with behavioral difficulties. These symptoms interfere with education, career, and relationships. And there is every level of severity in between these extremes.

Tourette syndrome may sneak up so gradually that you only have a vague suspicion that your child has a "problem." Perhaps he seems unusually hyperactive, impulsive, or quick to anger, but when you discuss your concerns with physicians, they offer reassurance and insist you have nothing to worry about. In others, Tourette syndrome appears with little or no warning when your child suddenly starts making peculiar movements or sounds. At first, you may think that your child's tics are deliberate, but eventually you realize that they are out of his control.

While your child's unusual movements and sounds gradually increase in number and frequency, you may spend months or years searching for the reason behind them. You may take your child to an eye doctor if he seems unable to control his blinking. He may have his tonsils removed if he continually clears his throat, or he may be diagnosed as having allergies if he constantly twitches his nose. Even when parents get a correct explanation from a doctor, the diagnosis means little to them.

Not that many years ago, most people had never heard of Tourette syndrome. Today, it's more likely that they are familiar with the term, but—thanks to TV and movies—think it means people who "bark" or shout curse words. (In fact, only a small percentage of people with Tourette ever exhibit these symptoms.) The reality is that most people with Tourette only develop mild tics that never even require medication.

If your child's symptoms are more severe—or even if you're just worrying that they may become so—there's no need to despair. There are medical and behavioral treatments that can help many children control their symptoms, and educational strategies that can help them around the learning problems sometimes associated with TS. There are also plenty of up-to-date facts about the nature and causes of Tourette syndrome that can help children and their families cope with the disorder, as well as to dispel public misconceptions. Also, we know that the symptoms usually improve in adulthood.

Tourette syndrome *is* a widely misunderstood and misdiagnosed disorder. You need current, accurate information at your fingertips to ensure that your child receives the treatment and education he needs. This chapter is designed to give you the basic understanding of Tourette syndrome—its symptoms, causes, treatment, diagnosis, and prognosis—you need to get started.

:: What Is Tourette Syndrome?

Tourette syndrome is a neurobiological (brain) disorder that causes involuntary movements (motor tics) and involuntary vocalizations (vocal tics). Motor tics can occur in any part of the body, and may include eye blinking, facial grimacing, shoulder shrugging, head jerking, and/or hand movements. Common vocal tics include throat clearing, sniffing, making loud sounds, grunting, or repeating words. Both motor and vocal tics may occur many times a minute, or only a few times a day. They may even disappear completely at times. Tics can be so mild that they're barely noticeable, or so severe that they're highly distracting, even disabling.

Tourette syndrome begins before the age of eighteen, usually at around six or seven, and typically peaks during early adolescence. A group of international researchers—including educational specialist Larry Burd and psychiatrist Jacob Kerbeshian, both of whom contributed chapters to this book— have been following the progress of several thousand people with Tourette syndrome for more than twenty years, and found encourag-

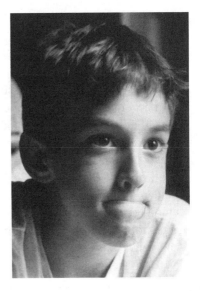

ing results. By adulthood, 75 percent of people with TS function well, have few tics, and find that TS has very little impact on their lives. Fifteen percent have ongoing problems of moderate difficulty that do affect their lives, but which are manageable and allow the individuals to be employed and married. Only 10 percent of people with TS have a severe disorder as adults. Unfortunately, for that one in ten, TS is a lifelong health problem that produces substantial impairment.

Tics must be present for at least a year for a diagnosis of Tourette syndrome to be made. Like other "syndromes," Tourette syndrome is so called because it is diagnosed on the basis of the physical signs and symptoms it produces, not with a specific diagnostic test. Both motor and vocal tics *must* be present for the diagnosis of Tourette syndrome to be made, but there are also a variety of other signs and symptoms that *may* be present. The following section reviews both the types of signs and symptoms that all children with TS have, as well as those that only some children have.

‼ The Signs and Symptoms of Tourette Syndrome

Tics

As explained above, all children with Tourette syndrome have tics—sudden, repetitive, and uncontrollable movements of muscles in the body. Tics in the muscles that control speech cause involuntary sounds such as coughing, hissing, snorting, or outbursts of words or phrases. Tics in other muscles of the body produce involuntary movements such as eye-blinking, grimacing, or leg-jerking.

Medical professionals classify tics as *simple* or *complex,* depending on how many parts of the body are involved. Brief, isolated movements of only one part of the body (head twitching, eye blinking, or shoulder shrugging) are considered simple motor tics. Likewise, simple noises—produced by air or sound moving through the vocal cords, throat, or nose (throat-clearing, sniffing, coughing, spitting)—are considered simple vocal tics. Complex tics involve more complicated, seemingly purposeful movements or sounds, and include hitting, pinching, poking, smelling objects, complex touching movements, and saying recognizable phrases.

Here are some examples of common motor and vocal tics:

Motor Tics	Vocal Tics
Simple	*Simple*
▪ blinking eyes (frequently or in an unusual pattern) ▪ jerking neck ▪ shrugging shoulders ▪ grimacing ▪ flipping head ▪ kicking ▪ tensing muscles ▪ sticking tongue out ▪ moving fingers rapidly	▪ throat-clearing ▪ sniffing ▪ coughing ▪ grunting ▪ spitting ▪ yelling (wordless) ▪ belching
Complex	*Complex*
▪ facial gestures (eye rolling) ▪ grooming behaviors (smoothing hair) ▪ smelling things ▪ touching ▪ jumping ▪ hitting ▪ biting ▪ echopraxia (imitating others' actions) ▪ copropraxia (obscene gestures—giving the finger) ▪ self-injurious behaviors (picking scabs, rubbing sores raw, biting, hitting self)	▪ animal sounds ▪ repeating words or phrases out of context ("Oh boy," "I don't know," or words from advertising jingles on TV) ▪ palilalia (repeating one's own words or sounds—"Do my work, work, work") ▪ echolalia (repeating the last sound, word, or phrase spoken by another person—saying "Come over here" after mother has just said, "Come over here") ▪ coprolalia (using obscene or other socially inappropriate words)

More than half of all children with Tourette syndrome develop an eye tic first. In other children, the first symptom may be other facial tics, involuntary vocal sounds such as throat clearing, or vocal and motor tics together. Additional tics usually develop in the weeks or months after the first tic. Common examples of early motor tics are grimaces, head jerks, or hand-to-face movements. The first vocal tics are often throat-clearing, grunting, sniffing, or snorting. Tics usually develop in upper extremities first, and then move down the body. Motor tics involving the trunk or legs usually occur fairly late in the course of the syndrome, as do vocal tics such as coprolalia.

To receive the diagnosis of Tourette syndrome, children must have at least two motor tics and one vocal tic. (There are other types of tic disorders in which children may only have motor *or* vocal tics.) In addition, their tics usually change over time. New ones appear, replacing or adding to old ones. Bear in mind, however, that no child develops all, or even most, of the tics listed.

Although television dramas may give the impression that everyone with Tourette syndrome has coprolalia, in reality, only a small minority does—current estimates are 15 percent or less. Likewise, only a small percentage of people with Tourette syndrome develop self-injurious behavior such as biting or hitting themselves, or violent motor tics that may injure muscles.

Although scientists do not understand exactly what causes Tourette syndrome, they do have a good idea about what causes the tics that accompany the condition. Presently, researchers believe that tics are caused, at least in part, by nerve cells in the brain that are "sensitive" to the brain chemicals *dopamine* and/or *serotonin*. These two chemicals are neurotransmitters, meaning they ordinarily help transmit signals from one nerve cell in the brain to the next. Dopamine is a key brain chemical in the parts of the brain that control movement, and serotonin is another brain chemical that regulates a number of brain activities including pain, emotions, and movement. Tics are involuntary and reflect the "misfiring" of nerve cells involved with movement.

Your child is not deliberately making movements or sounds to seek attention, to annoy others, or for any other conscious reason. He may be able to suppress or hold back some tics for short periods of time, but eventually the need to give in to them will be overwhelming. (Just as you can temporarily prevent yourself from blinking, but you'll eventually have to give in.) Many people with TS report that this "need" is felt as a

conscious awareness of tension building up within themselves, sometimes in the part of the body where the tic occurs. They may "hear" a
word or sound coming into their mind, and feel that they "have" to say
it. Along with this build up of tension, anxiety may increase, muscles
may tighten, and a child may feel like "exploding." When the "explosion"
comes it discharges the anxiety, muscle tension, and pent up tics. (See
Chapter 10 for more information about what it feels like to have tics.)

Tic Severity

Tourette syndrome varies great-
ly from child to child. Your child's tics
may be mild, moderate, or severe, depending on their frequency and the degree to which they disrupt day-to-day
activities. For example, they may
range from a mild, easily disguised
nose-wrinkling tic to loud, violent,
disruptive full body movements.

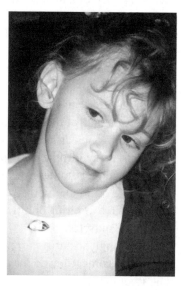

Within each child, symptoms
will also wax and wane—or vary in
intensity and frequency—from hour
to hour, day to day, and year to year.
There may be times when there are no
tics, and then times when many tics
occur many times a day.

Often the severity of tics increases during early adolescence (ages
twelve to fifteen). To add to the difficulties, teenagers with TS may become
increasingly self-conscious about their tics, and less tolerant of their own
differences. Fortunately, tics often diminish significantly around the ages
of sixteen to eighteen, as adolescents move toward adulthood. No matter
how severe tics were in childhood, there is usually at least some improvement in adulthood, although improvement is not as notable in the more
extreme cases. Some environmental factors can increase or decrease the
intensity of tics. For example, they occur less frequently during sleep or
activities that absorb a child's concentration (e.g., video games), but a child
may "bust out" with many tics when the absorbing activity is finished.

Caffeinated drinks and chocolate (which contains small amounts
of caffeine and other chemicals that stimulate the brain) may increase
symptoms in some children with Tourette syndrome. If a child with TS

takes stimulant medications to treat attention-deficit/hyperactivity disorder (AD/HD), the tics sometimes may worsen—an effect that may be temporary, or may necessitate the stimulant medication being stopped.

Many parents find that tics can occur more frequently during a bout with hay fever, allergies, or infections. Unfortunately, cold and allergy decongestants such as pseudoephedrine, as well as the non-sedating antihistamines such as Claritin and Zyrtec, can also increase tics. (See Chapter 3 for more information on medications.)

Intense emotions such as anxiety, fear, frustration, or anger can cause tics to increase. Stress, too, can make tics worse. For this reason, it's usually a bad idea to ask your child to try to suppress a tic, as this only puts increased stress on him and may cause his tics to become even more pronounced.

If increased stress makes tics worse, it stands to reason that you can help control your child's tics by reducing stress as much as possible. Ignoring the tics, helping your child manage time, providing clear expectations for behavior, and working with teachers to develop an educational plan that gives your child the best chance at success are just some of the ways you can make the environment less stressful. At the same time, you don't want to unconsciously reinforce tics by showering your child with attention when he tics. Chapters 3 to 5 will go into detail about different ways you can help your child, including stress reduction, behavioral interventions, and medications.

:: Tourette Syndrome "Plus"

In addition to tics, the majority of people with Tourette syndrome have symptoms of one or more other neurological disorders, such as AD/HD or obsessive-compulsive disorder. When a person with TS has "co-morbid" (co-existing) symptoms, it's often referred to as "Tourette Syndrome Plus" or "TS+."

Attention-Deficit/Hyperactivity Disorders

Attention-deficit/hyperactivity disorder (AD/HD) is a neurological condition that makes it more difficult for a child to focus his attention, control his impulses, and/or behave appropriately. As is the case with tics, these problems are caused by a chemical imbalance in the brain. More than half of all children with Tourette syndrome have some type of ADHD.

Symptoms of AD/HD fall into three areas:
1. inattention
2. hyperactivity
3. impulsivity

Inattention

Symptoms of inattention that may indicate that a child has AD/HD include:

1. overlooking details or making careless mistakes in schoolwork
2. having trouble focusing and sustaining attention on work or play activities
3. seeming not to listen
4. having trouble finishing assigned schoolwork or chores
5. organizational difficulties
6. being distractible
7. being forgetful

It's important for parents to understand that a child with AD/HD may be able to concentrate well during certain activities that he finds engaging. In fact, *hyperfocus*—concentration so intense that the child loses track of time and finds it hard to shift his attention—occurs frequently in people with AD/HD, as it's just another result of the disorganized attentional system in the brain. So the fact that a child spends hours reading a novel, surfing the Internet, or playing a video game does not mean he is faking concentration problems in school.

Hyperactivity

Some symptoms of hyperactivity that may be present include:

1. fidgeting or squirming
2. not staying seated when appropriate
3. running or climbing when it is inappropriate
4. excessive talking

Note, however, that symptoms of hyperactivity are not always present in children with AD/HD. Children who have the inattentive form of the disorder may actually appear to have low energy compared to other children. (This form of AD/HD is officially known as attention-deficit/hyperactivity disorder, predominately inattentive type.) And adolescents with AD/HD who were hyperactive when younger may seem more restless than hyperactive as teenagers. Children who do have symptoms of hyperactivity will be diagnosed either with attention-deficit/hyperactivity disorder, predominantly hyperactive-impulsive type or attention-deficit/hyperactivity disorder, combined type (if they have both inattentive and hyperactive symptoms).

Impulsivity

Symptoms of impulsivity in children with AD/HD include:
1. blurting out answers
2. having trouble waiting turns
3. interrupting or intruding on others

Diagnosing AD/HD

To determine whether your child does indeed have attention-deficit/hyperactivity disorder, the doctor will not only evaluate how well he is able to concentrate and control impulses, but also how your child's abilities compare with other children's of the same age. For example, just because your two-year-old has trouble waiting his turn does not mean this is a symptom of AD/HD. *Most* two-year-olds have trouble waiting their turn. If, however, your child has problems taking turns when he is eight, this difficulty could very well be due to AD/HD. As guidance in diagnosing your child, the doctor will refer to the *Diagnostic and Statistical Manual of Mental Disorders* of the American Psychiatric Association. This book lists the symptoms and official diagnostic criteria for AD/HD, as well as many of the other comorbid disorders children with TS may have.

In children with Tourette syndrome, symptoms of AD/HD often appear before motor or vocal tics do. Studies show that AD/HD symptoms are usually noticeable by age four or five. As a result, doctors may begin by treating attention-deficit/hyperactivity disorders as they would in any other children—by prescribing stimulant medications intended to make it easier to concentrate and control impulses. But in some children with Tourette syndrome, these medications may actually make tics worse or hasten their appearance. Fortunately, there *are* medications that may reduce symptoms without worsening TS symptoms. Chapter 3 describes these appropriate medical treatments for children with Tourette syndrome and attention-deficit/hyperactivity disorders. In addition, Chapter 5 offers some guidance in handling AD/HD on a day-to-day basis within the family, and Chapter 8 gives practical help for dealing with AD/HD in school.

Obsessive Thoughts and Compulsive Behaviors

In addition to having tics, at least 50 percent of children with Tourette syndrome have obsessive-compulsive disorder (OCD) or some of its symptoms. Examples of OC behavior include insisting on wearing clothing that is a certain color; repeatedly checking that doors are locked or the stove and lights are off; always having to be first in line or to sit in the same place; or erasing a sentence over and over until the paper tears in an effort to get the letters "perfect."

■■ Common Obsessions and Compulsions

Compulsions or Rituals
- Placing objects "just right"
- Touching things*
- Checking and rechecking
- Smelling*
- Licking*
- Excessive erasing
- Washing hands repeatedly

Obsessive Thoughts
- Mental echolalia—repeating words or phrases to oneself*
- Obscene thoughts
- Mental counting or grouping of items
- Sexual thoughts
- Thoughts about forbidden actions, such as standing on a desk at school, kissing a teacher, touching others sexually, exposing oneself
- Fear of hurting someone

*These same behaviors can appear as tics. The difference is that, with a tic, the child feels a physical urge to perform the behavior. With a compulsion, either the child performs the behavior as an attempt to relieve an obsessive thought (e.g., smelling objects to check for contamination) or in response to a set of strict, self-imposed rules (for example, "I can't get into the car until I've locked and unlocked the door four times.")

To understand what is behind these actions, it is essential to understand what medical professionals mean by the terms "obsession" and "compulsion." An obsession is a thought, idea, impulse, or image that, at first, seems intrusive or senseless to the person experiencing it. For example, a child may continually repeat words or thoughts in his mind, mentally count or group objects, or think about forbidden actions such as touching strangers or standing on a desk. The child experiencing these obsessions understands that they're a product of his own mind. That is, he doesn't think he is hearing "voices," or that he is getting the obsession from some other outside influence.

A compulsion is a repetitive behavior (thought or action) designed to stop the obsession, reduce anxiety, keep a dreaded event from occurring, or prevent discomfort. Examples include placing objects "just right," smelling hands, touching things three times, or turning the lights off and on many times.

Adolescents and adults with OC behaviors are usually aware of the unusual nature of their obsessions and compulsions. They may try to stop or ignore their obsessions and compulsions. But because this effort can trigger extreme anxiety, they may not succeed in stopping the OC behavior. Young children with OC symptoms, on the other hand, may not realize that their behavior is inappropriate. They may not be able to verbalize what their obsession or compulsion is, and may therefore see it as normal.

Obsessions and compulsions can greatly disrupt daily life. To begin with, they are often time-consuming. Other activities frequently fall by the wayside. For example, if a child feels compelled to turn a circle after each step, he frequently may be late for class. Obsessions and compulsions can also interfere with school or work performance. A child may check and recheck answers so often that he is unable to complete it in the allotted time, or he may lose his concentration if he is constantly counting the objects on the teacher's tie. In addition, OC behaviors are distressing to the child, family members, and others. The child may feel weird and out of control, while parents and siblings may be at a loss to understand and deal with the behaviors.

When obsessions and compulsions significantly interfere with a child's abilities to perform schoolwork, job, or other aspects of daily life, the child is diagnosed with obsessive-compulsive disorder. As Chapter 3 discusses, medications can often help control OC behaviors. There are also daily behavioral strategies, explained in Chapter 4, that can help reduce OC behaviors, or, at least, reduce their impact on your child's life.

Asperger Syndrome

Because Asperger syndrome (or Asperger's disorder) was only added to the psychiatric diagnostic manuals in the mid-1990s, the research on how much overlap there is between TS and Asperger's is limited. But the hallmark characteristics of Asperger syndrome (AS)—obsessive interests and difficulty with empathy and social interaction—are often seen in children with Tourette syndrome. Some children with AS also exhibit *stereotypies*—repetitive motor mannerisms such as hand flapping—which can be hard to differentiate from motor tics.

While OCD obsessions are disturbing for the child who experiences them, the obsessive interests of a child with Asperger syndrome are actually a source of joy or comfort for him. It's common for a child with AS to be so preoccupied with a certain subject area that he builds up an astounding, encyclopedic knowledge of the topic. And he may like to "share" the joy, lecturing others *ad nauseam* about that special interest—which could be anything from video games or cartoons to far more obscure topics such as train schedules, dentistry, or deep fat fryers. Unfortunately, that preoccupation with one subject can interfere with school work, social relationships, and many other aspects of daily life.

Just as TS symptoms vary tremendously from person to person, so do Asperger's symptoms. On the one extreme, you have the quirky, eccentric genius who may be socially inept, but makes millions of dollars writing groundbreaking software programs. On the other end, someone may be so disabled by his disorder that he can't hold a job or live independently. Most people with Asperger syndrome fall somewhere in between.

Asperger syndrome, which is far more commonly diagnosed in males than females, is considered an autism spectrum disorder, albeit on the high-functioning end of the spectrum. All autism spectrum disorders are characterized by difficulties in social interaction and the presence of extremely repetitive behaviors, interests, or activities. But while children with classic autism may have mental retardation and/or delayed or nonexistent speech, children with Asperger syndrome have IQs in the average to above average range and generally normal speech development before age three. In fact, children with AS often have expansive vocabularies, but their speech may be "off" in some other way. They may quote a favorite movie or TV show whenever asked questions. They may talk like "little professors," lecturing with words and phrases far more "grown up" than those used by their peers. They may have trouble modulating their tone of voice—always too loud or too soft. Or they may speak with exaggerated emotion—or no emotion at all.

Similarly, children with AS may have trouble interpreting the messages others are trying to communicate. Very literal minded, they may find it difficult to:

- "read between the lines" in a story,
- understand idioms (e.g., why does the teacher say "you're driving me up a wall," when she's obviously still on the ground?),
- interpret nonverbal cues such as facial expression, body posture, or tone of voice.

That same literal-mindedness means children with AS may say things that get them in trouble socially. Often honest to a fault, they may not understand why they shouldn't, for example, call someone "fat" or "smelly," if they are. (Keep in mind that a child with Tourette may say the same thing—not because he doesn't understand the social implications, but because he lacks the impulse control to refrain from verbalizing the thought when it pops into his head.)

On top of their social communication difficulties, children with Asperger syndrome are often very rigid, and can become upset easily when their normal routine is disturbed. They may want to dictate rules to their playmates, even "scripting" the dialogue the other children must use in a game. Children with AS may view the world as one of extremes and absolutes: If something isn't wonderful, it's terrible; it's either right or it's wrong. Where we see shades of gray, the child with AS may see only black and white.

Put all those symptoms together and you get a child who very likely has trouble making and keeping friends. When small, the child may not recognize the lack—in fact, he may think every classmate is his "friend," even the ones who tease him or ignore him. As he gets older, though, the child with Asperger syndrome often desperately yearns for a real friend, but is clueless on how to fit in with the other kids his own age. This social isolation can sometimes lead to struggles with depression in adolescence and young adulthood.

Diagnosing and Treating Asperger Syndrome

Although it's neurologically based, Asperger syndrome is typically diagnosed by a psychiatrist, rather than a neurologist. There's no medical test for AS at this time. Instead, the psychiatrist will base the diagnosis on interviews with the parents, observations and interactions with the child, and questionnaires about the child's behavior filled out by parents and teachers. Because children with Asperger syndrome are frequently misdiagnosed with everything from AD/HD to schizophrenia, if you suspect your child may have Asperger syndrome, you'll want to find a psychiatrist with significant experience in autism spectrum disorders.

There's also no one specific treatment for Asperger syndrome. Therapies must be tailored to the individual child's needs. Most children with Asperger syndrome benefit from social skills training—a form of group therapy in which they're taught the unwritten rules of behavior that other children seem to know implicitly. Cognitive behavioral therapy may help the more explosive, depressed, or anxious child with AS manage his emotions, as well as cut back on some detrimental repetitive routines. If the child has motor clumsiness or sensory sensitivities—as many with Asperger's do—he may benefit from occupational therapy (see below). If carrying on a back-and-forth conversation is very difficult for him, pragmatic speech therapy may be in order. Other therapies that were developed for treatment of autism—such as ABA (Applied Behavior Analysis), TEACCH (Treatment and Education of Autistic and related Communication-handicapped Children) and Floortime/DIR (Developmental, Individual Differences, Relationship-based approach)—have been adapted to treat children with Asperger syndrome.

Asperger syndrome, per se, isn't treated by medication at this time. But the psychiatrist may prescribe drugs to treat other related symptoms such as stimulants for attention difficulties or hyperactivity, atypical neuroleptics for aggression or obsessive-compulsive symptoms, or selective serotonin reuptake inhibitors (SSRIs) for depression. See Chapter 3 for more information about these classes of medications.

Aggression

For about 25 to 35 percent of children with Tourette syndrome, controlling their anger and aggressive behavior is a problem. They may appear to have a "short fuse" and get into fights for little or no reason. In the most extreme cases (which are sometimes referred to as "rages" or "rage attacks") they may attack other people or destroy property without provocation or turn their aggression on themselves, perhaps by impulsively punching themselves or a wall. Often, the target of their aggression is a parent or someone not likely to harm them in any way. Usually, children who have these types of problems with aggression greatly regret their explosive outbursts. Between outbursts they are reasonable, and feel guilty about their behavior.

Aggression mostly occurs in children with TS who also have hyperactivity, impulsivity, and concentration problems. Some studies indicate that the more co-morbid (co-occurring) conditions a child has, the more difficulties he may experience controlling aggression. In addition, irritability and aggression may increase when tics increase. Sometimes children with more severe tics have greater difficulty controlling their temper.

The connection between Tourette syndrome and increased aggression is still being studied. It may partly result from the increased pressure of dealing with TS on a daily basis. But scientists also believe that there may be an underlying neurological problem that makes it more difficult for children with TS to regulate anxiety and aggression. Some parents also report that certain medications have triggered aggressive behavior in their children with TS.

When a person with Tourette syndrome has a rage attack, he experiences a triggering of his "fight or flight" response, even though there is no objective reason for such a strong response. When a rage attack is coming on, a child may feel panicky and experience very unpleasant physical changes such as a rapid pulse, hyperventilation, sweaty palms, and nausea. When these changes are not observed and limits are not set, explosive behavior is likely to follow. It is essential to check for such signs and symptoms so you can help your child develop effective strategies to manage these problems.

As with attention-deficit/hyperactivity disorders, Asperger syndrome, and other neurological disorders, tantrums and aggressive behavior may arise in toddlers with Tourette syndrome *before* any tics develop. This type of behavior can also develop months or years *after* tics appear. Often, a child's aggressive behavior is worse in some settings than others. For example, a child may be able to control aggression at home or in the classroom, but have difficulty in the neighborhood or on the playground.

Treatment involves first helping the child learn that fighting and destructive behavior must be curbed, and then helping learn to handle aggressive impulses without losing control. Sometimes a psychologist or other mental health professional can help the child learn to recognize when he is about to lose control by keeping track of physical signs such as a faster heart rate or increased muscle tension. A child can then avoid an impending explosion by taking a time out break to calm down and regroup. A psychologist might also help the child develop better social skills to head off conflict with siblings and classmates. Social skills groups, too, can help children learn better ways of dealing with others and increase their success in relationships. Relaxation therapy and biofeedback are techniques to help relax the muscles, slow the heart rate, and reduce inner tension. In addition, medications are sometimes helpful in reducing anxiety, irritability, and aggression. Chapter 3 discusses the medical treatment of aggressive behavior in more detail.

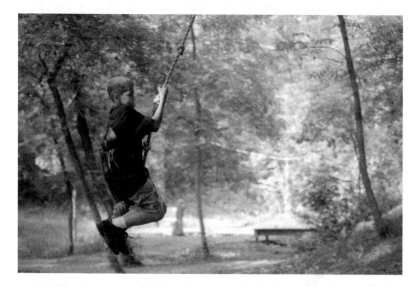

Sensory Processing Problems

The terms "sensory processing" or "sensory integration" refer to the way our brains organize and process information received from the senses of sight, hearing, smell, touch, movement, and balance. Some children with TS may have problems with sensory integration. As a result, their brain has difficulty processing incoming sensory information or stimuli. They may be over- or under-sensitive to input from one or more of their senses, or be unable to use sensory information efficiently. For example, they may over-react to touch (tactile defensiveness), and consequently be distressed by the feel of certain fabrics on their skin or the texture of certain foods in their mouth. Or they may have difficulty telling where parts of their body are in space, and therefore appear clumsy. Sensory integration problems can also contribute to problems with speech, muscle development, hyperactivity, aggressiveness, and learning problems.

Sensory processing disorder is best treated by an occupational therapist with expertise in sensory integration therapy. An occupational therapist is skilled in using special exercises and activities to help children overcome problems in development that interfere with their activities of daily living. Chapter 7 goes into sensory processing in more detail.

Learning Problems

Tourette syndrome has no effect on intelligence. Some children with Tourette syndrome have mental retardation and some score in the "gifted" range on IQ tests, but most have about average intelligence. This is as it is in the population as a whole.

Even though most children with Tourette syndrome have average intelligence, they are more likely to have learning problems. In fact, about one fourth have specific learning disabilities—delays or difficulties in learning to use one or more specific types of information. Children with learning disorders may, for example, have unusual difficulty with reading, spelling, handwriting, or mathematics. They may also have problems with auditory processing (i.e., reacting appropriately to information they hear), because their ears and brain don't fully coordinate. That can result in various difficulties in school or at home, such as problems following spoken instructions. Children with learning disabilities don't do as well in an area as expected, given their intelligence level. By definition, learning disabilities are not the result of other causes such as mental retardation or sensory disorders such as hearing and vision loss.

Tics, distractibility, or obsessive-compulsive symptoms can also contribute to learning problems in children with Tourette syndrome. For example, eye blinking or head jerking can impede reading; hand jerking can make writing impossible. Likewise, if a child has a compulsion to count mentally, concentration can be reduced. Medications used to control tics can also interfere with learning or memory, or make children too sleepy to pay attention in class.

Learning problems most often become apparent when a child enters school and has difficulty reading or understanding math concepts. At this point, a thorough professional assessment of the type discussed in Chapter 8 can help determine the best way to deal with the learning problems. For example, if a reading problem is found to be related to head jerking tics, reducing or eliminating the tics through medication would likely be the simplest strategy. But if the reading problem is not related to any TS symptoms, then the child might benefit from special educational strategies. In any case, if you are aware of your child's specific learning disabilities, you and the teachers can plan ways to help overcome these problems. Chapter 8 explains how you can work to discover how your child learns best and incorporate that knowledge into the educational program.

■■ What Causes Tourette Syndrome?

For many years, Tourette syndrome was believed to be the result of underlying psychological problems. Anger was thought to be central to the development of tics. And unfairly enough, parents were sometimes blamed for causing the mental conflicts that led to these anger problems. Today, however, researchers have proven that this simply is not true. Nothing you did caused your child's tics, obsessive-compulsive behavior, or other symptoms, nor does your child have a mental illness. Although the precise cause of Tourette syndrome has yet to be pinpointed, studies suggest that it is related to a neurobiological disorder linked to problems in brain chemistry and physiology.

The first clue that Tourette syndrome is caused by neurobiological factors came in the early 1960s. Researchers found that tics were sometimes reduced or eliminated by using Haldol™ (scientific name: haloperidol). This medication keeps the brain chemical dopamine from reaching a receptor where it can "deliver" its message; hence medications like Haldol are called dopamine blockers. As mentioned earlier, dopamine is a chemical that acts as a *neurotransmitter,* or messenger between brain cells, and is involved in the control of motor movements. Serotonin, norepinephrine, and acetylcholine are several other neurotransmitters that play a role in control of movement. Studies are currently underway to discover the specific roles that these and other brain chemicals might play in Tourette syndrome. Researchers are also investigating specific parts of the brain to determine what role they play in TS. The Tourette Syndrome Association (TSA) supports this ongoing research into the specific cause of TS, in hopes that determining the cause will lead to a cure.

By the late 1970s, researchers discovered that Tourette syndrome runs in some families more than others. In other words, an alteration in the normal genetic make-up can lead to the development of the tics.

Genes are basic units of genetic material found in all the body's cells. Genes, which are made out of long chains of DNA, play a role in all of a person's traits—from eye and hair color to foot size and special talents. With just four chemicals called nucleotides, DNA creates the building blocks of the genetic code that drives the work of our cells. The change of just one of these nucleotides in a gene can have a profound effect on how the brain works.

Just as your child's genes determine whether he will be tall or short, musically gifted or tone deaf, they also largely determine whether or not he will have tics or obsessive-compulsive symptoms. As with other genetic disorders, the predisposition to develop Tourette syndrome is sometimes passed on within families, from one generation to the next. (Geneticists call this predisposition "vulnerability.") Mothers or fathers who are themselves vulnerable to Tourette syndrome may pass the tendency on to their sons or daughters. When one parent has a Tourette syndrome gene, each child he has will have a 50 percent chance of inheriting the vulnerability for Tourette syndrome.

Not all children who inherit these genes go on to develop TS. For reasons that are not fully understood, about 30 percent of girls who inherit the vulnerability show **no** symptoms at all, whereas the figure for boys is only 1 percent.

When the Tourette syndrome genes *do* cause symptoms, they can vary greatly from person to person. For instance, some children develop both OCD and the vocal and motor tics associated with Tourette syndrome. Others have just one condition or the other. This is because genetic research indicates that the same gene(s) that cause the tics of TS may also be related to OC behaviors. Some children, too, may have one of the other tic disorders described below in the section on "Getting a Diagnosis." In general, boys are more likely to have tics, and girls are more likely to have obsessive-compulsive symptoms. Both boys and girls, however, can have any of the symptoms of Tourette syndrome, in any combination, and in any degree of severity.

Although Tourette syndrome is usually attributed to genetic causes, sometimes it may be caused by other factors. For example, brain damage resulting from an auto-immune reaction, viruses, lack of oxygen at birth, or other prenatal problems may also be involved in causing TS.

❚❚ How Many People Have Tourette Syndrome?

Tourette syndrome is more common than once believed, but estimates are difficult to make because the disorder is frequently undiagnosed or misdiagnosed. Currently, the Tourette Syndrome Association estimates that at least 200,000 people in the United States are affected, while the Centers for Disease Control estimates that approximately 3 to 5 in 10,000 individuals has TS. Tourette syndrome is more common in boys than girls.

❚❚ Having Other Children

If you already have one child with Tourette syndrome, any other children you have will have a fifty-fifty chance of inheriting the Tourette syndrome vulnerability as well. And, as explained above, any daughters that inherit a TS gene will have a 70 percent chance of developing symptoms; any sons, a 99 percent chance.

At present, there are no prenatal tests to determine whether a baby will carry the gene(s) or develop symptoms. There are also no tests to determine which parent passed on the gene (although it may be obvious which side of the family has a tendency toward tics or OCD) or whether a younger sibling also inherited the gene(s) or will develop symptoms. However, genetic research on Tourette syndrome is progressing rapidly. Once the responsible genes have been discovered, not only will genetic testing for Tourette syndrome be possible, but better treatments and perhaps a cure can eventually be developed.

In the meantime, it is important to remember that symptoms of Tourette syndrome can vary widely from child to child. If your other children *do* inherit a genetic vulnerability for Tourette syndrome, their symptoms may be much milder *or* more severe than either their sibling's or their parent's. A genetic counselor can explain your chances of having additional children with Tourette syndrome and the possible range of symptoms. He can also help you cope with your feelings about embarking on another pregnancy that may produce a child with Tourette syndrome. You may also find it helpful to talk to other parents who have chosen to have additional children and then wound up with more than one child with TS. The final decision, of course, is up to you.

■■ Getting a Diagnosis

Getting a firm diagnosis of Tourette syndrome can be difficult for several reasons. First, because of the tendency of tics to wax and wane and change over time, it may take a while before your child's doctor gets a complete picture of his symptoms. Second, children often suppress their symptoms when they are around strangers, including doctors. And third, there are a variety of other conditions with similar symptoms that can sometimes be confused with Tourette syndrome. Provided your child sees a specialist or specialists with training and experience in tic disorders, however, the diagnosis process should be fairly straightforward.

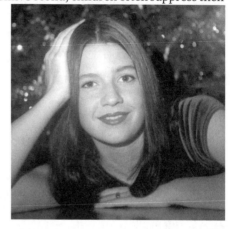

To reach a diagnosis, the doctor follows guidelines in a book called the *Diagnostic and Statistical Manual of Mental Disorders,* fourth edition, text revision (DSM-IV-TR). As mentioned above, this book, published by the American Psychiatric Association, outlines the "official" criteria for conditions commonly diagnosed and treated by psychiatrists. The DSM-IV-TR lists the following criteria for diagnosing Tourette's disorder (Tourette syndrome):

A. Both multiple motor and one or more vocal tics have been present at some time during the illness, though not necessarily concurrently. (A tic is a sudden, rapid, recurrent, non-rhythmic, stereotyped motor movement or vocalization.)

B. The tics occur many times a day (usually in bouts) nearly every day or intermittently throughout a period of more than 1 year, and during this period there was never a tic-free period of more than 3 consecutive months.

C. The onset is before age 18 years.

D. The disturbance is not due to the direct physiologic effects of a substance (e.g., stimulants) or a general medical condition (e.g., Huntington disease or postviral encephalitis).

[Reprinted with permission from the Diagnostic and Statistical Manual of Mental Disorders, Fourth Edition, Text Revision (Copyright 2000). American Psychiatric Association.]

In addition to checking your child's symptoms against these criteria, the doctor will also perform a *differential diagnosis*. A differential diagnosis involves comparing your child's behavior with the behavior of children with other disorders that might produce the same symptoms. In other words, it is a way of ruling out what disorders your child does not have, and determining what disorder he does have.

In making a differential diagnosis of Tourette syndrome, several similar tic disorders, as well as other conditions, must be ruled out. The tic disorders include:

1. chronic motor tic disorder;
2. chronic vocal tic disorder;
3. transient tic disorder; and
4. tic disorder not otherwise specified.

In contrast to Tourette syndrome, the two other chronic tic disorders cause only motor *or* vocal tics, not both. Transient tic disorder may cause both one or more motor tics *and* one or more vocal tics, but the condition lasts less than twelve consecutive months. Tic disorder not otherwise specified is a catchall diagnosis for all other types of tic disorders. For example, the name may refer to a disorder that causes both motor and vocal tics but begins *after* age eighteen. Or it may refer to a disorder that causes vocal tics and just one motor tic, in contrast to the multiple motor tics in Tourette syndrome. Most researchers believe that these tic disorders are milder variations of TS, possibly due to the same cause, but this has not yet been proven.

Other conditions with symptoms similar to Tourette syndrome that must be ruled out include: Duchenne muscular dystrophy, head trauma, brain tumors, epilepsy, and autism spectrum disorders. The doctor must also make sure that tics and other symptoms are not due to overexertion or drug use.

The Diagnosis Process

Observation plays a large role in the diagnosis of Tourette syndrome. Medical professionals will want to look not only at the type of tics your child has, but also at their severity and frequency, and the extent to which they disrupt your child's daily activities. Because your child may suppress his tics or have fewer than usual in the doctor's office, the doctor will also question you about your child's behavior in the past. You can help a great deal if you prepare a list of all your child's past tics or OC behaviors ahead of time. You may also want to document your child's tics by taking home videos. In addition, you might suggest that the doctor follow your child into the waiting room if your child suppresses his tics in the office. Determining what factors make your child's symptoms change is especially important. In addition, the doctor should ask about your family's history of tics, obsessive-compulsive behavior, hyperactivity, or other health conditions.

Before your child receives the diagnosis of Tourette syndrome (and any related disorders), he ideally should see a variety of specialists with differing expertise. Ideally, these specialists will consult with one another and share their observations about your child with one another in order to arrive at the best possible understanding of your child's disorder. When specialists from different disciplines work together in this manner, they are known as an interdisciplinary or multidisciplinary team. Multidisciplinary teams are often involved in diagnosing children with mental retardation, autism, cerebral palsy, and other developmental disorders. Unfortunately, the concept of using multidisciplinary teams to diagnose TS has not yet caught on in some areas. If a team with expertise in TS is not available in your area, it will be up to you to coordinate the efforts of each specialist, making sure each knows about test results and conclusions reached by other specialists. Specialists with expertise in diagnosing Tourette syndrome include:

Pediatric Neurologist: A pediatric neurologist is a medical doctor specializing in diagnosing and treating neurological disorders in children. Neurological disorders—disorders of the brain, spinal cord, or nerves—include epilepsy, cerebral palsy, and Parkinson's disease. The neurologist will also talk to you to get a picture of your child's medical history.

Neuropsychiatrist: A neuropsychiatrist is a medical doctor with expertise in diagnosing and treating mental disorders of neurological origin, including OCD, depression, bipolar disorders (manic-depression), and neurological disorders such as AD/HD with behavioral symptoms. Although both the neuropsychiatrist and pediatric neurologist are qualified to diagnose TS, the neuropsychiatrist is generally more familiar with child development and medications used to treat associated difficulties such as obsessive-compulsive behaviors or AD/HD.

Psychologist: A psychologist is not a medical doctor, but has a Ph.D. in psychology. This professional is trained in understanding human behavior, emotions, and how the mind works. Psychologists cannot diagnose Tourette syndrome or prescribe medication, but can help your family cope with the diagnosis and help your child with self-esteem or emotional issues related to living with TS. Psychologists can also diagnose some of the coexisting disorders such as AD/HD or learning disabilities. Some psychologists are trained in habit reversal and other behavioral therapies that may help reduce tics, obsessive thoughts and/or compulsive behaviors, and conquer some organizational challenges (see Chapter 4).

Occupational Therapist: An occupational therapist specializes in helping people with neurological impairments or other movement problems improve the motor skills (particularly the fine motor skills involving the hands and fingers) needed to carry out their daily activities. During the diagnosis process, they perform evaluations to find specific motor problems that may relate to a neurological impairment. Some OTs specialize in diagnosing and treating sensory integration difficulties.

If you are lucky enough to be able to work with a multidisciplinary team, after each member of the team has completed his evaluation, you will be given a summary of the team's findings, together with their treatment recommendations. If a team is not involved with your child, you should work with the professional you consider to be your child's primary physician to discuss the different findings and develop a treatment plan.

Diagnostic Studies

In diagnosing TS, the physicians will do a number of tests to rule out other neurological disorders and to look for specific neurological impairments or weaknesses. Tests may include blood tests and perhaps an electroencephalogram (EEG)—a test that measures the electrical activity of the brain and helps identify seizure activity. A physician may also do brain imaging studies, such as CT (computerized tomography) scans or MRI (magnetic resonance imaging) scans to rule out other causes of Tourette-like symptoms. (Chapter 3 discusses diagnostic studies in more detail.)

■■ The History of Tourette Syndrome

For most of history, Tourette syndrome has been grossly misunderstood. Centuries ago, people with Tourette syndrome were thought to be possessed. Often, they were kept isolated from others; sometimes they underwent extreme "treatments" such as flogging, lobotomies, or even being burned at the stake. Later, medical professionals theorized that the condition was due to mental or emotional problems arising within the child himself, or triggered by "bad parents." People with TS were sometimes committed to insane asylums, or went through psychoanalysis to work through the past emotional traumas they were believed to have suffered. And, as recently as the 1970s, Tourette syndrome was frequently misdiagnosed as schizophrenia, obsessive-compulsive disorder, epilepsy, or just plain "nervous habits."

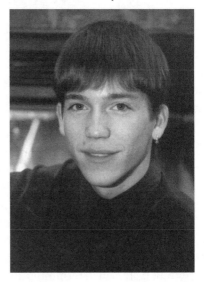

These misconceptions persisted even though the idea that Tourette syndrome was a genetic disorder had been around since at least 1885. In that year, Georges Gilles de la Tourette, a French neurologist, first identified Tourette syndrome as a distinct syndrome and suggested that the disorder was hereditary.

Since that time, medical researchers have written many reports and made many systematic studies. Today, although the cause of Tourette syndrome is still somewhat of a mystery, much progress has been made in understanding the condition, as well as in developing effective treatment strategies. As mentioned earlier, there is a very real hope that researchers will eventually be able to pinpoint the exact cause of TS, and that a cure will not be far behind.

Unfortunately, Tourette syndrome is still sometimes misdiagnosed or misunderstood, even by medical or mental health professionals. If you feel your child meets the criteria for Tourette syndrome and/or affiliated disorders and you're being told that the problem is discipline or anxiety-related, it may be wise to get a second opinion from a physician who specializes in TS.

■■ Your Child's Future

Many of the barriers that previously prevented people with Tourette syndrome from reaching their full potential have now fallen. Federal and state regulations and laws guarantee your child the right to a public education tailor-made to his unique learning needs. By prohibiting discrimination against people with disabilities, state and federal laws also ensure your child's right to work and participate in community activities. And, although misunderstanding and prejudice may still be encountered, growing awareness and public understanding of the disorder are helping to reduce negative attitudes. The Tourette Syndrome Association, in particular, has taken a leading role in combating misconceptions, as well as in providing essential support services and advocacy for people with Tourette syndrome.

How well your child will eventually flourish in this new climate of acceptance and opportunity depends on many factors. Some of these factors are out of your control. For example, the severity of your child's tics, the presence of associated disorders such as AD/HD or OCD, the way his body responds to different medications and even his intelligence can all affect his ability to adjust. Continued difficulties with mood, aggression, or handling frustration can also contribute to problems in adulthood.

But other factors vital to your child's adjustment *are* under your control. Your child's level of maturity as an adult and his ability to cope with the stress of having Tourette syndrome are perhaps *the* most important factors in determining how happy and fulfilling his life will be. These are things that you, as a parent, can help nurture with a steady diet of support and encouragement. You can learn to foster your child's independence and mastery without neglecting any special needs. Your child's school program, too, can play a large part in helping him achieve the successes he needs to feel good inside and develop skills, talents, and interests. In fact, no matter how severe your child's symptoms are, his future should be as bright as any other child's, as long as he has the right attitude and effective coping skills.

Most children with Tourette syndrome go on to lead normal, independent adult lives. As with other children, how far they can go in school is limited only by their intellectual abilities and drive. Most graduate from high school; many go on to complete college and even graduate school. People with Tourette syndrome are equally successful on the job—provided personal strengths and preferences are taken into account in choosing a career. Someone with loud coprolalia, for example, probably shouldn't choose a job in a library, any more than someone who has claustrophobia should choose to work in a coal mine. As long as your child has a healthy acceptance of both his strengths and weaknesses, however, he will find his place in society.

∷ Conclusion

Tourette syndrome is a chronic condition that can—but won't necessarily—have a major impact on your child's psychological development and relationships with others. Depending on the severity and the presence of associated disorders, it may also make it harder for your child to develop skills in certain areas. But unlike many other disabilities, which often place very definite limits on what a child is able to learn and achieve, Tourette syndrome in itself rarely prevents children from reaching their potential. Many highly successful people have had Tourette syndrome, including Dr. Samuel Johnson, one of the greatest English writers of the eighteenth century.

In short, remember that Tourette syndrome is only one small part of your child. And although it is a part that cannot—and should not—be ignored, it is also a part that both your child and your family can learn to work around. Like every child, your child with Tourette syndrome deserves to be given the chance to make the most of life. With proper medical treatment, appropriate education, and support from your family, your child should be well on their way to reaching that goal.

∷ Parent Statements

Finally getting a diagnosis of TS was scary, but at the same time a relief because we finally had a name for what was happening, and now we could start doing something about it.

❧

When my husband was in his late forties, he went with us to the neurologist, because I suspected that the "funny" things I was told he did as a child just might have been due to TS. I was right. He was misdiagnosed as a child, put on all types of strange medications, and never understood by his family and friends. His TS symptoms faded in his late teens and he forgot all about them until our daughter was diagnosed.

❧

*Because there is still so much misinformation out about TS, parents **must** become educated and not rely totally on the doctor.*

❧

The TS and OCD caused problems when my kids were younger. Constant touching, loud vocalizations, broken items, compulsions to have the last word. It didn't help that my second child also had OCD issues!

❧

It is characteristic with TS that tics often disappear when the person is focused on some activity. Our daughter has never had a tic during a vocal or theatrical performance, or when modeling. Rare are her tics when giving presentations or speeches. If you know what to listen for, you may hear her when she is off stage but never when she is on.

❧

*When I took my quirky, twitchy, fussy child to an occupational therapist, she told me he had sensory integration dysfunction. When his tics worsened, we went to a neurologist, who diagnosed Tourette syndrome. After I read an article about Asperger syndrome on the Internet, I took my son to a psychiatrist, who said he had a textbook case. A few months later, the school psychologist told us he also had AD/HD. The fact is, our son has **all** these challenges—but not one of the specialists ever suggested we might want to seek additional evaluations by others.*

❧

When Joan was seven, her tics were causing her lots of problems. She had this cough—she did it fifty or a hundred times a day. She would also squint her eyes and jerk her shoulder. This was enough of a problem, but on top of that, she had this hand-washing routine. I couldn't count how many times a day she washed her hands. She had to have a clean towel each time and she was wild over germs. She thought everything had germs: we had to cover the plates before each meal, and if someone coughed or sneezed in the kitchen or at the table, she wouldn't eat.

❧

When Derek was four, he had this sniffing thing which lasted for four months. Then it went away. He then started to blink his eyes, and after a couple of months he started clearing his throat. It's been like that ever since—one thing starts and then goes away, and then another starts. Sometimes he has three or four tics at once.

❧

I knew he was "hyper" from the time he was a toddler. From six in the morning until eleven at night, he was like a motor you wind up. It was go, go, go. I wish I could bottle and sell some of Dave's energy.

❧

Allen is creative, bright, loving, caring, and affectionate. He has many facial hand-to-face, and vocal tics. He exhibits SIB (self injurious behavior) and aggressive behavior much of the time.

❧

We knew about Tourette syndrome, the lip smacking, and the way he flipped his head like he was trying to get the hair out of his eyes, but we didn't know about the echoing. He started repeating the last two or three words of each sentence. At first it was a whisper and then out loud. We had four very tough months before someone told us that the repeating was also part of the TS. He got in so much trouble at school because of this, and we weren't able to help him at home because we didn't know.

❧

I am always amazed at how interesting Sharon's obsessions can be. She is able to transfer her unusual thoughts into very creative art, games, and puzzles.

❧

Our son's symptoms began around age five with prolonged sniffing, which we thought was a habit. If we told him to stop, he would then start clearing his throat. The throat clearing lasted for months and then he began repetitive movements—head to shoulder, hand to nose, eye, and ear. That's when we brought him to the doctor.

❧

It was a long journey to diagnosis, but when we found out, it was as if somebody had opened a window. Everything Brad did made sense.

❧

When Sierra was diagnosed, the first thing I did was join the TSA support group. What they were saying fit Sierra to a tee. It seemed like they were all talking about my child.

❧

I will never forget the day my son was diagnosed. I felt relieved and sick to my stomach at the same time; also guilty. My heart began to break. These feelings are still with me.

❧❧

Developing a sense of humor will go a long way in helping you to live with Tourette syndrome.

❧❧

We would ask ourselves, concerning the latest behavior. Is it the TS? The OCD? Just being a teenager? During the teen years, a lot of behavior cannot be defined clearly. We spent a lot of time in separate rooms, relaxing and calming ourselves down.

❧❧

Every characteristic of your child, TS or not, has both a positive and negative interpretation and application. Concentrate on the positive. Your child may come up with some wild ideas of what he or she wants to do, but give it a chance—you may be surprised!

❧❧

*My oldest daughter has Tourette syndrome, and, like most kids with TS, she was made fun of and had only one or two close friends. One of her tics was a singing one. She would hit a high operatic note as she strolled through the house. Music became her release. Last year she auditioned for the show **American Idol** and made it to the Hollywood round. She has also had success on other shows. When she was little she asked me why God gave her this and I told her that he gave her a pure heart, a brilliant mind, beauty, and a fantastic voice, but with all that, he had to give her something to keep her humble. She laughed and told me she thought she had been humbled enough. I am so very proud of her. Her tics are milder now but she is almost 18 and so I think she has figured out how to deal with them. I think she is really a good inspiration for younger ones with Tourette syndrome.*

2

ADJUSTING TO YOUR CHILD'S DIAGNOSIS

Tracy Marsh

There is really no such thing as a "typical" case of Tourette syndrome. In addition to mild to severe tics, your child may have associated disorders with symptoms of hyperactivity, impulsiveness, obsessive-compulsive behaviors, or attention deficits, in any combination of symptoms and in any degree of severity. Her symptoms may have unfolded overnight or developed so gradually that you were scarcely aware of their arrival. They may have appeared as early as infancy or as late as adolescence.

But despite the countless forms Tourette syndrome can take, most parents' experiences shortly before and after their child's diagnosis are quite similar. Often parents spend months or years desperately seeking an explanation for their child's puzzling behaviors. They get conflicting advice from family, friends, and doctors. Often, they are blamed for the very behavior they would do anything to understand. And depending on how their child is doing and what the latest doctor says, they may be alternately buoyed up by hopefulness or paralyzed by dread. Then, when their child finally receives a diagnosis of Tourette syndrome, they are flooded by a fresh torrent of emotions and experiences.

If your child has just tics and none of the associated disorders such as AD/HD, OCD, or rage problems, your story will be different from mine. I don't want to scare you when I tell my story, since my son has many associated disorders and they were a bigger issue for us than his tics were. But if your child does have TS Plus, our family's story may sound very familiar to you.

Our son, Jeffrey, was born in August, 1981. An active, happy baby, he walked early and was soon into everything. He seemed very excited about the world and needed to touch and experience everything. In marked contrast to his older sister, he kept me very busy chasing after him, trying to keep him out of danger. I began asking our pediatrician about Jeff's activity level before he was two. The doctor said that Jeff was "all boy," and gave me the impression that he thought I was just a nervous mom. I thought maybe he was right. (Remember, associated disorders such as AD/HD typically show symptoms years before tics start.)

By the time Jeff was three, my concerns had deepened. He just couldn't seem to control his behavior as well as other three-year-olds could. For example, no matter how many times we warned him not to, he would impulsively run into the street or hit other children and grab their toys. He seemed unable to anticipate how others would react to his behavior. For example, whenever he hit other children, he always seemed very surprised when they got angry.

Jeff was also very rigid about changes. Once he got an idea in his head, he could not be swayed. He would only wear green clothes, demanded that certain routines be carried out, and insisted on playing with particular toys. In addition, he was impossible to discipline. He just could not seem to understand that his behavior was inappropriate, no matter how many times we corrected him. Jeff needed constant supervision, and we couldn't take him into malls, restaurants, or many other public places without him running wild.

Frustrated and exhausted, we turned to a local psychologist. During a one-hour session, the psychologist focused only on our parenting skills. He told us that Jeff had probably picked up hostility from something in our home. Although my husband and I were convinced that Jeff acted this way not out of hostility, but because there was something wrong in his brain, we still felt guilty. The psychologist never told us he wasn't qualified to do neurological testing and he offered no suggestions. With no idea what to do next, we felt helpless and powerless. It seemed no one would listen to us or take our situation seriously.

When Jeff was four, we took him to the public school for pre-school screening. Jeff ran around the room from one activity to another and couldn't pay attention to the testing. Although his behavior was embarrassing to me, it qualified Jeff for a special education evaluation.

The school referred my son to a pediatric neurologist, who diagnosed Jeff with attention-deficit/hyperactivity disorder (AD/HD). Jeff had a slightly abnormal electroencephalogram (EEG), which meant he couldn't take the stimulants usually prescribed for AD/HD. The doctor suggested that we try behavior modification and special education services.

For the next two years, we worked hard to understand our son's needs and to help him learn to behave in more socially acceptable ways. We learned that a calm, relaxed environment helped Jeff to be more in control. He still had no friends, however, and because we could not get a babysitter, my husband and I had no social life, either.

At times we believed that Jeff would outgrow his hyperactivity. At other times we were overwhelmed and depressed. We tried special diets and explored allergy theories. We were desperate for solutions.

Jeff's first-grade year began with problems. He couldn't get along with the other children, and he had trouble following the teacher's directions. On the school bus and at the bus stop, Jeff did impulsive, inappropriate things, and the older kids began making fun of him. The behavior modification program the teacher and I tried didn't work. As a result of all these failures, Jeff's self-esteem was sinking fast. He also seemed to be developing "nervous habits"—clearing his throat, blinking, pushing hair out of his face, and making meaningless noises. All year long, whenever the phone rang, I feared it would be one of Jeff's teachers venting their frustration on me. The pain of watching my child suffer was overwhelming and I felt like no one understood. As a parent, there is no pain worse than being unable to help your child.

Near the end of first grade, the school psychologist observed Jeff in class. I will never forget his phone call. He said that he suspected a neurological problem and did not think Jeff's behavior problems were deliberate. A breakthrough at last! We returned to the pediatric neurologist, who diagnosed Jeff with Tourette syndrome. I had never heard of TS before, but was very relieved to have a doctor validate what we had believed for so many years—that there was a medical explanation for Jeff's behaviors. And when the doctor told me that medication could be used, I felt very optimistic.

▪▪ The News Sinks In

When my son was diagnosed in the 1980s, few people had ever heard of Tourette syndrome. My initial relief at having a medical diagnosis faded quickly as the realities of living with TS Plus hit me. I thought that having the medical name for Jeff's problems would mean all his symptoms would be helped by medicine. I quickly learned that professionals still didn't have good treatment or understanding for the complicated symptoms we were dealing with. Medications helped my son's symptoms somewhat, but I was acutely aware that there was no

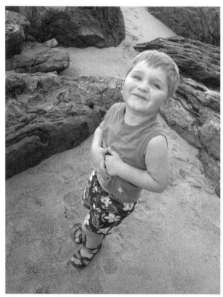

cure for Tourette syndrome. I was told that TS is lifelong, and that things would probably get worse before they got better. And teachers, neighbors, and other children *still* didn't understand me or my child. Like my child's TS symptoms, my worry, frustration, and sorrow would wax and wane, at times almost overwhelming me.

Depending on the severity of your child's symptoms and the way the diagnosis was presented to you, you may have felt as relieved as I did to hear that there was a medical explanation for your child difficulties—especially if you had been dealing with hyperactivity, obsessive compulsive symptoms, or behavioral problems for years before the actual tics developed.

Your situation may be somewhat different if your child's Tourette syndrome came on suddenly and you were fortunate enough to get an immediate diagnosis. Instead of relief, your initial reaction may have been shock, denial, or anger. If so, the emotional fallout from your child's diagnosis may hit you even harder and sooner than it would have if you had had the opportunity to adjust to the news more gradually. Fear that your child will develop coprolalia and other severe tics may be keeping you awake at night, even if your realize that the odds are against this.

If your child has mild TS symptoms, coping will probably be easier. Your child and your family will generally have fewer problems inside and outside the home, and you may not even think of your child as having a disability. But then again, there may be times when the reality of your child's neurological impairment and the changes that it brings seem very difficult to face.

No matter how and when you get the news of your child's TS, you could face a long, complicated adjustment process. This is because you, like most parents, probably had idealized expectations for your child's life. When your baby was born, you had hopes and dreams that she would be happy and successful. But once your child is diagnosed with Tourette syndrome, you may fear that you will have to let go of some of those hopes and dreams. Instead of hoping that your child will one day become a doctor, athlete, or lawyer, you may now wonder (rightly or wrongly) how she will make it through high school. These feelings are part of the mourning process for the "perfect" child that will never be. Often it awakens intensely painful emotions in every member of the family.

No two families handle the adjustment process in quite the same way. But it is easier to handle if you are prepared for some of the emotions you may have and understand why you feel the way you do. This chapter is designed to give you that understanding, as well as to suggest some strategies to help you get on with your life.

▪▪ Your Emotions

In coming to terms with your child's diagnosis, it is normal to be besieged by a variety of emotions: shock, fear, helplessness, guilt, anger, grief, and resentment, to name a few. You may feel a number of these emotions simultaneously, or may move in stages from one to another. Occasionally you may seem to get "stuck" in one emotion for a while. Even after you think you have conquered one emotion, something may happen to set it off again. For example, whenever Jeff's symptoms began to worsen, I would re-experience the grief and helplessness I felt right after his diagnosis. Or when I saw a young boy shopping cooperatively with his mother, I would grieve over the many years I'd lost struggling with Jeff in stores, instead of enjoying our time together. Even now that Jeff is a young adult, when I see him being misunderstood because of his symptoms, my anger can resurface.

Regaining your equilibrium can be tough. There are no foolproof coping methods, and sometimes it can seem as though you take three steps back for every two forward. But with time, most parents learn to master their emotions and enjoy the good things their child and their life have to offer. To help you sort out what you might be feeling, the sections below describe some of the most powerful emotions parents typically have en route to acceptance.

Shock and Denial

Many parents react to the diagnosis of Tourette syndrome with shock. This reaction is especially common if your child's TS came on abruptly and you had no clue it was anything serious. But even if you have been searching for answers for years, hearing the words "Tourette syndrome" is shocking. To learn suddenly that something is wrong inside your child's brain is a tremendous jolt. You may go numb, and might not feel or think anything other than "this is not really happening to me."

Shock, in fact, serves a useful purpose. It helps insulate us from the total blow of a painful experience. It gives us a grace period before we must face reality and begin to actively deal with our problems. If you get stuck in this phase too long, however, you may have trouble accepting the reality of TS in your family. Because of the waxing and waning of symptoms or their subtlety, you may easily fool yourself into thinking that the tics are just "bad habits" and fall into the trap of long-term denial. This could make it harder for you to recognize and do something about your child's needs. In this situation, it may help to talk to other parents of children with Tourette syndrome and see that many otherwise "normal" families are in your situation.

Fear

Today, the term "Tourette syndrome" is much better known than when my son was diagnosed. That can be both a blessing and a curse. Thanks to the way it's been portrayed in popular media, many people think Tourette syndrome is simply a disorder that makes people yell curse words. Hopefully, the doctor who diagnosed your child has explained that only a very small percentage of people with TS develop coprolalia, while many *do* manifest other symptoms that the general public has no idea are associated with the disorder—AD/HD, obsessive-compulsive tendencies, etc. It's important that you don't let Hollywood screenwriters warp your perspective. Most children with Tourette syndrome never develop symptoms beyond the mild stage. But if your child does, there will be help available.

It's only natural to worry about your child—how bad her tics or other symptoms may become, how much they'll affect her future, whether she'll be teased or ostracized. We all want to protect our children and shield them from pain. Unfortunately, that's not always possible. The fact is, at this point, no doctor can predict how bad your child's symptoms will become. But you can take comfort in knowing that most children's tics subside at least somewhat by late adolescence/early adulthood, and for many, they disappear completely.

Helplessness

As the shock wears off, a feeling of overwhelming helplessness may set in. Your child's problems may seem so numerous or complicated that you don't know how to begin helping her. Especially if teachers and other professionals have previously tried and failed to improve her symptoms, you may wonder if there are any real answers. And just the thought of dealing with the platoons of doctors, problems at school and in the neighborhood, medication side effects, and daily care of your child may make you want to run away. Worst of all, when you think about the future, you see no end to the constant drain on your time and energy.

When I first realized the extent of Jeff's needs, I cried for three days. I felt unequipped to handle the present problems, and looking into the future brought overwhelming worry. Advice from well-meaning friends who didn't understand what I was going through only made matters worse. In trying to make me feel better, some denied Jeff's TS or tried to minimize my pain. My feelings of powerlessness did not begin to lift until other parents of children with Tourette syndrome showed me that it really could be done. It was especially helpful to talk to parents of older children and to adults with TS and hear their success stories.

Guilt

Guilt is another emotion that can really run you through the emotional ringer. After you learn that TS is genetically transmitted, you may scour through family histories, looking for other family members who may have had Tourette syndrome. You then may blame yourself or your spouse for not knowing that TS runs in the family. Whether or not a genetic link is found, you may feel terribly guilty for somehow "causing" your child to suffer so much. If one parent has TS and knows the child inherited it from her, she may feel an added burden of guilt, knowing first-hand what problems their child will likely endure.

Often parents fault themselves for their treatment of their child before diagnosis. They may feel guilty for punishing their child for tics and other behaviors that were out of her control. My husband and I, for example, felt guilty about the behavior modification we had used to try to stop Jeff's tics. We had had him wear a rubber band on his wrist and snap the rubber band whenever he had a tic. Although this method stopped one tic, two new tics appeared to take its place. We also felt guilty about our frustration over his behavior, once we learned that he definitely could not control it. Sometimes parents think back to the many times people made fun of their child's tics and feel guilty about not intervening. And then there is the lingering guilt about being a "bad" parent, even though you know in your heart you didn't cause your child's TS. For example, any time a professional, friend, or relative suggests that something might have been my fault, I felt angry and guilty at the same time.

Remorseful as you may feel, it is important to realize that you are not to blame for your child's troubles. Tourette syndrome may be genetic, but there are no pre-natal tests that could have predicted that your child would have the condition. You are also not to blame for failing to realize that your child's symptoms were out of her control—even the best specialists sometimes have difficulty recognizing Tourette syndrome. Your energies are far better spent in helping your child today, than in blaming yourself or your spouse for what happened yesterday.

Anger

There is a lot to be angry about in dealing with Tourette syndrome. We are angry at all the doctors and professionals who misdiagnosed or minimized our child's Tourette syndrome, and angry that they can't make our child "better." We are angry with all the people who blamed us as parents for the TS symptoms. We are angry with the schools, churches, and social organizations for the way they may have misunderstood and mishandled our child. We are angry at the comedians who think "Tourette syndrome" is a big joke. Often we are angry at God for allowing this to happen, and at our families and friends for minimizing our situation or for not giving us support.

For my part, I was outraged at the ignorance of people who constantly misunderstood our son and judged him mercilessly. My husband

and I were also furious at the medical insurance system when they refused to pay Jeff's medical bills, claiming that TS was a mental illness, not a neurological impairment.

Anger is a powerful emotion. If you can channel it in the right directions, it can be a great impetus for needed change. My anger over the public's ignorance about TS motivated me to become involved with my local TSA as a parent advocate. I now try to educate people about TS whenever possible. And our anger about the insurance issue propelled us to take the insurance company to an appeal board. We won the appeal, and they had to pay our claims. But when your fury is out of control or you become "stuck" in your anger, it can lead to roadblocks in communication with school staff, doctors, and others who could help you with your child. You may enter a conversation with a hostile, defensive attitude, which impedes open communication and makes it difficult for you to understand what people are saying. Getting mired in anger can also make you sick or depressed. In these situations, it's essential to vent your anger with others—your spouse, the parents in a support group—who understand what you're going through.

Grief

Grief is the deep sense of loss we feel when we lose something or someone dear to us. It is a lonely, empty, painful feeling that seeps into your very being like a poisonous gas, altering your whole outlook on life. In the early days, your grief can be all-encompassing when you think of the idealized child—the perfect family life—that will never be. As my husband and I did, you may grieve about losing years of your life to constant stress and struggle. Later, grief can intrude on you when you least expect it, rekindled by everyday experiences that remind you that your family is different than average. Watching two girls amiably playing together in the park, for instance, you may suddenly be overcome with sadness that TS will always set your child apart from other children. I had trouble accepting that typical vacations and many normal family activities were not feasible for our family.

Although it is almost inevitable that you will feel some sense of loss when your child is diagnosed with Tourette syndrome, grief does lessen with time. At first when you look at your child, the TS may be all you are able to see. As you learn more about your child and about Tourette syndrome, however, your main focus will shift away from TS. Like all parents, you find out what your child is capable of and adjust your expectations. Your idea of the perfect child is replaced by a more realistic view. And although you may still feel occasional twinges of grief, you recognize them for what they are: expressions of your love and concern for your child and of your desire that she have the opportunity to live the best possible life.

Resentment

Everything can seem so *unfair* when you have a child with Tourette syndrome. Other families can go out to eat or to a movie and melt right into the crowd; you and your child may immediately become a magnet for stares if you venture outside. Other parents can just assume that their child will adapt to her teacher and the classroom; you may have to trudge to the school for meeting after meeting to work out your child's educational problems. Other children have sleepovers and go on outings with friends; your child may not be able to handle these situations. Thinking about how much harder your family has it than other families can naturally lead to strong feelings of resentment.

Often, your resentment doesn't stop with people who take normal family life so much for granted. For example, you can also resent people who say insensitive things about your child. I sometimes resent society in general for being so narrow minded and intolerant as to look at people who are different as freaks. And even though you know that your child cannot control her tics and other symptoms, you may even resent her for making your life more difficult. I found that if I spent too much time caring for my son by myself, I was much more apt to feel resentful toward him for his disability. I'd lose my perspective, get tired, and my resolve would get worn down by constant demands and interventions. Eventually, I learned that I needed a break now and then from the stress of raising a child with Tourette syndrome. I *needed* support from others—husband, friends, and family. And then sometimes I resented being different from other families and needing help.

Although all these types of resentment are normal and understandable, it is important not to let it rule your life. Dwelling on your resentment can come between you and your child, lead to self-pity, and drive away the very people you need for support. To keep from getting stuck in resentment, it helps to be aware of these feelings, and to remind yourself of the good things in your life. For me, a growing spiritual life helps to keep my life in perspective. I have learned to be grateful and thankful for all the blessings in my life and that helps counteract resentment. I know that at times my emotions can be overwhelming, and it is good to know that I have a higher power I can lean on. I find that reading inspirational books such as *When Bad Things Happen to Good People,* which is included in the Reading List, helps me put my feelings in perspective. This may seem like small consolation at the moment, but most people have felt at one time or another that their lives, too, are unfair.

:: How to Adjust

Acknowledge Your Feelings

When you're hurting, it's senseless to pretend that you're not. You cannot make rational decisions when your mind is a jumble of painful and conflicting emotions. Nor can you see things as they really are when your thoughts are colored by despair, anger, or guilt. Getting the support you need from other people can also be more difficult if your feelings short-circuit open communication.

Looking back on my own situation, I think fear kept me in a state of anxiety too long. My fear was in imagining the worst case scenario for my son's future. In retrospect, I realize that the worst time for him was early adolescence and if I had not had so much fear and anxiety 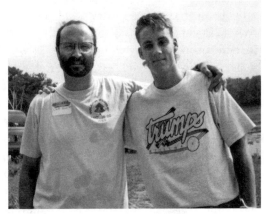 about the future, I would have had more internal resources to work with the present. His situation never got anywhere near as bad as I feared. And these unconscious fears led to pain, worry, and grief. I wasn't always aware of my inner fears but they stole too much of my peace of mind for too long.

Obviously, you must first come to terms with your own emotions if you are to be effective in meeting the needs of your child and the rest of your family. This means you must first honestly own up to everything you are feeling. In the beginning, this can be difficult: you may have so many emotions at once that you aren't sure *what* you're feeling. You may also feel ashamed of certain feelings you are having, and worry that you must be an awful person to be having such "bad" feelings. For example, I thought that feeling resentful was a selfish thing to do, and that feeling helpless was "weak." It can help to remember that any feeling you're having has probably been shared by thousands of parents before you. Your feelings are a normal reaction to hearing devastating news, and are neither good nor bad.

Everyone has their own way of coping with difficult emotions. Some find it helpful to work out their frustrations through exercising or concentrating on a hobby. Others cry, talk to a friend, or seek help from professional counselors. My personal way of coping is by talking things over many times. A friend of mine copes by swimming laps every day. Do whatever seems right to you. Remember, you have a right to have whatever emotions you are feeling *and* to express them.

Take Your Time

Following your child's diagnosis, you may feel as if you should rush right out and try to solve all her problems immediately. You don't want to waste a moment discovering the medication that will best control her tics or devising the educational strategies that will best help her learn. In fact, my husband and I began experimenting with medications and trying to set up a special education program for Jeff right away. But coming on top of everything else you are feeling, the very thought of everything that needs to be done may be overwhelming.

Take your time. If you don't feel emotionally ready to handle major decisions yet, then by all means, put them off until you do. Just like broken bones, emotional wounds take time to heal. You cannot rush or force the adjustment process. But if you're good to yourself, you *can* make things easier on yourself. Make whatever changes to your lifestyle you can to make this time less stressful. For example, simplify things or cut back on stress-producing family activities or social events. Look at your short- and long-term goals for your family, and set priorities. For instance, is it more important to sell pies at the PTA fund raiser or to spend relaxed time at home with your family? Is it more important to attend family social gatherings, or to find less stimulating activities for your child that won't send her behavior out of control?

It *is* important for your child to receive the right medical treatment and educational program and to become an accepted part of the community. But it is also important that you be emotionally ready to give your child the support she needs to make the most of her opportunities. I would suggest taking it easy before you plunge into a whirl of activities. Later on, when you and your child with TS have developed better coping skills, there will be time to make decisions and to take part in activities. (See Chapter 5 for practical methods of coping with community activities.) Remember, you can be your child's most powerful ally—if you allow yourself time to grow stronger.

Get the Facts

When it comes to Tourette syndrome, there are no stupid questions. People with TS have been misunderstood and mistreated for so long that there are all kinds of erroneous bits of information floating around out there. Then, too, because Tourette syndrome is such a complex disorder, you will probably have many questions even if you have access to the most accurate and up-to-date information.

Becoming informed about Tourette syndrome is the best way to put needless worries to rest. It helped my family immensely to learn about the expected outcome of TS. We could mentally prepare ourselves for coping with the next six to eight years of worsening symptoms. And we could prepare for the changes as a family. Information is also essential to being able to deal effectively with school staff and doctors. In addition, knowledge about TS can boost your confidence in your abilities as a parent because you will be better able to interpret your child's behavior and needs. You also need the facts about TS so you can help your child understand and deal with her symptoms.

To gather information about your child's symptoms in particular, it is essential to find a doctor who is not only knowledgeable about TS, but also accessible to parents. As problems arise, you may need to contact your doctor for immediate advice.

For information about TS in general, contact the national Tourette Syndrome Association (TSA) at the address in the back of the book for information about their many helpful pamphlets, booklets, and videos. Your local TSA should also be a great source of information. In addition, it may be helpful to contact the Obsessive-Compulsive Foundation, learning disabilities organizations, or ADHD associations, which are listed in the Resource Guide. The Reading List also suggests useful books and journals that may be available through your library. Finally, you may want to attend one of the conferences on TS held throughout the

U.S. and Canada. My husband and I have found these conferences to be a great way to learn the latest TS findings, and meeting other parents and hearing their experiences is enriching. Information on conferences can be obtained through your local TSA.

Seek Support

Meeting other parents of children with Tourette syndrome can be a lifeline for exhausted and bewildered parents. Better than anyone else, other parents are equipped to tell you about what lies ahead and how to deal with it. They can help you out with everything from inside information about your school system, to practical strategies for dealing with specific problems at home or in public. Best of all, they can offer an understanding ear when something is troubling you.

My husband and I felt nervous at our first support group meeting. But people were so understanding and accepting that we soon felt comfortable. In fact, we found that talking about our family was therapeutic. Who better to tell your story to than people who are going through, or have been through, the same experience?

Your local TSA chapter most likely sponsors a TS support group. To make contact, call the national Tourette Syndrome Association or go to their website. (Contact information is listed in the Resource Guide at the back of this book.)

Besides sponsoring support groups, most state TSA chapters put on social events for families of children with Tourette syndrome. Not only do these social events allow you to meet and swap information with other parents, but they also allow you to truly relax without worrying that someone will criticize your child's behavior.

If your family takes part in your local TSA activities, your child can meet older role models with TS, as well as children their own age. It has helped Jeff to realize there are others in the same boat as he is and to accept his TS. "Normal" siblings are also welcome at TSA activities. They can vent their frustrations about their brothers and sisters (and they do!). Our daughter has become good friends with several other siblings of children with TS, and the whole experience has helped our family immensely. Everyone in the family now realizes that they are not alone with their feelings and frustrations about Tourette syndrome.

▪▪ Telling Your Child

As the person most directly affected by TS, your child deserves to know why she has tics and other behaviors. Just like you, she has probably agonized over why she cannot seem to control certain sounds and movements no matter how hard she tries.

How you break the news to your child will depend somewhat on her age. It was pretty easy telling our seven-year-old that he had TS, because he was well aware of his "hyper" behavior and problems with friends. We explained to him that there was a problem in his brain that made it harder for him to control his behavior and calm down. If your child is somewhat older, she may want more factual information on the neurology of TS. For help explaining your child's diagnosis, you can contact the national TSA. 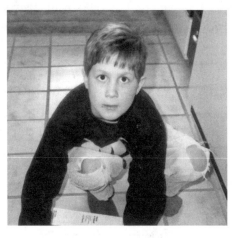 They offer videotapes and pamphlets which explain TS to all age groups, from very young children to adults. Several useful children's books about TS and ADHD are also available. These can be found in the Reading List at the back of this book.

Whatever your child's age, you don't want to overload your child with more information than she is ready for at this time. But it is often helpful to reassure her that as she grows older, she will probably be more in control of her Tourette syndrome, and chances are good that symptoms will improve. It is also imperative to give honest answers to your child's questions about TS. Many young children want to know if they will die from TS or whether it is contagious. When specific symptoms occur, your child may wonder, "Is this TS, or am I crazy?" If you don't know the answers to questions, talk to other children or adults with TS, as well as their parents. You might also urge your child to make a list of questions for the doctor to encourage her to begin taking responsibility for her own care.

In our family, we felt that merely learning *facts* about TS was not enough. We thought it was also important to learn how it *feels* to have TS by getting to know adults with TS. This knowledge pays off every day. I cannot tell you how many times my son has complained of feeling "different" or "weird" only to discover that his feeling is a typical TS symptom. One day, for example, Jeff was concerned about how "grossed out" he was at the feel of the gooey glue they were using in school, when the other kids seemed to enjoy it. Because of my knowledge of TS Plus symptoms, I recognized that Jeff's disgust was caused by tactile defensiveness—a type of sensory problem which causes a strong, adverse reaction to some touch sensations. I was able to allay Jeff's fears and explain that people with TS often have this reaction. He felt much better.

Once you break the news to your child, you can expect that she will go through the same grieving process that you experienced. When we first told Jeff about his diagnosis, he crawled under a blanket and said he didn't want to hear about it. We watched him slowly progress through each phase until he, too, reached acceptance. Eventually, he was able to tell TS jokes and talk openly about his latest tics or compulsions. If your child is somewhat older when you get the diagnosis, she may have more difficulty coping. During the early adolescent ages of eleven to fifteen, children all want to be exactly alike, and peer pressure is exceptionally strong. Because of your child's "difference," she may feel overwhelming denial and anger at first.

In addition to her feelings about the diagnosis, your child will also have to cope with feelings resulting from years of being misunderstood. Because your child was probably blamed, shamed, and humiliated because of her symptoms, her self-esteem may be very low by this time. She may have little trust in adults or teachers because no one would believe her or help her. You must reassure her that her symptoms are not her fault, and that people who make fun of them are wrong. You will also need to educate everyone in your child's world—at school, around the neighborhood—so that teasing or punishing is stopped. Family counseling, too, may help your child develop higher self-esteem, as well as cope with feelings such as anger and frustration that have built up over years of being misunderstood. Chapter 5 provides more information on boosting your child's self-esteem.

◼◼ Your Family and Friends

It is not enough for you to love and accept your child. If she is to grow up feeling like a valued member of society, others around her must also treat her with caring and understanding. The logical source of this added emotional support is your family members and friends.

Most family members and friends gladly rally to the support of a child with Tourette syndrome. But before they are able to do so, they usually must go through their own process of adjusting to the diagnosis. Like you, they will have many questions and concerns and will have to work through their feelings in their own way. Often, however, they will follow your lead. For this reason, the following sections offer some suggestions for gently guiding others toward acceptance.

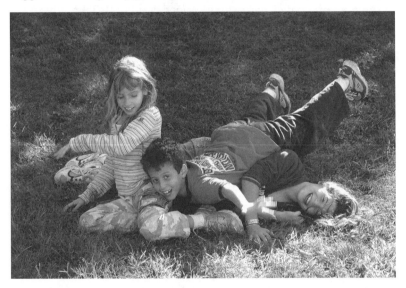

Brothers and Sisters

If your older children are old enough to ask "Why?" they have probably noticed at least some differences in their sibling with Tourette syndrome. Whether or not they've actually articulated their questions, you can be sure an explanation about TS would be welcome. In our family, Jeff's nine-year-old sister had stored up a lot of anger about how he treated her. Jeff could not seem to lose a game graciously and often hit or kicked her. In addition, his behavior at school often embarrassed her. Understanding that he didn't do these things on purpose helped her cope.

In explaining Tourette syndrome to brothers and sisters, there are several basic points to cover. First, you must help them understand that their sibling cannot control certain sounds and movements even though most people can. It may help if you compare having tics to having hiccups or sneezes or to having your knee tapped with a mallet by the doctor. Second, you should tell your other children that their sibling's tics increase if she is stared at, so they should ignore the symptoms whenever possible. Most children are very good at ignoring tics once they have this understanding.

If your child has more than simple tics and noises, explaining TS will be more complicated. Some obsessive-compulsive rituals or aggressive or impulsive behavior may appear purposeful, especially in the eyes of a child. For example, your child with TS might insist that her siblings follow a bedtime ritual or might have a compulsion to spit at family members. Telling siblings that their brother or sister with TS "can't help" behavior like this brings up many concerns about fairness and what to expect from siblings. At first, you may have to explain TS as each puzzling incident occurs. Counseling by a psychologist experienced in working with TS can also be a great help in coping with these family issues. Chapter 3 provides more information on psychological counseling.

After your other children have absorbed the information about your child's TS, they will probably go through many of the same stages you did in adjusting to the diagnosis. They may be angry and resentful because you seem to spend more time with their brother or sister. Or they may worry that they somehow caused their sibling to get Tourette syndrome. Like your child, they will need to be reassured that people do not die from TS and it is not contagious. Of course, if your other children are still quite young, there is a possibility that they, too, may develop TS, because of its genetic nature. It is probably *not* a good idea to bring this possibility up, as young children would not be able to understand genetics and there is no sense awakening needless worries.

Try to give your other children what they need—whether it is information about how TS will affect their sibling, or someone to talk to about their worries. Especially at first when you are busy with doctor appointments, school meetings, or TS support groups, take care that their emotional needs don't fall by the wayside. We fell into this trap when Jeff was first diagnosed. Our daughter—who is usually pretty independent—let us know in so many words that she resented the neglect. Be sure you set aside some special time to spend with your other children doing activities they enjoy. And by all means, arrange for your children to get to know other siblings of children with Tourette syndrome.

Grandparents and Other Relatives

How grandparents, aunts, uncles, and other relatives initially react to your child's diagnosis will likely depend on how aware they were of your earlier concerns. If relatives have been involved with your family and are aware of your concerns about your child, they may feel relief at having an explanation. If they were not previously aware of any problems, they may react with shock or disbelief. We experienced both of these reactions by relatives. Some had been concerned about Jeff for years, as we had. These relatives were relieved when we finally had a name for Jeff's problems. Others, who had had less contact with Jeff, denied and minimized the diagnosis, and again hinted that our parenting (or lack of discipline) must be the problem.

After the news has sunk in, your relatives are sure to have similar emotions to yours—perhaps with a new twist. Grandparents, for example, may blame themselves for passing on "defective" genes to your child. Aunts and uncles may worry that they, too, may have inherited the TS gene and will pass it on to their own children. This is a legitimate concern, and they need to become educated themselves on the genetic vulnerability that may run in your family (see Chapter 1). Your relatives may blame your spouse for giving your child Tourette syndrome, and your spouse's relatives may blame you. Everyone—especially grandparents—will probably grieve. Grandparents may grieve not only about the loss of their "perfect" grandchild, but also about the pain that you are going through.

You can help relatives adjust by reassuring them that their feelings are normal. Realize that this is a difficult time for them, too, and try not to be upset by questions and comments that seem insensitive or off the wall. Instead, volunteer information you think will help them and encourage them to ask questions. Try to allow for individual coping styles; don't expect them to come to terms with Tourette syndrome overnight. Let them know how important their understanding and acceptance is in reassuring your child that she is a welcome member of the family and of the human race. Also tell them how much *you* value their support. Chances are, you will find, as we have, that the relatives who take the time to really know your child will become great allies in her life.

Friends

Finding out that your child has Tourette syndrome can strengthen or disrupt old friendships. Some friends may feel genuinely uncomfortable around your child. Others may stay away for fear of doing or saying the wrong thing. Then again, friends may think that you have your hands full just caring for your child and that they would be in the way.

On the other side of the coin, you may send your friends subtle or not-so-subtle messages that you wish to be left alone. For example, you may think that your friends cannot possibly understand what you are going through, and therefore avoid them. Or you may stop attending parties and other social events because you feel you must devote yourself totally to your child. In our family, we cut back on socializing because Jeff became overly excited whenever we had company. I also sometimes found it very hard to be around my friends because I resented their normal lives. They would talk about their children's sports activities or family social events, and seemed insensitive to the way our lifestyle would have to change because of Jeff's TS.

Obviously, there is much room for misunderstanding. You may think your friends are "deserting" you, at the same time they think that you are shutting them out of your life. The best solution is usually for everyone to be honest with one another about how they feel and what they have been going through. With enough background information, many of your friends will probably adapt well and be eager to help out however they can.

Often, parents discover new friends through Tourette Syndrome Association activities or through special education. As mentioned earlier, other parents of children with Tourette syndrome can offer you unparalleled understanding. I don't know if I could have survived the first year after Jeff's diagnosis without the support of friends I made through TSA.

❏❏ Your Marriage

The first few months after your child's diagnosis can really be taxing. In addition to coping with your emotions, you may need to try out new medications and monitor their side effects, work on setting up an educational plan for your child, learn how to manage your child's behavior, and deal with medical insurance problems. Through teamwork, however, most parents find that the physical and emotional drain becomes more manageable.

In our case, it took some time to work out a smooth-running system. At first I was overwhelmed with all the new responsibilities and all

I needed to learn. My husband, Clyde, had to take a great deal of time off from work to help me at home and to meet with school personnel and doctors. Eventually, we each settled into doing what we did best and started working as a team. Clyde's strong point turned out to be organizing household jobs and activities. I handled daily care, school meetings, and doctor appointments. Because I spent so much time with Jeff during the day, Clyde took over at night to give me free time to go out with friends. When Jeff's needs were more intense, meal preparation and household duties often took a back seat, and we both became more flexible in our roles around the house.

While you and your spouse are working out ways to handle the practical aspects of raising your child, do not neglect each others' emotional needs. No one understands you as well as your spouse does, and no one can help you cope with your feelings quite so well. It is important to remember, however, that everyone copes in a different way, at a different rate. Your spouse may be feeling guilty the day you are feeling angry, or may seem to skip right over an emotion that engulfed you for weeks. The important point is to listen to your spouse without judging and to acknowledge that he or she has a right to feel that way.

Finally, try not to let your marriage revolve around Tourette syndrome. It *is* necessary and important for you and your spouse to discuss your concerns about your child, but this should not be your sole topic of conversation. Nor should all your activities be related in some way to TS. After all, your child with Tourette syndrome is not the only one in the family with special needs and interests. To recharge your batteries, you and your spouse must occasionally take a break and do something *you* enjoy. All parents need to learn to balance their time and energies between family and self, and you are no exception.

▪▪ Keeping Your Perspective

Having a child with Tourette syndrome is certainly no laughing matter. TS can complicate almost every aspect of your child's life and challenge your family's coping abilities to the utmost. But believe it or not, developing a sense of humor about TS can be an integral part of coping. Almost every adult with TS I know says that their ability to laugh at themselves and others with TS has been a lifesaver. They often tell the funniest stories about tics (especially vocal tics) and people's reactions to them. One person with TS told me, for example, about a TS conference

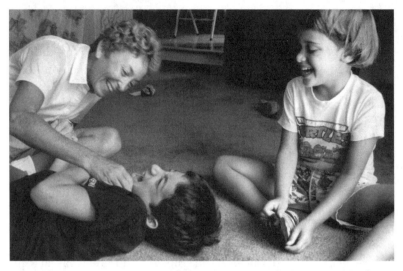

in which a speaker was talking about the Statue of Liberty. Suddenly, an audience member with TS let loose a hilariously appropriate vocal tic: "BIG MAMA!" The audience greeted this tic with a hearty laugh, which is actually the best way to cope with funny vocal tics. I don't mean that you should laugh *at* someone for having TS, but you may want to laugh along with her. A friendly laugh can sometimes do more than anything else to ease a potentially awkward situation.

For me, remaining open to the genuine humor in everyday situations is only part of the sometimes difficult task of keeping my perspective. It is also important to remember that TS, in and of itself, is not going to rob your child of her potential to succeed in life. As long as she develops effective coping strategies, there is no reason to believe your child will not achieve her personal, academic, or career goals. Today there are adults with TS pursuing successful careers in almost every profession you could mention, from doctor and lawyer, to professional athlete and musician. Samuel Johnson, the great eighteenth-century British writer and compiler of the first English language dictionary, is believed to have had Tourette syndrome with OCD. Dan Aykroyd, the hugely successfully comedian and entrepreneur, has come forth and said that he has TS (although his tics disappeared during adolescence) as well as Asperger syndrome.

As I have said earlier, my son's symptoms were worst in early adolescence. Now he is a young man with two daughters and a long-term relationship. He works and supports his family, and his symptoms are not obvious to anyone who doesn't know him well. His tics are mild and not noticeable. And he was diagnosed with the most severe associated disorders. The great majority of people with TS grow out of most of the symptoms. I knew many people with TS who were counselors in our TSA camp when they were teenagers and they are all now successful adults.

You may also be heartened to know that research has shown that people with TS develop some valuable skills other people don't ever have to develop. These include the skills of being empathetic to others with problems, knowing how to laugh at themselves, being more aware of their own body and their inner mind, and using excess energy to develop special skills such as drumming. I know from personal experience that a great sense of humor is a common special skill that people with TS develop.

∷ Conclusion

Right now, your child's diagnosis of Tourette syndrome may seem to hover overhead like a monstrous thunder cloud. It overshadows everything else in your life and makes the years ahead look long, dark, and hopeless. Even when a ray of sunshine manages to pierce the gloom, it only seems to spotlight your child's latest tics and behaviors. Maybe you feel that you will never be happy and carefree again. This is how I felt when my son was diagnosed.

I want you to know that there *is* life after Tourette syndrome! The clouds disperse and everyone in the family gets on with their lives. True, the life you have after the diagnosis will likely be different than the life you knew before. But do not assume that these differences will be for the worse. In our case, we moved from a relatively expensive house into a more affordable one, enabling me to quit my job. This meant we had to give up some of our material goals—to let go of the American Dream of enviable prosperity and success. But because the smaller house required less upkeep, it also meant we both had more energy to devote to our children. And because we had moved into a school district known for the highest quality education, we had more assurance that Jeff would have his special needs met at school.

Through our experiences with TS, we have been stretched, as people, in so many ways. I have learned, for example, never to look askance at a child who is acting up in a restaurant or mall. (And, because not everyone is so enlightened about behavior problems, I've learned to be tough skinned about criticism when my family is on the receiving end.) Along the way, I think I've developed a heightened sensitivity for all people who are being judged in ignorance. In addition, as my gut feelings and instincts about my son have proven correct time after time, my trust of my own instincts has been reinforced. We learned that the experts are not always the people with a Ph.D. behind their name. My daughter, I believe, has learned to accept differences in others with great tolerance, and Jeff—now a father himself—has learned that people love him and understand him just the way he is. Together, we have faced up to the fact that we will never be a perfect family. We have loosened up and accepted that we will always be different than the norm. And as TS has pulled our family closer together as a team, we have also discovered our own private brand of happiness.

Eventually, your family, too, will adjust to Tourette syndrome. You will learn to appreciate the "waning" times, and to cope with the "waxing" times. And as your love and acceptance grow, you will realize that what your child *does* is not nearly as important as who she *is*. One day you will see that whatever tics, rituals, attention deficits, or other symptoms she has are just part of the total package that makes her the unique and special child that she is. You will see her not as your child with Tourette syndrome, but simply as *your* child.

▪▪ Parent Statements

We have gone through many emotional stages since our son was diagnosed with TS two years ago. Counseling has helped us to sort through our feelings. Although we still feel great sadness that our son has a disability that will affect him all his life, we are coming to understand that he can have a good, fulfilling life despite having TS.

❧

There are many paths to happiness, and our daughter will find hers.

❧

It is devastating to have family, friends, and neighbors—not to mention doctors, counselors, and teachers—accuse you of bad parenting. I went it alone—in anguish—until I went to my first TSA meeting. The problems and stories told by the other members were so totally similar to my experience I could hardly believe my ears.

❧

When I chaperoned my son's field trip last spring, I noticed that he was having large motor tics, running, and swinging his arm up behind his head. I was terrified that the other children would tease and ridicule him. But you know what? No one paid any attention. The other kids were totally accepting. I felt like a huge weight had been lifted off me.

❧

If it hadn't been for the support and affiliation of other parents (and TS camp), I don't know what would have happened to me.

❧

Sometimes the condemnation of so-called "well-meaning" others is so hurtful it's impossible to convey in words.

❧

After years of looking for a diagnosis, we finally found a child neurologist who said my daughter had Tourette syndrome. I was shocked and grief-stricken. Yet at the same time, this doctor and his very sensitive nurse were the first to assure me that I was in no way responsible for her symptoms.

❧

When my son was first diagnosed, I lay awake at night, worrying about his future. Now I go days at a time without even thinking about his Tourette syndrome.

❧

I'm still learning to adjust to the fatigue that hits me when Robby's going through a trying phase. I try to forget the outside world's expectations of me. If I don't feel I can have relatives over or go to social events, I don't.

❧

Going to TS summer camp was very enlightening. Seeing all these loving parents with their children, it was obvious that these parents were not causing the problem behaviors.

❧

No one understands like other parents of kids with TS do. Not even the very best of the "TS doctors" in our area understands to the fullest. I wish he did, though.

❧

As a parent, I got to the point where what I needed more than anything was understanding. Everyone blamed me for Avery's TS, AD/HD, and OCD behaviors until his diagnosis.

❧

*The TS support group people don't doubt my observations or experiences. They **know** there is no hidden agenda. TS parents are the true professionals when it comes to this disorder.*

❧

And then there are the people who want to know if you drank or did cocaine during the pregnancy. Explaining to friends and neighbors that NO, he has TS, seems to fall on deaf ears.

❧

People thought I was wrong to deal with the hyperactivity. They said I should punish it. You get a lot of so-called well-meaning criticism. I'm so glad I followed my own instincts.

❧

After she'd watched the tapes on Tourette syndrome, my son's grandmother was overheard saying, "I still wonder if he could have caught it from the dog."

❧

When I told my parents about our daughter's TS, they said, "It couldn't have come from our side of the family, by God!"

❧

We have a pretty strong faith and have tried to help instill it in our children, but that hasn't solved everything. Kelsey still asks, "Mom, why did God make me this way?" It makes you pause as you think up that perfect answer when you yourself are trying to ask God, "Why did you do this to our baby?"

❧

My sister and niece were with our children at the local McDonald's eating when Kelsey nonchalantly mentioned that a boy in her class told her, "Kelsey, stop doing those tics." I immediately felt threatened that my baby was being treated badly in school and had all the rushes of emotion that I must begin to battle to save Kelsey from her classmates. So, I'm sitting there thinking up my reply to make sure I'm going to be fair and wise and help teach our child to stick up for herself when my sister said, "So, what did you tell that boy?" And she said, "Oh, I told him that he already knows I can't help making them and to just go away. You know (ugh noise) he is a BOY." And that was that. No big deal—no need for Mom to swoop in and save the day. You know, sometimes kids can deal with things on their own.

❧

I was so relieved to finally get the diagnosis of TS. We thought he just had habits and tried to make him stop, but one would stop and another one start. He had the tic of throwing his head back, like his hair on his forehead was bothering him. We had his hair cut super short and he kept up the head throwing. Now we don't even notice the tics anymore.

❧

A sense of humor is mandatory! Once while walking to class, some boys were imitating my daughter's noises and movements. When she came out of class, they were still there, still laughing at her. She stopped, and in front of everyone, told the boys she was disappointed in them! She thought they were doing a very sloppy job of imitating her. She wanted them to go home and practice, and come back next week at the same time, and she then wanted to see a much better performance. Needless to say, they never returned.

3

MEDICAL TREATMENTS AND HEALTHCARE PROFESSIONALS

Jacob Kerbeshian, M.D.

The good news about Tourette syndrome is that most people with TS never require treatment for their tics. In the majority of cases, the tics stay mild enough that using medication to prevent them doesn't make sense. In fact, it's more likely that a child with TS will require treatment for an associated disorder such as AD/HD, rather than for the tics themselves.

Unfortunately, there's no way to predict the course of Tourette syndrome in a particular child. Obviously, some do require medication or other treatments, either because the tics are physically uncomfortable for them, are socially unacceptable, or make the child self-conscious. While there's no cure for TS yet, there are many different treatments available today that can be effective. The tricky thing is that different treatments are effective for different symptoms in different patients. Simply put, what works well for one child may not work for another.

The route to the best treatment for your child will probably be through teamwork. At the beginning, the "team" will consist of at least you, your child, and a physician specialist—probably a neurologist, psychiatrist, or developmental pediatrician—who can diagnose Tourette syndrome.

:: Diagnosing Tourette Syndrome

The basic criteria for diagnosing Tourette syndrome are pretty straightforward: the child must have had a number of motor tics and at least one vocal tic frequently for at least a year.

However, we also know that children with Tourette syndrome are more likely than other children to have certain other neurologically based disorders such as AD/HD, obsessive-compulsive disorder (OCD), or learning difficulties. (Medical conditions that occur together like this are called "comorbidities.") So when diagnosing a child with Tourette syndrome, the doctor needs to focus on more than just the tics. She needs to look at the whole child, and how his tics and other symptoms contribute to who he is and how others see him.

A good diagnosis, therefore, isn't simply a tally of symptoms on a checklist. It should be an analysis of the many different physical, neurological, behavioral, and emotional patterns in your child, and how they interact. The more thorough the diagnosis, the easier it is to pinpoint the best treatment options for your child.

:: The Medical Team

If you suspect your child may have Tourette syndrome, you'll want to make an appointment for him to be evaluated by a specialist as soon as possible. Many parents are shocked to find that the wait to see some specialists can be several months long—and the first appointment is usually harder to get than a follow-up appointment. Even if your child's symptoms are fairly mild, it's wise to have a knowledgeable specialist evaluate him. Then, if his symptoms worsen later, the wait for an appointment shouldn't be as long.

Who's the best specialist to diagnose and treat your child? That depends on a few factors. Typically, you'll want to start with a pediatric neurologist, a child and adolescent psychiatrist (or neuropsychiatrist), or a developmental pediatrician. Any of these physicians can diagnose and treat TS, but some, obviously, will have a greater interest—and more expertise—than others. Your local branch of the Tourette Syndrome Association (or parents in a local TS support group) may be able to give you names of local specialists who have a particular interest in TS.

Each specialty has particular strengths in diagnosing and treating children with Tourette syndrome:

A **pediatric neurologist** is a physician who has done at least a two-year residency in pediatrics and an additional residency in neurology with an emphasis in the diagnosis and management of children with neurological disorders (disorders of the brain, spine, and/or nerves). A neurologist is usually the best choice to evaluate and treat a child who may have an additional complicating neurological condition, such as a seizure disorder, or another associated movement disorder. Your pediatrician (or 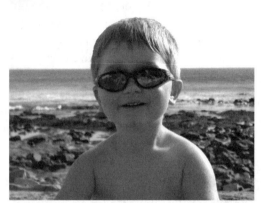 insurance company) may want you to have a neurologist do the initial diagnosis of your child, just to rule out any other possible neurological problems. A neurologist can prescribe medications, order and interpret diagnostic tests, and coordinate and integrate the findings of other developmental specialists. A neurologist does not do psychotherapy.

A **child and adolescent psychiatrist** is an M.D. with five or more years of post-graduate training in the diagnosis, treatment, and prevention of mental disorders (disorders that affect or are manifested in a person's brain) and emotional problems in children and teenagers. Because psychiatrists have training in both medicine and psychology, they often are the best choice to evaluate and treat a child with Tourette syndrome who may also have a related disorder such as AD/HD, OCD, or Asperger syndrome. While a psychiatrist is trained to do psychotherapy, in some cases (especially if you have managed care insurance), the psychiatrist may do the diagnosis and medication management, but send your child to a psychologist, clinical social worker, or counselor for therapy.

A **pediatric neuropsychiatrist** is a physician who has had post-graduate training and/or extensive experience in pediatrics, neurology, *and* psychiatry. A neuropsychiatrist can be an excellent choice for the child with both Tourette syndrome and other mental or behavioral disorders, if you have such a doctor in your area (or are willing to travel to see one).

A developmental and behavioral pediatrician is an M.D. who has received an additional two to three years of specialized training in child development and behavior, beyond the required three years for pediatrics. This physician may be the best specialist to evaluate and treat a child who has other ongoing long-term healthcare needs or a chronic illness such as a metabolic disorder.

Whatever her specialty is, you want a specialist who will work as part of the team involved in the care of your child. Depending on your child's issues, other members of the team could include clinical or developmental child psychologists, special educators, occupational therapists, physical therapists, and communication specialists. If you're lucky, the specialist may take the lead in pulling together all these professionals and keeping communication running among them. If not, that job may fall to you. But ultimately, *you,* as the parent, are the team captain. No one cares more about your child than you do. You may not have the technical expertise that the others do, but you *do* have the right to understand and approve all elements of your child's care. If at first you don't understand—ask questions. If the doctor doesn't want to take the time to answer them... she may not be the best choice for your team.

What to Expect at the Specialist's Office

Let's say your pediatrician has referred your child to a specialist because she suspects Tourette syndrome. The first thing the specialist will need to do is a basic medical workup for TS. That should include:

- **A thorough history (medical, psychological, and behavioral) of your child.** Beyond the basics (childhood illnesses, etc.), it's a good idea to bring a list of any unusual difficulties or behaviors your child has had during his lifetime, as well as any symptoms you're noticing now.
- **A family history.** Before your appointment, talk to relatives on both sides of the family to find out whether they remember anyone having tics or twitches, obsessions and/or compulsions, AD/HD, or similar symptoms.
- **A thorough physical exam.** The doctor will check weight, height, ears, eyes, and throat, listen to the chest, palpate the stomach—you know this routine.
- **A neurological exam.** This is a totally noninvasive exam, and nothing that should scare your child. The doctor

will have him do various movements or exercises to test his reflexes, muscle strength, eye and mouth movement, coordination, and alertness. A psychiatrist may ask the pediatrician to perform the physical exam and the neurological exam for her.

- **Blood work.** The nurse may draw your child's blood in the office, or you may have to take your child to a lab to have a CBC (complete blood count) and blood chemistries workup done.

If there's a strong history of tic disorders, Tourette syndrome, or OCD in either the mother's or father's family and no other red flags, the doctor may decide just the basic workup is necessary. About two-thirds of children diagnosed with Tourette syndrome have such family histories, and the majority of children diagnosed with Tourette syndrome do not have other diagnosable causes of their symptoms.

However, a number of other medical conditions can cause motor and vocal tics, including drug abuse, hormone abnormalities, or other neurological disorders or infections. If your doctor thinks there's any possibility that one of these other conditions may be present, she may run additional tests. A few examples include:

- If a child had apparent lapses in consciousness while having tics, the doctor would order an electroencephalogram (EEG) to investigate whether seizures might be present.
- If there were other neurological symptoms, such as a weakness in just one area of the body, she might order a CT or MRI scan of the brain.
- If the child exhibited other abnormal movements in addition to tics, or if he had mental retardation, she might order more extensive laboratory tests.
- If the child had a flare up of symptoms after an infection, she might do a throat culture to check for strep.

The Rest of Your Child's Team

Although only a physician specialist should diagnose Tourette syndrome and prescribe medication for it, other professionals can make a great contribution to your child's team. Not only can they provide useful services themselves, but they also can give the specialist important data on how your child's symptoms—and the treatments he's receiving for them—are affecting his development.

Pediatrician. Unless your specialist is a developmental pediatrician, your child will need a pediatrician (or family practitioner) for his general healthcare (checkups, sore throats, etc.). If your family belongs to a managed care organization, this doctor will be his primary care physician, who may need to sign off on referrals to any specialists. Ideally, your child's pediatrician should have a developmental perspective. That is, she should feel that not all delays or problems a child might have should be seen as an illness, nor should they be dismissed as something the child will "grow out of."

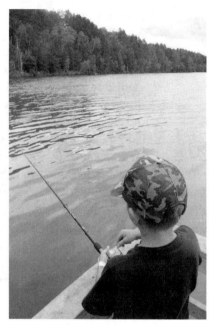

Child Psychologist. A child clinical psychologist has a Ph.D. rather than a medical degree, and has extensive training in child development, mental disorders, psychological and cognitive testing, and psychotherapy. A child psychologist may diagnose Tourette syndrome within the scope of her specialty, but this would not be a medical diagnosis of the condition. A psychologist could also:

- Give your child an IQ test and other evaluations to root out any learning disabilities.
- Set up a program to track tics and other symptoms (so the team can tell whether treatments are working).
- Diagnose any comorbid mental disorders such as AD/HD, obsessive-compulsive disorder, bipolar disorder, etc.
- Teach him special techniques for anxiety reduction or anger management.
- Provide supportive psychotherapy ("talk therapy") if he's struggling with low self-esteem or depression.
- Offer a "social skills group" if your child has trouble interacting with other children.
- Suggest behavioral techniques and/or changes to your child's environment that might lessen some AD/HD

symptoms. While some behavior modification programs that bring attention to a child's tics may actually worsen them, some psychologists today are learning to use techniques such as *habit reversal training* to help reduce tics (see Chapter 4).

Speech-Language Pathologist. In a sense, any vocal tic—whether it's a simple grunt or, at the other extreme, coprolalia—is a speech/language disturbance, because the sound coming from the child's mouth or vocal cords doesn't actually communicate a message that he means to send. But this breakdown in communication is more significant for some children with TS than for others. In fact, it's not unusual for a child to be referred to a speech therapist for stuttering, before anyone realizes he has Tourette syndrome with *palilalia* (repeating his own words). But in addition to vocal tics, some children with TS are saddled with other speech and language disorders as well, such as true stuttering; speech articulation difficulties; word finding problems; and hesitations during speech, which actually may be a type of vocal tic. A speech and language pathologist can help evaluate and treat these conditions.

Educational Specialist. Children with Tourette syndrome—especially those with comorbid diagnoses—are at higher risk for learning difficulties. Obviously, if a child has a specific learning disability in addition to TS, he will have extra challenges in the classroom. Most people also understand that AD/HD can lead to an ineffective style of learning. But other issues can arise as well that may not be so obvious. Tics may interfere with the flow of a child's writing, reading, speech, attention... or really, any learning activity. A child with OCD may get "stuck" reading a passage over and over again, erase his handwriting until he wears a hole in his paper, or be unable to finish a test or paper because he's so focused on getting it "perfect."

An educational specialist (usually, but not always, a teacher with a graduate degree in special education or educational psychology) can evaluate your child's specific learning challenges and engineer behavior and educational programs to overcome some of these obstacles. The educational specialist can also help your child's teacher educate other students and faculty regarding Tourette syndrome. (See Chapter 8 for more information on learning-related issues.)

Occupational Therapist. An OT's job is to evaluate how a disorder or injury might be interfering with your child's daily life, and in particular with tasks involving the fingers and hands, and then design a plan to help him overcome those obstacles. Depending on your child, an OT might prescribe specific therapies, exercises, classroom accommodations, and/or special equipment. For example, if your child has trouble with handwriting, the OT will evaluate whether the problem is being caused by tics or some other difficulty and then develop a specific plan to tackle the problem.

Some OTs specialize in *sensory integration therapy*. Often, a child with TS has sensory processing difficulties, including subjective phenomena known as *sensory tics* (e.g., feeling something brush against the skin when there's nothing there). He may over- or under-react to sensory input (noise, light, smell, taste, or touch). He may appear clumsy—banging into things frequently. Or he may seem to "need" a certain sensation such as spinning, swinging, or being wrapped tightly in a quilt. An occupational therapist with sensory integration expertise can be helpful in evaluating and treating all these difficulties.

Physical Therapist. The physical therapist can evaluate (and if necessary, suggest or provide treatment for) any neuromuscular problems your child may have. While an OT addresses specific life skills, sensory processing issues, and fine motor skills (such as handwriting), a PT looks more at gross motor functioning (e.g., walking, running), pain, strength, and range of motion. The most common neuromuscular problem a child with TS might experience would be muscle fatigue or soreness caused by a motor tic (e.g., a sore neck from head rolling). Infrequently, one muscle or muscle group may become enlarged because of an excessive motor tic.

In a few, very rare instances, individuals with TS have experienced "pseudohemiparesis"—a partial paralysis or weakening on one side of the body (although, upon medical examination, the muscles respond as if no paralysis is present). There have also been reports of sensory tics where the person with TS experiences a sudden, distinct sensation of pain—for instance, feeling as if he's been slapped.

Dentist. A pediatric, developmentally oriented dentist would be a good choice for a child with Tourette syndrome, especially if his tics involve the mouth, teeth, or jaw. For example, bruxism (teeth grinding) can wear away the teeth over time. Vigorous tics of the jaw could contribute to TMJ disease. Clacking of the teeth occasionally will lead to unusual patterns of wear, or even to dental fractures. Dentists can mold protective dental appliances that may be helpful for some of these children. On the other hand, because the tics of many children with TS are set off by sensory input, braces or a retainer in the mouth could *trigger* a motor tic. A dentist who's aware of these issues would be most helpful.

Your Role as Team Member and Case Manager

Remember, you, as the parent, are the team captain. Although other team members may change over time, you and your child will be the constants. You're the one who can tell the rest of the team how your child's symptoms, development, and treatment have changed over time. Unless you have a professional case manager or a very coordinated team, you will probably be the one who makes sure that each member of the team gets copies of the other members' evaluations and recommendations.

Ultimately, *you* will be the one who has to sift through all the information and recommendations to make the best decisions on behalf of the child. And *you* will be the one who must advocate for your child if his needs aren't adequately met by the healthcare systems, schools, or community.

Sure, it sounds intimidating at first, but parents rise to the challenge every day. No one will expect you to have the same medical knowledge as a physician. But you *will* need to keep up to date (at a layperson's level) with the state of the art in the diagnosis and treatment of Tourette syndrome and associated disorders. You may want to join the Tourette Syndrome Association or another patient or parent support group that will send you regular updates on TS-related news.

❚❚ The Medical Treatment of Tourette Syndrome

The most common—and typically most successful—medical treatment for tics is medication. But the decision of *whether or not* to treat with medication is as important, if not more important, than the decision of *which* medication to use. If a child has one or more comorbid conditions (AD/HD, depression, etc.), the decision becomes all the more complex.

As far as treating the tics of Tourette syndrome is concerned, keep this in mind: The medications we have available today for TS and related disorders primarily treat *symptoms*. They do not cure the underlying neurological problem, nor do they change the course of the condition over time.

Whether or not you treat those symptoms, therefore, should depend not so much on the severity or frequency of tics as on the effect the tics are having on your child, his development, or the family and community. For example, you may want to consider medication if:

- the tics involve self-injury, such as poking at his eye;
- the tics are socially disabling, such as screeching in public;
- the tics make learning difficult, such as eye-blinking that interferes with reading;
- the tics cause personal distress, such as a feeling of being out of control;
- the tics disturb family harmony, such as if your child repeatedly touches others.

Some physicians are more enthusiastic about treating tics (or AD/HD, or OCD) with medication, while others are more conservative.

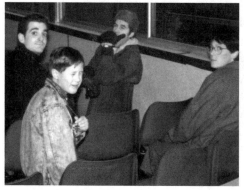

Before consenting to a medication for your child, you need to do a risk-benefit analysis. What are the potential benefits of the medication? The potential risks and possible side effects? What other treatments are available? And what might be the consequence of *not* treating?

You also need to take your child's feelings into account when making a decision about medication. These wishes often change as the child grows. For example, a younger child may object because he's afraid of having to swallow a pill—but that's a hurdle that usually can be overcome. (See box, below.) Sometimes a teenager may see the use of medication as a parent's attempt to gain too much control in their relationship. On the other hand, a teenager might be more self-conscious about tics than a smaller child would be, and therefore more anxious to get rid of them. A child of any age may resist once he's started taking a medication, if the side effects bother him.

Ultimately, when making a decision about a possible treatment, you need to look at how the disorder is affecting your child's development. Together as a team, you need to discuss not only how the symptoms are affecting your child right now, but also what effect they may have on his unfolding future. The same may be said about the side effects of the treatments.

∷ TEACHING YOUR CHILD TO TAKE A PILL

Some children (and even some adolescents and adults) have great difficulty swallowing a pill or capsule. If the normal approach ("Put this on your tongue, then swallow it with a sip of water") doesn't work for your child, try one of these tricks:

- Have him fill his mouth with water first, then drop the pill in and swallow. (He's less likely to taste the pill or feel it on his tongue.)
- Have him chew up a piece of bread or cookie, then drop the pill in just before he swallows. (Make sure he doesn't bite down again!)
- Have him put the pill on his tongue, then drink liquid through a straw. He may concentrate so hard on the straw that the pill goes down easily.
- Have him build up to taking a real pill. Start by having him swallow a tiny candy sprinkle with a sip of water each day for a few days. Next, have him do the same with a slightly larger candy, such as a miniature M&M, for several days. (Don't let him chew the candies, or he may try to chew a real pill. Yuck!) Then move up to the smallest vitamin you can find, followed by slightly larger vitamins, until you reach vitamins as large as any pills he's likely to take. (Obviously, this is a long-term plan—not one to start on the day your child needs to start taking a prescription.)

If none of these approaches work, talk to your child's doctor about an alternative way of getting the medication into your child. Some drugs are available in liquid form or as dissolvable tablets. Some pills can be crushed or capsules opened to sprinkle the medication onto applesauce, yogurt, or ice cream—but others will burn the mouth if you do this, so ask the doctor or pharmacist first! Others taste so bad that there's no way to disguise them in food or drink.

Sometimes, the doctor may choose to prescribe a different medication, if the child has a pill-swallowing aversion. If the particular medication is vital, some parents resort to having a compounding pharmacy create a liquid form of the pill or capsule—but that's an expensive option, and not always possible.

Anti-tic Medications: Taking Aim at Moving Targets

Tics come and go unexpectedly. Their severity and frequency wax and wane. John might wrinkle his nose 200 times a day for two weeks, and then suddenly... no more nose wrinkling. Sarah's mother might call the doctor for an urgent appointment because she's suddenly developed a painful neck tic... but by the time they get in to see the neurologist, the neck tic is gone, her old eye tic is back, and a new coughing tic has appeared.

Occasionally, we can point to something that seems to have brought on tics or made them worse—a bout of the flu, perhaps, or the stress of studying for a big test. Most of the time, though, tics seem to change at random. And that very randomness is what makes tics difficult to treat. Or, to be more specific, what makes it hard to judge a treatment's effectiveness. The doctor is truly taking aim (with the medication) at a moving target.

When are you most likely to take your child to the doctor? When his symptoms are causing him the most trouble, of course. In the case of Tourette syndrome, that means when his tics are most frequent and most severe. But given the waxing and waning course of TS, it is more likely that even without treatment, his tics would improve, rather than get worse. But it is precisely at this point that medication is likely to be started and likely to appear successful.

On the other hand, let's say you take your child in to see the specialist once every six months. Your appointment may happen to fall at a time when your child's tics have been mild for several weeks. At that time, odds are that the tics will soon wax again, increasing in frequency and severity. If the doctor prescribes a new medication at this checkup, when the tics worsen again it may look like the medicine isn't working. But it's very possible that the symptoms would have gotten much worse, much faster, had the medication not been started.

Of course, your doctor may prescribe a medication for your child that quickly makes most of his tics diminish or disappear. If so—wonderful! But don't be discouraged if it doesn't happen that quickly. Some medications must build up in the system over a period of days or weeks before they're fully effective. Likewise, any attempt to discontinue an anti-tic medication has to be done gradually, with a downward tapering of doses. Stop them too rapidly, and your child may experience a "rebound," in which tics may become worse than they were before the medication was started.

It's hard to be patient when your child is in distress. If tics are hurting him or upsetting him, your instinct is to demand the doctor do something to fix them NOW. But when prescribing or changing medications for tics, a doctor has to give priority to safety over speed. We'd all love for there to be a magic pill that would just make our children's symptoms disappear. But actually, the goal of any antitic medication is to achieve a major and significant improvement in tics—but not to suppress them completely. Why not? Because you don't want your child overmedicated. If the tics are completely suppressed, the doctor can't tell if the tics are improving over time, in which case a much lower dosage of medication would be just as effective. Ideally, a doctor wants to treat tics to a point of 80 percent to 90 percent improvement, giving her a guidepost to increase medication as tics worsen, and decrease medication as tics improve or disappear. Of course, that treatment strategy is easier to use with children whose tics have a slower rate of change, as compared to those with a more rapid change in pattern.

Fortunately, for most children, the tics of Tourette syndrome will diminish or disappear by late adolescence or early adulthood. (The exception is that small group of individuals with significant tics persisting into adulthood.) Odds are, therefore, that by the time your child is grown, he will need less medication—or none at all.

The Biochemistry of Tourette Syndrome

Scientists haven't totally unraveled the mysteries of Tourette syndrome yet. But we're getting closer every day. One thing we do know is that the motor and vocal tics of Tourette syndrome are caused, at least in part, by a subtle chemical imbalance in the brain.

All the thoughts, movements, sensations, and feelings a person experiences are caused by signals passing rapidly through the cells of his brain—the neurons. In order for a signal to be communicated from one neuron to the next, the first neuron fires chemicals into the synapse (space) between the cells. These chemicals, called neurotransmitters, are then picked up by the next neuron's receptors. The signal is transmitted across that next cell, which in turn fires neurotransmitters downstream toward the third neuron, and so on.

The neurotransmitters involved in Tourette syndrome act in the parts of the brain that coordinate movement and speech. When brain cells in these areas fire neurotransmitters in an organized pattern, the

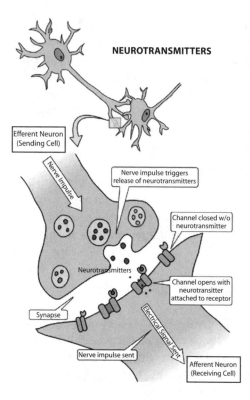

result is in a predictable, fluid physical movement or sound. However, if those same neurotransmitters are out of balance—say, too many of one and/or too few of another—it can result in the spasms of movement and vocal sounds we call tics.

We know today that the neurotransmitters dopamine, serotonin, norepinephrine, and glutamate all seem to influence tic activity. Medications that increase or decrease the activity of these neurotransmitters, therefore, can affect the brain's production of tics.

Tourette Syndrome and PANDAS

PANDAS is an acronym for "Pediatric Autoimmune Neuropsychiatric Disorder Associated with Strep." PANDAS refers to a small subgroup of children with Tourette syndrome and/or OCD who some scientists believe may have acquired their symptoms as the result of a strep infection.

Typically, the body reacts to a bacterial infection, such as a strep throat or a strep ear infection, by generating antibodies. These antibodies attach themselves to the bacteria, enabling white blood cells to destroy the bacteria. If the PANDAS hypothesis is correct, in some genetically predisposed individuals, the antibodies generated to attack strep bacteria also mistakenly attack the parts of the brain that are involved in Tourette syndrome or OCD. This *autoimmune response* causes a change in the way the brain functions, making it produce tics and/or OCD symptoms.

Of course, strep throat is a very common childhood ailment—the fact that your child has had strep infections does not necessarily mean they were the cause of his TS. If theories are correct, the onset of PAN-

DAS-related Tourette syndrome or OCD is very sudden and dramatic, and occurs during or following a strep infection. It is only believed to occur in children who haven't yet reached puberty, and may be associated with other neurological symptoms as well. Repeated strep infections could reactivate and worsen the symptoms.

If you believe your child's TS or OCD may be related to a strep infection, you should discuss it with your specialist. As of the writing of this book, research into PANDAS is ongoing, and treatment recommendations are not agreed upon by the experts and are still evolving.

■■ Medications Used to Treat Tourette Syndrome

Several different kinds of medication can be prescribed to alleviate tics and associated symptoms.

Alpha-Adrenergic Agonists

For a child with mild to moderate tics, the first drug a specialist will prescribe is frequently an alpha-adrenergic agonist—a medication usually prescribed for high blood pressure. That's not to imply that there's a link between Tourette syndrome and hypertension. Instead, these drugs happen to help reduce tics because they decrease the amount of norepinephrine released by the neurons. Less norepinephrine in turn decreases the activity of dopamine. And less dopamine activity often results in milder or less frequent tics.

Clonidine (Catapres™)

Clonidine is often the first drug a physician will prescribe for tics. That's not because it's the most effective treatment, but because it has a relatively low risk of side effects. (Neuroleptics, which we discuss later in the chapter, actually tend to be better tic fighters, but come with bigger risks.) Studies show that about 25 percent of patients with TS respond well to clonidine. In addition to reducing tics, clonidine also may reduce the hyperactivity or inattentiveness associated with AD/HD—all the better for a child with that comorbid diagnosis. A small dose at bedtime can be especially beneficial if your child suffers from the sleep disturbances that often accompany TS.

Typical Dosage: From 0.1 mg in younger children to 0.6 mg per day in older children and adolescents, divided into three or four doses. A dose of 0.1 mg to 0.2 mg at bedtime is appropriate for sleep difficulties. Clonidine can also be administered in the form of a slow release transdermal skin patch, which must be changed every five to seven days. It may take a week to ten days after starting the medication or changing the dosage before you'll be able to judge whether the medication is helpful.

Common Side Effects: Sedation, daytime napping, lightheadedness, headache, dry mouth, irritability, sleep disturbance, and depression. With gradual dosage increases, these side effects often can be minimized. Even though this is a blood pressure medication, any decrease in a child's blood pressure is usually negligible. Of greater concern is the possibility of slowing of the heart rate. The skin patch can sometimes cause an irritating skin rash, which often necessitates returning to the oral form of medication.

Additional Notes: If your child is prescribed clonidine, you should take his pulse occasionally and contact the physician if it drops below fifty-five beats per minute. Clonidine should not be stopped suddenly, as rebound high blood pressure may result.

Guanfacine (Tenex™)

Guanfacine is similar to clonidine, but is longer acting and less sedating. Like clonidine, guanfacine may help with the hyperactivity or inattentiveness of AD/HD. Given at night, guanfacine often aids sleep.

Typical Dosage: From 0.5 mg twice per day for the younger child to 1.5 mg twice per day for the older child and adolescent.

Side Effects: Similar to clonidine, although guanfacine tends to produce less sedation or less lightheadedness and is less likely to slow the heart rate. May cause sleep disturbance.

Additional Notes: Guanfacine should not be stopped suddenly, as rebound high blood pressure might result.

Neuroleptics

Neuroleptics, which are sometimes referred to as major tranquilizers or antipsychotics, are often very effective in treating the tics of Tourette syndrome. Of course, TS is *not* a psychotic disorder, so don't let the term throw you. These drugs were originally developed to treat psychoses, but doctors later found that, in smaller doses, they also could be useful in treating movement disorders. Scientists believe they are effective in treating TS because they block the action of the neurotransmitter dopamine in areas of the brain that affect the flow of movement and speech.

Neuroleptics are powerful drugs which, even in small doses, often have significant side effects and risks, so your doctor probably won't prescribe one unless your child's tics are in the moderate-to-severe range. Weight gain is a common side effect, and may be greater for some medications in this class than for others. Neuroleptics can also have a sedating effect, which may interfere with a child's ability to function in school. Infrequently, a child treated with a neuroleptic for Tourette syndrome may develop a pattern of school avoidance (phobia) which will stop if the medication is discontinued.

While it is rare, you should discuss the risk of *tardive dyskinesia* with the doctor before she prescribes a neuroleptic medication for your child. Tardive dyskinesia is a neurological disorder that causes involuntary movements of the mouth, tongue, and lips, and, sometimes, quick, jerky movements of the trunk and limbs. (It can, in fact, be difficult to distinguish from Tourette syndrome.) The longer a child is on a neuroleptic, and the higher the dosage, the greater the risk of tardive dyskinesia. The risk also is higher in those with mental retardation. Once brought on by a neuroleptic drug, tardive dyskinesia can be permanent, even if the medication is stopped.

Tardive dyskinesia is an *extrapyramidal side effect (EPS)* of neuroleptic drugs (the extrapyramidal system is a neural network in the brain that is involved in the coordination of movement). Other EPSs can include akathisia (restlessness), dystonia (abnormal muscle positioning or spasms in the head, neck, limbs, or trunk), and parkinsonism (tremors, muscular rigidity, and/or slowed motor movement—resembles Parkinson's disease). These side effects typically are reversible, and go away if the medication is stopped.

There are two major classes of neuroleptic drugs— *typical* (first generation or conventional) neuroleptics and *atypical* (second generation). First generation neuroleptics, as the name implies, have been around longer, but they also have greater risk of serious side effects, including tardive dyskinesia. Doctors, therefore, often prefer to try the second generation, or atypical, neuroleptics first.

Atypical Neuroleptics

Atypical neuroleptics have varying degrees of dopamine blocking activity, but unlike first generation neuroleptics, they also block the activity of the neurotransmitter serotonin. Serotonin, scientists believe, may play a role not only in tics, but in the obsessions and compulsions that often occur in people with Tourette syndrome as well. While they carry less risk of extrapyramidal side effects than first generation neuroleptics, atypical neuroleptics may increase the risk of developing obesity and diabetes (so be sure to tell the doctor if diabetes runs in your family).

Risperidone (Risperdal™)

Of all the atypical neuroleptics, Risperdal has been the most studied in the treatment of Tourette syndrome. It may reduce tics anywhere from 21 percent to 61 percent. Risperidone may also be helpful in other symptoms associated with Tourette syndrome, such as outbursts of rage or impulsivity.

Typical Dosage: 0.5 mg in the younger child to 8 mg per day in the older child or adolescent, in one single or two divided doses.

Side Effects: The most frequent side effects of Risperdal are tiredness, sleepiness, and moderate weight gain. Occasionally, Risperdal may cause a rapid heart rate. In the lower dose range, it is far less likely than the typical neuroleptics haloperidol and Orap to cause symptoms such as shakiness, stiffness, or restlessness. Its risk of causing tardive dyskinesia appears to be less than that of typical neuroleptics.

Olanzapine (Zyprexa™)

In addition to reducing tics, Zyprexa can be helpful in reducing the outbursts and shifts in mood which may accompany Tourette syndrome.

Typical Dosage: 2.5 mg in the younger child to 10 mg per day in the older child or adolescent, in one single or two divided doses.

Side Effects: Zyprexa can be sedating, and frequently results in an increase in appetite and significant weight gain. Zyprexa may increase an individual's risk for type II diabetes more than the other atypical neuroleptics. As with Risperdal, the risk of side effects such as shakiness, stiffness, restlessness, and tardive dyskinesia is less than with first-generation neuroleptics.

Quetiapine (Seroquel™)

Seroquel is unique among the neuroleptics in that it is only a weak blocker of dopamine, but a potent blocker of serotonin.

Typical Dosage: Can range from 25 mg in the younger child to 300 mg per day in the older child and adolescent, in one single or two to three divided doses.

Side Effects: Light-headedness, dry mouth, and sedation are the most common side effects. Weight gain may be an issue. There is less of a likelihood of EPS with this medication than with the other atypical neuroleptics.

Ziprasidone (Geodon™)

Geodon may be helpful in stabilizing mood, as well as reducing tics.

Typical Dosage: 20 mg per day in the younger child to 80 mg per day in the older child and adolescent, given in one single or two divided doses.

Side Effects: Geodon is far less likely than the other atypical antipsychotics to cause weight gain or increase the risk for type II diabetes. Shakiness, stiffness, or restlessness are less common than with conventional neuroleptics. Geodon does carry the risk of triggering heart rhythm disturbance in individuals at risk for long QT syndrome (which is determined by an electrocardiogram).

Additional Notes: A baseline EKG should be done prior to starting Geodon, and periodic EKG's thereafter. Doctors need to be cautious about prescribing additional medications that may affect long QT syndrome.

Aripiprazole (Abilify™)

Abilify is one of the newest atypical neuroleptics being used to treat Tourette syndrome. Scientists are particularly intrigued by its unique effect on dopamine. In those parts of the brain linked with excess dopamine activity (including the areas associated with Tourette syndrome), Abilify acts to block dopamine, as do other neuroleptics. But in those parts of the brain linked with *deficient* dopamine activity (e.g., the areas associated with AD/HD), Abilify acts as a dopamine *enhancer*, increasing the neurotransmitter's activity. It also has a stabilizing effect on serotonin, and in turn can have a mood stabilizing effect on the child or adolescent.

Typical Dosage: 2.5 mg per day in the younger child to 15 mg per day in the older child and adolescent. Usually given once per day.

Side Effects: The risk of shakiness, stiffness, or restlessness is less than that of the conventional neuroleptics. Sedation with Abilify appears to be dose dependent—the higher the dose, the more sedating the effect.

Conventional Neuroleptics

Haloperidol (Haldol™)

Haloperidol was the first medication found to be useful in treating Tourette syndrome, and it is still one of the most effective. Unfortunately, the side effects—especially at higher doses—are often so troublesome that many patients choose to stop taking it in spite of the improvement in their tics.

Typical Dosage: Significant reductions in tic severity may occur with doses as low as 0.25 mg to 0.5 mg per day. Older children and adolescents rarely require doses of more than 5 mg to 10 mg per day. Usually given once per day.

Side Effects: Side effects may include tiredness, sleepiness, weight gain, depression or irritability, dullness in learning, shakiness, stiffness, or restlessness. School avoidance and aggressive outbursts have also been seen as possible side effects of haloperidol. Infrequently, tardive dyskinesia may develop. The abnormal movements of tardive dyskinesia may continue, even if the medication is stopped.

Pimozide (Orap™)

Orap was the first and is currently the *only* drug the FDA has approved specifically for treating Tourette syndrome. Although Orap works much like haloperidol, blocking the actions of the neurotransmitter dopamine, it may also have a beneficial effect on attention and learning.

Dosage: Orap is usually started in the dose range of 0.5 mg to 1 mg per day, with a maximum dosage in the older child and adolescent of no more than 8 mg to 10 mg per day, in one single or two divided doses.

Side Effects: The side effects of Orap are similar to those of haloperidol, but seem to be less prominent in the middle dosage range. An important concern with Orap is its potential to cause serious heart rhythm disturbance, as is the case for Geodon, particularly when there's a family history of long QT syndrome. When combined with other drugs with a similar potential, the risk increases.

Additional Notes: The doctor should obtain an EKG, or heart tracing, prior to starting a child on Orap, and from time to time afterwards.

Fluphenazine (Prolixin™) and Trifluoperazine (Stelazine™)

Prolixin and Stelazine are other conventional neuroleptics occasionally used to treat Tourette syndrome. Their general side effect profiles are similar to those of haloperidol and Orap.

Benzodiazepines

Benzodiazepines are a group of medications that reduce the strength of some central nervous system functions. They are often prescribed as anti-anxiety medications, muscle relaxants, sedatives, and anticonvulsants. They may be beneficial for some adults with Tourette syndrome, but less so for children and adolescents.

Clonazepam (Klonopin™)

Clonazepam's effectiveness is generally considered on a par with clonidine or Tenex when it comes to alleviating tics (i.e., it's not as powerful as neuroleptic medications), but it's not usually prescribed for children. Clonazepam can be physically addicting, and it may impair attention and concentration, especially in children with comorbid Tourette syndrome and AD/HD. Sedation and decreased reaction time are the most common side effects. Due to similarities in the names, rarely a pharmacist may mistakenly fill a prescription for clonidine with Klonopin.

Other Medical Treatments for Tics

Other treatments, less commonly used, but possibly helpful in selected cases of Tourette syndrome, include:

Nicotine patches may be used to increase the effectiveness of neuroleptics in the treatment of tics. Issues of concern would include the effect of nicotine on blood pressure, and the possibility that the child could become tolerant to the effects of nicotine.

Pergolide (Permax™) in higher doses is used in the treatment of Parkinson's disease. In lower doses it may be helpful in treating the tics of Tourette syndrome, particularly in children with nighttime restless legs syndrome. Common side effects include stomach upset and insomnia.

Baclofen (Lioresal™) is a skeletal muscle relaxant, most often used in treating people with spastic muscles due to spinal cord and brain disorders such as cerebral palsy. It may be helpful for some children with Tourette syndrome. Stomach upset, fatigue, and sleepiness are more common side effects.

Botulinum toxin (Botox™) is best know for smoothing the brows of aging movie stars and society ladies, but it may have a place in treating children with severe tics, particularly ones associated with self-injurious behavior. When injected into the muscle involved in a specific tic, this poison can weaken the transmission of nerve activity to that muscle for up to three months at a time, resulting in fewer and less severe tics. Common side effects may include drowsiness, weakness, nausea, or muscle weakness.

Tetrabenazine, which currently isn't available in the U.S., but is sold in Canada, acts by decreasing the supply of dopamine in a nerve cell. As a result, it decreases the transmission of dopamine from one nerve cell to another. It may be helpful in the treatment of Tourette syndrome and other movement disorders.

Metoclopramide (Reglan™) is most often used in medicine to treat gastrointestinal disorders such as nausea and vomiting, or gastroesophageal reflux disorder. It is a weak blocker of dopamine and benefits some individuals with Tourette syndrome. Long-term use may be associated with a lower risk of tardive dyskinesia.

Topiramate (Topamax™) is most often used as an anticonvulsant (seizure medication). It is also used in psychiatry as a mood stabilizer. It is fairly unique among the mood stabilizers in that it decreases rather than increases the appetite. Topamax may be helpful in treating the tics of Tourette syndrome, as well as in reducing mood swings.

Donepezil (Aricept™) is used primarily to treat the memory problems of Alzheimer's disease and other dementias. It increases levels of the neurotransmitter acetylcholine, which in general would counter the effects of dopamine. It has been tried in the treatment of Tourette syndrome without any convincing benefit.

Mecamylamine (Inversine™) is a high blood pressure or anti-smoking medication which initially received much fanfare as an effective treatment for Tourette syndrome. Unfortunately, studies have indicated that it is not effective for the tics or the spectrum of other symptoms associated with Tourette syndrome.

Invasive and Experimental Procedures

The following procedures would rarely be used to treat Tourette syndrome in a child or adolescent. In fact, the only time they would even be considered would be if the child had suffered from a severely self-injurious tic for a long period of time. (And even then, only after consulting with a team of expert physicians.) Because Tourette syndrome typically improves by late adolescence to early adulthood, it makes sense to avoid invasive procedures if possible.

Deep Brain Stimulation

Guided by modern imaging techniques, a neurosurgeon precisely places one or more electrodes into the deep structures of the brain where neural activity is producing tics. These electrodes—connected by wires under the skin to a pulse generator implanted in the chest—emit a continuous, high-frequency electrical current that stimulates the tic-producing brain cells. This stimulation has, in some cases, markedly improved tic severity, including self-injurious behavior.

Psychosurgery

In years past, psychosurgery meant prefrontal lobotomy. Today, procedures are much more subtle and precise. A skilled neurosurgeon using imaging techniques can make very tiny, exact permanent cuts in the brain tissue, interrupting the neural pathways associated with severe self-injurious behavior or obsessive-compulsive symptoms. Unfortunately, all too often, improvements are temporary, and the problematic behaviors return later.

Electroconvulsive Therapy (ECT)

Also known by the more negative term "electroshock," this procedure—in which an electric current is briefly applied to the brain, through the scalp, to induce a seizure—is actually one of the oldest and most effective biological treatments for severe depression and other mood disorders. ECT is not used as a treatment for Tourette syndrome, per se. However, there have been individual case studies where tics and obsessive-compulsive symptoms decreased when individuals who had both significant mood disorders and TS were effectively treated with ECT. That's not surprising, since Tourette symptoms often parallel the course of other comorbid conditions. For example, tics may worsen when an individual is very depressed, and ease up when the depression lifts. There could be times when it would be appropriate to use ECT to treat an older adolescent with tics and a mood disorder, if the mood disorder has not responded to other medical treatments.

Alternative Treatments

Complementary and alternative medicine is very much in vogue today, and it's only natural that parents might hope for an alternative therapy that could cure or at least lessen their children's symptoms. But, to date, no alternative therapy has been scientifically proven to be as effective as the conventional medical treatments for Tourette syndrome. This is despite decades of fads: elimination diets; salicylate-free, preservative-free, dye-free, and insecticide-free diets; allergic desensitization; megavitamins; trace mineral supplementation; amino acid precursors of neurotransmitters; lecithin; choline; and heavy metal elimination and chelation.

More recently, attention has turned to omega-3 fatty acids. There does appear to be some evidence that omega-3 supplements are helpful in treating mood disorders. Whether there would be an overlap with comorbid Tourette syndrome remains to be seen.

Some alternative treatments could, at least in theory, *worsen* symptoms. For example, St. John's Wort has an enzyme activity that could increase levels of neurotransmitters, and, in turn, increase tics.

The most important caveat in the use of alternative and complementary therapies is to inform your child's physician that your child is taking them. Some of these therapies have been associated with central nervous system toxicity, or may affect the metabolism of more conventional medications your doctor might prescribe.

Cannabinoids (Marijuana)

The use of marijuana in the treatment of Tourette syndrome bears mentioning, although it is hardly a bona fide alternative or complementary therapy, since it's illegal in the United States. Studies have suggested that, in adults with Tourette syndrome, cannabinoids (the psychoactive components of marijuana) may improve tics, as well as associated mood and impulsivity difficulties. Many have argued that the use of "medical marijuana" should be legalized for treating individuals with Tourette symptoms that haven't responded to other treatments. Research into how and why cannabinoids affect TS is still ongoing.

Regardless, marijuana should never be used to treat children or adolescents with Tourette syndrome. Because their central nervous systems are still actively developing, children and adolescents would be particularly vulnerable to any unknown toxic effects of the drug on the nervous system. In addition, marijuana bought illegally in the United States is often contaminated with pesticides or fertilizers, infected with molds or bacteria, or laced with other drugs, making it especially risky for someone with a neurological disorder such as Tourette syndrome.

Medications That Can Make Tics Worse

Certain medications, both prescription and over-the-counter ones, can worsen tics. In particular, be wary of cold or allergy medications containing decongestants for stuffy nose and sinuses, such as Sudafed™ (pseudoephedrine), Actifed™, Dimetap™, etc. Decongestants act as mild stimulants, and may worsen tics in some children, just as the stimulants used to treat AD/HD may. (Caffeine can worsen tic symptoms, as well.) One clue that you should check the label for a decongestant is if the brand name ends in "-D" (Claritin-D™, Zyrtec-D™, Allegra-D™, etc.).

Dextromethorphan, another medication often found in cough suppressants, should also be avoided for similar reasons.

That doesn't mean that your child must suffer through a cold untreated. Other cold/allergy medications that usually *don't* make tics worsen include antihistamines (which treat the sneezing and runny nose), and guaifenesin (an expectorant, which relieves congestion by thinning and loosening mucus secretions).

As you've probably realized by now, though, the way children react to different medications can vary tremendously. If you notice *any* unusual symptoms after your child has started a new medication—physical, emotional, psychological, or behavioral—call your doctor immediately. And keep in mind that, while some side effects of medications appear immediately, others can emerge over time as the medication builds up in your child's body.

∷ Treating Associated Disorders

Having Tourette syndrome puts a child at greater risk for learning disorders and other developmental psychiatric disorders or symptoms including attention-deficit/hyperactivity disorder, obsessive compulsive disorder, anxiety disorders, depressive disorders, autism, Asperger syndrome, and bipolar disorder. Among these, the most common are AD/HD, OCD, and rage attacks. Let's take a look at how these comorbid conditions affect the medical treatment of Tourette syndrome.

Attention-Deficit/Hyperactivity Disorder

An estimated 3 to 7 percent of all school children have attention-deficit/hyperactivity disorder—but at least 25 percent of children with Tourette syndrome have AD/HD. In clinical samples—that is, children

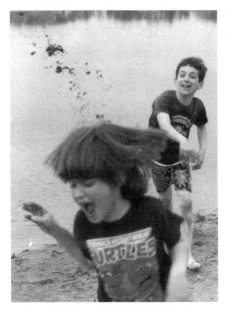

whose Tourette symptoms were significant enough that they sought medical treatment—at least 50 percent have AD/HD.

The reason so many children with TS also have AD/HD is probably because both disorders are caused by an imbalance of neurotransmitters. But while TS seems to be related to *too much* dopamine activity in some areas of the brain, AD/HD seems to result from *too little* dopamine activity in other areas.

Contrary to the stereotypes, not all kids with AD/HD are hyperactive, noisy, and impulsive. Some are, certainly, but others have primary trouble with concentration, distractibility, and *executive function* (organization and planning skills). And some kids, of course, face challenges in all of the above. See Chapter 1 for a fuller description of AD/HD.

Stimulant Medications

Typically, the symptoms of AD/HD are treated with stimulant medications such as methylphenidate (Ritalin™, Metadate™, Concerta™, Methylin™), dexmethyphenidate (Focalin™), dextroamphetamine (Dexedrine™), and mixed salts of amphetamine (Adderall™). All increase dopamine activity, which in turn can lesson AD/HD symptoms.

For years, doctors recommended against prescribing stimulant medications for a child with Tourette syndrome, for fear the influx of dopamine would increase his tics. Today, that question is more controversial. Some children can take a stimulant without their tics increasing significantly (or with tics increasing initially, but then subsiding). But many parents still report that their children have more tics—or develop new ones—when they take stimulant medications. Other possible side effects can include headache, loss of appetite, trouble sleeping, a decrease in the growth curve, fatigue, or a worsening of hyperactivity. Some children with a vulnerability to mood disorders may experience mood swings, irritability, or elevation in mood.

Stimulant medications take effect quickly. If a stimulant at a particular dose is going to be effective for a child's AD/HD, it should be obvious within a week. If it's not effective, or if a child reacts badly to it, it can be stopped quickly (no need to "wean" a child off it).

Some children may experience a rebound effect as a stimulant wears off at the end of the day. That is, some may exhibit more intense hyperactivity for an hour or two and others may experience withdrawal fatigue and tiredness.

Alpha-Adrenergic Agonists.

In the case of children with Tourette syndrome and AD/HD, many doctors prefer to try clonidine or guanfacine before a stimulant. These medications are often effective in treating both AD/HD and tics (see more on these drugs under "Medications Used to Treat Tourette Syndrome," earlier in this chapter). They may be of more use in treating the impulsiveness and hyperactivity of AD/HD than the inattentiveness and distractibility.

Atomoxetine (Strattera™)

Strattera is a nonstimulant medication—the first nonstimulant developed specifically for treating AD/HD—which is also less likely to worsen tics. It can be effective with both hyperactivity/impulsiveness and inattentiveness. Side effects of atomoxetine include stomach upset, nausea, and dizziness. There have been rare cases of sudden onset liver failure with atomoxetine.

Antidepressants

Two of the newer generation antidepressants on the market, bupropion (Wellbutrin™) or venlafaxine (Effexor™), may also improve AD/HD symptoms (both inattentiveness and hyperactivity/impulsivity) without activating tics. If, in addition to his other symptoms, your child is depressed, one of these medications might be particularly helpful. In a very controversial advisory, the FDA has recommended that children, adolescents, and their parents be made aware of the possibility that any antidepressant medication might increase the risk of suicidal thoughts and behaviors. Close follow-up is recommended when starting the medication or changing the dosage.

Common side effects of Wellbutrin include headache, sleep disturbance, nausea, or diarrhea. For individuals already at risk for seizures, Wellbutrin could increase the risk, but that's less likely with the extended or slow release form. Side effects for Effexor can include headache, nausea, diarrhea, or an increase in blood pressure. Typically these medications should be decreased and discontinued gradually in order to minimize withdrawal effects.

In the past, the tricyclic antidepressants desipramine (Norpramin™) and clomipramine (Anafranil™) were frequently prescribed for children with comorbid Tourette syndrome and AD/HD or obsessive-compulsive disorder, but far less so today due to concerns about side effects and the possibility of heart rhythm disturbances. Anafranil is still occasionally prescribed when a child has comorbid obsessive-compulsive disorder that has not responded to other treatments.

Other Options in Treating AD/HD

If an AD/HD medication is necessary for your child, but they all seem to worsen his tics, your doctor may try adding clonidine, guanfacine, or one of the atypical or first generation neuroleptics to one of the medications above.

If your child can tolerate stimulants, but they don't provide sufficient relief from the AD/HD symptoms, studies have shown that behavior therapy *in conjunction with* stimulants may be more effective than stimulants alone. (Behavior therapy in the absence of stimulants is not effective.)

Unfortunately, treatment of AD/HD, other than the milder cases, typically requires the use of prescription medications. Of course, you always have the option of not treating the AD/HD, just as you have the option of not treating the tics. Some psychoeducational approaches (see Chapter 8), including a one-on-one paraprofessional, may help your child manage better in the classroom (and make his behavior more tolerable to others), but they are not as likely to be as effective as stimulants.

Obsessive-Compulsive Disorder

About 60 percent of children with Tourette syndrome have OCD or some of its symptoms. An *obsession* is an unwanted and inappropriate thought, desire, or mental image that a person can't get out of his head—one that he finds upsetting or disgusting. A *compulsion* is a behavior that he performs repeatedly in an attempt to prevent or reduce distress. This behavior may be related to an obsession—for example, washing hands repeatedly because of an obsession with germs. Often the compulsion involves very rigid, specific rules that must be applied. For example, a child might feel he can't leave his room unless his set of Matchbox cars are lined up evenly in a specific order. Obsessions with violence or aggression, as well as compulsions for symmetry, "evening up," and having things "just right," are more common in people who have both TS and OCD than in those with OCD alone.

The distressing nature of the thoughts and behaviors in OCD differentiates them from those in Asperger syndrome, in which children get enjoyment or comfort from their all-encompassing interests and repetitive routines (see Chapter 1).

Just like TS symptoms, OCD symptoms are repetitive, intrusive, and may wax and wane over time with one symptom replacing another. In fact, when Tourette syndrome and OCD run in the same family, scientists believe they may both be caused by the same genetic defect, which shows up more often as OCD in females and Tourette syndrome in males.

Selective Serotonin Reuptake Inhibitors (SSRIs)

OCD symptoms appear to be associated with decreased serotonin activity in certain parts of the brain. These symptoms often respond well to *selective serotonin reuptake inhibitors* (SSRI), a class of antidepressants that increase serotonin activity. Some of these medications commonly used to treat children with both OCD and Tourette syndrome include fluoxetine (Prozac™), sertraline (Zoloft™), fluvoxamine (Luvox™), paroxetine (Paxil™), citalopram (Celexa™), and escitalopram (Lexapro™).

As noted previously, there are concerns that the SSRIs and other antidepressants may increase the risk of suicidal thinking and suicidal behavior in children and adolescents, even if these medications are being used to treat depression. This concern remains controversial, but as per FDA guidelines, close follow-up is advised. Children and adolescents with OCD and Tourette syndrome may be less responsive to SSRIs than those with OCD alone. When that's the case, adding an atypical or typical neuroleptic to the treatment may be necessary.

The SSRIs' more common side effects include nausea, diarrhea, headache, sleep disturbance, shakiness, and restlessness. A rare but very severe complication that can occur is *serotonin syndrome*, in which excessive levels of serotonin cause high fever, high blood pressure, and complicated metabolic abnormalities. This usually happens because another drug the individual is taking, such as clomipramine (Anafranil™), prevents the SSRI from breaking down and being eliminated in the liver.

Other OCD Medications

The most effective medication for the treatment of OCD is the tricyclic antidepressant clomipramine (Anafranil). Doctors generally prefer to try SSRIs first, because clomipramine has a greater risk for significant side effects, including seizures or heart rhythm disturbances (so baseline and follow-up EKG monitoring is usually advised). Other side effects might include fatigue, blurred vision, constipation, light-headedness, dry mouth, and difficulties with urination. Doctors need to be particularly cautious when prescribing clomipramine together with another drug, such as Orap, that also might increase the risk of heart rhythm disturbance. Occasionally, an SSRI and clomipramine may be used together, which increases the risk of serotonin syndrome (see SSRIs, above).

Tourette Syndrome and Rage Attacks

A number of children with Tourette syndrome struggle with control of their impulses and regulation of their emotions. *Rage attacks*—sudden, uncontrollable outbursts of violent anger, totally out of proportion to the incidents that trigger them—may be a problem for some of these children. But before tackling this problem medically, the medical team needs to decide if these difficulties are part of the general lack of inhibition that many children with Tourette syndrome experience, or whether they are a product of another behavioral or mental problem coexisting with Tourette syndrome. For example:

- **A child with both Tourette syndrome and AD/HD** might experience anger and impulsivity due to the AD/HD. Treating the AD/HD with clonidine could lead to improvement in both impulsiveness and anger management.
- **A child with Tourette syndrome and OCD** may experience rage attacks when he's prevented from following through with a compulsion. In that case, treating the OCD with an SSRI could lessen the rages.
- **A child with Tourette syndrome and bipolar disorder** (what used to be called manic depression) may become hostile and aggressive during a manic episode. Treatment with a mood stabilizing anticonvulsant such as divalproex (Depakote™) might be helpful for this child. One of the tic inhibiting, mood stabilizing atypical neuroleptics such as Zyprexa or Geodon might also prove beneficial.

- In a child for whom the rage attacks appeared to be sudden, intrusive, and "tic-like," increasing the anti-tic medication might be helpful.

In addition to medical treatment, psychological and behavioral interventions can be helpful in tackling rage attacks.

■■ Future Directions in the Medical Treatment of Tourette Syndrome

Neuroscience researchers are delving into a number of promising clues that may lead to improved medical treatment of Tourette syndrome. Areas of exploration include:

- **Glutamate's role in brain activity.** Glutamate is one of the neurotransmitters involved in the expression of tics. Medications that affect brain glutamate activity might therefore reduce tics.

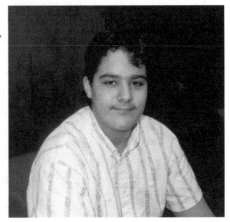

- **The role of the immune system in triggering Tourette syndrome.** Can viruses or bacterial infections bring on Tourette syndrome in someone who already has a genetic predisposition? Is a faulty immune system a cause? The phenomenon of PANDAS is still controversial, but scientists on both sides of the Atlantic are looking for answers.
- **The genetic or biochemical factors that cause tics to wax and wane.** If scientists can learn how the body triggers tics to increase and decrease naturally, they one day may be able to develop medical strategies to keep the tics waning longer or indefinitely.
- **Imaging studies of the brain.** MRI scans and PET scans already are showing us different chemical patterns

involved in Tourette syndrome. As they become more advanced, brain scans eventually may allow us to match the right medication to a child depending on his patterns of brain activity.

- **The search for specific laboratory biochemical markers for subtypes of Tourette syndrome.** As we've discussed, there's a great deal of variability in how children respond to medications for Tourette syndrome. Is this because there are different subgroups or "phenotypes" of TS? If so, and we could identify a biochemical indicator (such as the concentration of a certain enzyme) that would tell us which subtype a child has, we might one day be able to tailor medication choices to the individual child.

- **The specific genetic cause(s) of Tourette syndrome.** We already know that Tourette syndrome tends to run in families. Once we identify the specific genes involved in TS, it may be possible to correct the problems through gene therapy while the unborn child is still in the womb, or shortly after the child is born.

- **Further advances in psychology, education, and other allied health fields.** Drugs and other medical treatments are only part of the picture. A combination of, say, medications, therapies, and educational interventions could prove to be more helpful to children with Tourette syndrome than any of those elements on their own.

▪▪ Conclusion

When a child develops tics, a parent's first instinct often is to ask the doctor for a pill to make them go away. But rather than rush to medicate, you'll want to find a specialist who can do a thorough evaluation of your child—not just his tics, but his overall physical, emotional, and cognitive development. Often a child with Tourette syndrome has another associated disorder, such as AD/HD or obsessive-compulsive disorder, that may not be as obvious as the tics, but has a much bigger effect on development. Once you have a thorough diagnosis, your team (which will include you, your child, the specialist, and possibly other healthcare professionals) can work together to determine the best treatment approach.

If your child does require anti-tic medication, there are several different types available, including alpha-adrenoceptor agonists, and atypical or typical neuroleptics. There are also medications that can help with associated disorders such as AD/HD, OCD, rage attacks, or depression. Your specialist should discuss the pros and cons of any medication with you—including how it may alter your child's symptoms—before prescribing it. For example, some anti-tic medications may help with AD/HD symptoms, but certain AD/HD medications may worsen tics. Every child reacts differently to different drugs, so don't be discouraged if the first medication the specialist prescribes doesn't do everything you'd hoped.

Meanwhile, be sure to check with the doctor before giving your child any over-the-counter drugs—including any vitamins or supplements—as some can worsen tics and some can interact badly with prescription medications.

As a parent, your role in your child's medical treatment is crucial. Not only are you part of his treatment team, but you're its captain. It's important for you to stay up to date on the latest developments in Tourette syndrome treatments. Other team members may come and go over the years, but you'll always be there as your child's case manager and his biggest advocate.

▪▪ Parent Statements

We thought Zach's restlessness and pacing might be a side effect of medication. But then again, it could have been his AD/HD. Last fall he started having anxiety attacks, phobias, and OCD. We are seeing more physical expressions, so we can't be sure it's the TS or associated disorders or the side effects of medication.

◆◈◆

I have found that doctors diagnose according to their specialty. Dr X always says the mother is too involved and the father is too distant. Dr. Y always says the child has AD/HD, but no TS. And Dr Z always diagnoses TS with OCD.

◆◈◆

Some doctors are better than others, so parents must educate themselves to enable them to recognize the difference. It is best to get a referral from another TS family if you need someone who knows about TS.

◆◈◆

We took our teenaged son to see a specialist at a movement disorder clinic for a second opinion to determine whether he had a motor tic disorder or some other diagnosis. In preparation for the visit, we carefully filled in the clinic's forms with the requested several years' worth of history, taking approximately two hours to do so. Upon arrival, the resident didn't even look at the forms (if she had them at all) and expected us to regurgitate the information on the spot. To make matters worse, the doctor swept into the room and within a matter of a few minutes, announced that our son had a tic disorder. We were shocked to receive what we considered poor treatment at the hands of a highly regarded medical institution.

❦

Medication wipes Brad out. He gets so tired, and as soon as his body changes a little, the medication needs to be changed, too. Then we start all over again.

❦

It was a real blessing to have TS diagnosed with one referral and one visit. I know families that go from doctor to doctor not knowing what is wrong.

❦

Right now medication controls about 60 percent of Sean's tics. We don't go for total control because of the possible side effects.

❦

We've always been very conservative in our approach to medications and appreciated those like-minded doctors who treated our son. One, in particular, was very careful in his approach to monitoring medication treatments. When starting a new course of risperidone, he asked us to frequently monitor our son's blood pressure (easily done at the local drug store or grocery store), check in with him by phone in between appointments when changing the dosage or to report side effects, and warned us against suddenly ceasing the medication.

❦

Kids with TS often need counseling as they approach adolescence. An eleven- or twelve-year-old wants to be just like his peers, and having TS sets him apart. Lots of anger and frustration can build up. Counseling *gives them an outlet to express their feelings and it helps to build up self esteem and eventual acceptance of themselves.*

◆⚛◆

Jasmine seems to have a mental block against swallowing pills. I know she can easily swallow big chunks of food when she is eating, but give her a little pill to swallow, and she gags every time. We always have to give her medications that come in liquid form or crush pills up and mix them in yogurt or applesauce.

◆⚛◆

We tried some alternative therapies to help lessen Nathan's tics. Hypnotherapy held some promise for awhile. After the first session, my son's tics were noticeably absent for about an hour, and then slowly began to reappear. In a few hours, he was back to his normal tic rate. Nathan continued to see the hypnotist for a few more visits, and she provided him with a recorded tape of suggestions that he was to play just before going to sleep. He stuck with it for a couple of weeks, but the level of tics didn't seem to appreciably change. Still, the initial effect from the hypnosis was interesting to us.

◆⚛◆

Biofeedback was another approach we tried. Our son worked with a therapist for several weeks who taught him how to assess his arousal level and gave him relaxation tips. For whatever reason, it didn't seriously affect the tics. However, my son sometimes employs the deep breathing techniques to help him relax in stressful situations.

◆⚛◆

Remember the "Three M's" of TS. 1.) Medication: If you keep on trying, you will eventually find the right medication and method of dosage that will help to lessen the TS symptoms. 2.) Maturation: As your child matures, usually by his late teens, there's a good chance symptoms will decrease and his ability to control his symptoms will increase. 3.) Motivation: With maturity comes eventual awareness and desire to control the most disruptive behaviors of TS for inner reasons of self worth-inner motivation rather than punishment from outside of himself.

◆⚛◆

When our son was eight, we finally started him on a course of stimulant medication treatment for his AD/HD symptoms, primarily impulsivity and inattention. We were amazed at how well it worked. However, after about ten days, we noticed some unusual repetitive behaviors in him such as eye blinking and tipping of his head. He had never displayed anything like that before. All of our son's doctors (from psychiatrists to neurologists) claim that the stimulant medication did not "turn on" his tics, but still we wonder if that's true.

❧

The side effects of the medication (risperidone) our son took were alarming. He experienced dry mouth, fainting, and stomach ache. The worst part was how he was zombie-like a good bit of the time. He reported falling asleep in school, as did his teachers. He decided for himself that this was a case of "the cure being worse than the disease," and discontinued the medication.

❧

Through the years, we've tried risperidone and Strattera (the doctor said that some people taking it for other reasons report a lessening of tics), but nothing seemed to work for long. Sometimes, the tics would decrease, but they always returned. It could be that at the same time we were trying a new med, the tics were in the waning period of the typical waxing and waning cycle. After years of giving meds a good trial, we've decided that we're no longer interested in pursuing them as a treatment.

❧

Often when a professional doesn't understand your child, they don't refer you on to someone who will be able to help. They sometimes blame the patient instead of admitting they don't know the answers.

❧

As early as possible, we wanted our daughter to "own" her Tourette syndrome. Someday she was going to have to be her own advocate and make her own way. With small steps, beginning in fifth grade, she became involved in her medication decisions, developing and being responsible for her accommodations, sitting in on and then later running group meetings with her teachers. When she started college, the head of Disability Services said that they had never had a student so ready to be a self-advocate as my daughter was.

4

BEHAVIOR THERAPIES FOR TOURETTE SYNDROME

John Piacentini, Ph.D.

Medication is, by far, the most commonly used treatment for Tourette syndrome, and it can be very effective. Clinical trials have shown that medication can reduce tic symptoms by anywhere from 25 to 80 percent. However, medication doesn't work in all cases. Even when it is effective, unwanted side effects and other safety concerns can limit the use of some medications, especially with children (see Chapter 3).

Increasingly, researchers have been looking at behavior therapies—most prominently *Habit Reversal Training,* but also functional interventions—as alternative treatments for tic disorders. These are used either as an addition to medication or as stand-alone treatments. Much of this recent work has been conducted by members of the Tourette Syndrome Association Behavioral Sciences Consortium.[1]

---

[1] *Including John Piacentini, Ph.D., Chair, and Susanna Chang, Ph.D. (UCLA); John Walkup, M.D. & Golda Ginsburg, Ph.D. (Johns Hopkins University); Douglas Woods, Ph.D. (University of Wisconsin-Milwaukee); Sabine Wilhelm, Ph.D. and Thilo Deckersbach, Ph.D. (Massachusetts General Hospital/Harvard University); Alan Peterson, Ph.D. (University of Texas San Antonio Health Sciences Center); and Lawrence Scahill, MSN, Ph.D. (Yale University).*

▌▌ What Is Behavior Therapy?

Just about every parent knows the basic premise of behavior therapy (even if you've never put a name to it): Reward a child (or adult, or animal) for a given behavior, and she'll tend to repeat it. That's why handing your toddler a cookie every time she starts whining doesn't

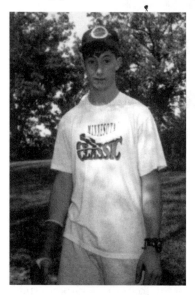

produce a well-behaved child—it produces a whiny, overweight child. You've taught (or "conditioned") her to whine by pairing the behavior with a reward.

Wouldn't it be great if we could eliminate tics just by withholding cookies? (That's a sacrifice most kids with TS would gladly make!) Unfortunately, it's a lot more complicated than that. Most behaviors are rewarded in subtle ways that might not be evident to either you or your child. A behavior therapist is a trained, objective third party (usually a psychologist) who can analyze the way in which a behavior is rewarded (or "reinforced"), and then come up with an alternate plan of reinforcement to modify the behavior.

Does lumping tics in with other behaviors that can be changed through behavior therapy imply that a child's tics are deliberate? Absolutely not! Although it may seem counterintuitive, scientists learned years ago that even *involuntary* behaviors can be influenced through behavioral conditioning. Perhaps the most common example of this is the development of a fear or phobia following a frightening situation. For example, someone who got stuck in an elevator may experience all the physiological symptoms of anxiety (e.g., rapid heartbeat, shortness of breath, sweating, muscle tension, etc.) the next time they need to ride one. Fortunately, the same conditioning process that created the fear can also be used to alleviate it.

Behaviorists look at two different types of reinforcement that may strengthen a behavior. *Positive reinforcement* occurs when a behavior is rewarded by something good—a word of praise, a cookie, or even some less tangible inner reward, such as a sense of satisfaction. *Negative reinforcement*, on the other hand, occurs when a behavior is rewarded by *removing* something bad or unpleasant. For example, if an annoying little brother goes away when your child punches him, the punching is being negatively reinforced. Or how about that the whining toddler… if she stops whining when mom gives her a cookie, then mom is receiving negative reinforcement for her own behavior!

A Word about Punishment

If rewarding a behavior makes it increase, than punishing it should make it decrease… right? Well, sometimes. *Punishment*—following an unwanted behavior with a bad/unpleasant response (e.g., a spanking or a dirty look)—can be very tricky. A child may associate the punishment with the punisher, rather than with the behavior. That is, she may attribute the punishment to the fact that the punisher is a "mean person," rather than the fact that she did something wrong. Or she may associate the punishment with getting caught, which just encourages her to hide the behavior. Alternatives to punishment used in behavior therapy include *extinction* (removing whatever reward is reinforcing the unwanted behavior) or *time out* (removing the child, for a limited period of time, from the circumstances that are reinforcing the unwanted behavior).

Punishment, we know, is not an appropriate approach to treating a tic disorder. Fear of punishment makes a child feel stressed and anxious. And what happens when a child with TS feels anxious? She tics. If she has obsessive-compulsive (OC) symptoms as well, she may increase her ritualistic behaviors. While a child may be able to suppress her symptoms for a short period because she is afraid she'll be punished for them, her worries about being punished for her tics will more than likely lead to more tics rather than fewer. In fact, behavioral theory would predict that the child's tics would be especially bad whenever she was around the person threatening punishment, since this would be such an anxiety-provoking situation. Unfortunately, the use of punishment often ends up making the problem worse rather than better. No child should ever be put in this position.

Fortunately, there are more effective ways of dealing with tics through behavior therapy. The most well-studied behavioral method, by far, is Habit Reversal Training.

❖ Habit Reversal Training

Habit Reversal Training (HRT) was first developed about thirty years ago to treat what was, back then, called "nervous habits" (hence the term "habit reversal"). This included not only tics—which were considered nervous habits by some clinicians and researchers at that time—but also nail biting, thumb sucking, compulsive hair pulling, skin picking or scratching, and nose picking. Over time, researchers and therapists found HRT often could be successfully used to treat all of these problems, as well as the tics associated with TS.

HRT is related to a strategy many people with TS already use: replacing a tic with a more socially acceptable behavior. For example, a person with an arm-jerking tic might run his fingers through his hair at the end to make the tic look like a more purposeful behavior. However, the ultimate goal of HRT is not simply to camouflage or hide the tics, but, rather, to greatly lessen, and in some cases, eliminate the premonitory urge and/or the tics altogether.

Not every tic is worth tackling. If a tic doesn't cause your child any injury, embarrassment, or social difficulties, the best thing you can do is learn to ignore it. Some tics can be more distressing for Mom and Dad—who are observing them—than for the child who's actually experiencing them. Therapy—be it HRT or pharmaceuticals—usually isn't advisable for a child who isn't bothered by her minor tics.

Awareness Training

The first step in HRT is to increase a child's ability to recognize the urge or feeling that she experiences just before a specific tic.

When a child with TS first starts having tics—often around the age of six or seven—she may not "feel them coming on." They "just hap-

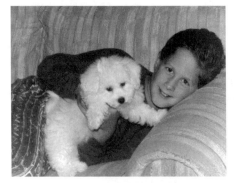

pen." That's typical, and for that reason, HRT isn't usually done with small children.

However, between the ages of eight and ten, the child with TS will probably start to recognize some signs when certain tics are going to occur. People with TS often describe these *premonitions* as either a building tension in the area of the body where the tic will occur, or a strong physical urge to perform the tic behavior. Performing the tic will relieve that tension or urge—temporarily. Generally, people with TS become better at recognizing these premonitions as they get older, but therapists have found that children can be taught to better recognize them through awareness training.

Depending on how aware the child already is of her tics and premonitions, the therapist may use any combination of these techniques in awareness training:

- Videotaping the child when she is having tics and/or having her reenact the tics while looking in a mirror;
- Assisting the child in detecting the tics by pointing out each tic immediately as it occurs during a set time period. (Note: This does *not* mean that it's beneficial for parents to mention a child's tics every time they occur at home!);
- Having the child count how many times a tic occurs during a defined period, either by keeping a tally in a notebook or using a wrist counter;
- Teaching the child an "early warning" procedure, where she learns to recognize and practices identifying the earliest signs that a tic is going to occur.

Interestingly, some children experience a temporary decrease in tics just as a result of the awareness training. Because this downturn tends to be short lived, though, awareness training is usually followed by *Competing Response Training*.

It's important to note, though, that not every tic is preceded by a premonition. Certain simple tics, such as eye blinking (the most common first tic in children with TS), appear to be direct expressions of neurobiological activity. They happen almost like reflex actions—the brain signals a muscle to move with no warning and no thought processes involved. These tics are harder to control with HRT, although the treatment can still be effective in some cases. The good news is that most simple tics tend to be less noticeable, distressing, and/or interfering, and as such are less likely to warrant intervention. However, HRT can still be used with simple tics if needed.

Competing Response Training

Once the child is able to reliably detect a specific tic and, hopefully, its premonitory urge, the therapist will teach her to use a competing response (CR) each time she feels that urge, and hold the CR until the urge passes. If the child doesn't experience premonitions, she'll be taught to use a CR as soon as she feels the tic occur.

What's a competing response? It's a more socially acceptable behavior that the child learns to substitute for the bothersome tic, ideally using the opposite muscles to the ones used in the tic (or at least different ones). The CR needs to be an action or position that the child can maintain for at least a minute, is inconspicuous, and is compatible with normal activity. Most people choose an isometric CR that involves the same part of the body as the targeted tic, but tenses the muscles in the opposite, or at least a different, manner than the tic would. For example, a child with a severe head-shaking tic might be taught to stare straight ahead while gently tensing her head or neck muscles, while a child with facial grimacing might be taught to simultaneously raise her eyebrows slightly and gently clench her teeth. A child with a frequent throat clearing tic might be taught to engage in slow rhythmic breathing whenever she felt the urge to clear her throat.

As these examples demonstrate, the goal of the competing response is to prevent the muscles involved in the tic from expressing themselves, or at least to make them express themselves in a less intense manner than dictated by the tic. For many children, the competing response is easiest to learn for big, troublesome tics. Not only will the child be more motivated to change tics like this, but she'll be more conscious of their occurrence, as well.

In the case of a simple tic, the child would be taught to implement the competing response at the first sign of the tic, rather than in response to the premonitory urge. For example, for a simple head or arm jerk, the CR would be gently tensing opposing muscles so as to keep her head or arm motionless until the need to tic dissipates. For eye blinking, the competing response might be a slow controlled up-and-down movement of the eyelids

Over time, with consistent and repeated use of a carefully chosen CR, the tic often lessens in intensity and/or frequency. It may even disappear completely. Although it sounds like a simple enough procedure, it's not always so. The brain is sending a message through the child's nervous system that her muscles need to tic—and that can be a very compelling urge to fight. And while substituting a CR is far more reasonable than trying to simply repress the tic completely, it's an approach that can take hard work on the child's part. In other words, parents, don't try this on your own—find a psychologist, psychiatrist, or other therapist who's skilled in behavior therapies to work with your child.

Often, CRs need to be implemented in a gradual manner using a "shaping" procedure (where incremental steps towards the desired CR are reinforced). Younger children, or those with more forceful tics, may feel overwhelmed at the prospect of completely blocking their tics—and they may actually be physically unable to do so. The goal of shaping strategies in these situations is not to completely block a tic, but rather to lessen the explosive aspects of it.

An initial or intermediate goal may be to "morph" the tic into a more socially inconspicuous behavior. For example, a child with a bad arm-jerking tic may not be able to perform a forceful CR such as pushing the hand down on the thigh or stomach and pushing the elbow in towards the hip. Instead, the therapist might help her perform a CR designed to slow down the behavior and make it look like she is smoothing her hair back. Then, as the child gains greater control over the targeted tic, the CR could become increasingly more forceful with the ultimate goal of greater tic control.

Given that the explosive aspects of a tic are typically the most noticeable, distressing, and physically damaging, helping the child to slow it down or "de-intensify" it may be more successful in some cases than trying to teach her to stop it completely.

How Does CR Training Work?

As mentioned earlier, many people with TS taught themselves to substitute more socially acceptable actions or sounds for their tics, long before CR training was formalized. Researchers are still learning about how and why it works.

In premonition-triggered tics, the tic normally relieves the muscle tension that builds up in the area of the body that's going to tic—it's a negative reinforcer. Each time the tension builds and the child responds with a tic, she (unconsciously) reinforces the behavior again. In other words, the more times the uncomfortable muscle tension disappears after a tic, the more likely the child is to tic (because the tic makes her feel better). On the other hand, if the child is able to substitute a CR in place of a tic, she is interfering with that negative reinforcement loop. Over time, because the premonition never gets reinforced, it is extinguished. But, because the premonition usually doesn't disappear right away, the child must learn to tolerate some level of discomfort during the process. Fortunately, HRT contains some additional elements to help children deal with this (see below).

Of course, that still doesn't really explain why CR training can work with a simple tic with no premonitory urge. Researchers speculate that when a person interrupts a simple tic by switching to a CR as it happens, she may be disrupting an automatic chain of neurological events. Disrupting this chain of events repeatedly appears to extinguish it over time.

Other Elements That Might be Included in HR Training

Awareness Training and Competing Response Training are the two primary techniques of Habit Reversal Training, but therapists often find it helpful to include other elements as well:

Social Support. Habit reversal training is hard work, and no fun. One factor that can make it a little easier is if family members, teachers, and even friends provide praise and support to the child when she successfully uses her awareness techniques and CRs, manages tic-free intervals, or sticks with the treatment protocol.

Anxiety Management Techniques. Since stress and anxiety can lead to an increase in tics, it would seem a logical assumption that stress management training would lead to decreased tics over time. Unfortunately, researchers haven't found that to be the case. Nevertheless, a child who experiences a lot of anxiety or stress may benefit in other ways from relaxation techniques such as deep breathing, progressive muscle relaxation, and guided imagery.

Reward Systems. Sure, the child who participates in HRT should be motivated to stop a tic that bothers her. But that's a rather intangible goal, and can take weeks to achieve (and there are no guarantees). A systematic rewards program can help keep a child motivated and on track. The therapist, parents, and child should all work together to come up with an incentive plan and schedule that will work for the individual child—whether it's extra video game time, new books, or trips to the ballpark. These rewards should be linked to the child's participation in the therapy, not to her successfully replacing a tic with a CR. That way, she'll be more willing to keep at it, even when results aren't immediate.

Cognitive Strategies. HRT can be difficult for adults to grasp, much less children. Therapists sometimes find it useful to put the therapy into "kid speak." For example, the "Habit Reversal Training

Program," becomes the "Tic Busters Program." Analogies can provide the child with a better understanding of her tics and the rationale underlying HRT. At UCLA, where kids are never far from the beach, therapists compare HRT to surfing. The urge to tic and the eventual expression of the tic are described as a wave breaking on the beach. The child can either try to "stop the wave" (completely block the tic urge), which is more difficult, or else "ride the wave" by controlling it with her HRT "surfboard" (express the tic, but in a controlled and less conspicuous manner).

‼ Functional Intervention

Functional Intervention (FI) is based on a number of studies conducted over the years that have shown that certain situations and/or social consequences of having tics (for example, being teased) can make tics worsen. The goal of FI is to identify these situations and consequences and attempt to change them so the tics aren't made worse unnecessarily. For example, a child whose tics worsen when she is nervous about taking a test would be taught stress management or other calming techniques as part of treatment. Or, if it was determined that teasing by siblings makes her tics worse, her brothers and sisters would be taught better ways to respond to their sister's tics.

As we mentioned earlier in the chapter, behaviors—even involuntary ones—often continue or increase because they are in some way reinforced. Reinforcement can be positive—a reward of some type—or negative—the removal of something unpleasant. Let's take a look at how this might affect a child with Tourette syndrome.

Example: How Tics May Be Reinforced

Jennie comes home stressed out from a tough day in middle school. She goes to the den, where her sister is watching TV, and begins tic-cing loudly. Her sister gets upset, screams for Mom, and teases Jennie. Jennie's tics get even louder. How might the family respond?

Scenario #1:

- *Mom yells at the sister.* Being a normal adolescent, Jennie finds it rather satisfying to see her sister get in trouble. Her tics and related behaviors are positively reinforced.
- *Mom comforts Jennie.* Hmm, attention and sympathy from Mom. That's another positive reinforcement.

- *Sister stomps off to her bedroom.* Not only does Jennie get the TV to herself (positive reinforcement), but she gets rid of her annoying sister as well (negative reinforcement). Bonus!

Scenario #2

- *Mom yells at Jennie.* Mom figures this is a punishment, so it shouldn't reinforce her daughter's tics.
- *Mom sends Jennie to her room.* She's removed from the place/situation where her tics occurred.
- *Jennie's sister gets the TV to herself.* The sister's teasing and screaming are reinforced both positively (sole possession of the TV) and negatively (removal of annoying sister). Odds are, she'll use the teasing and screaming tactic again in the future.
- *Jennie now feels persecuted.* While, granted, Mom's responses didn't reinforce the tics, they did increase Jennie's negative feelings (and she'd already had a difficult day at school). These bad feelings may cause Jennie's tics or other associated problems to worsen.

Does the whole situation remind you of *Catch 22*? Positive consequences reinforce tics BUT negative responses lead to distress, which leads to more tics

Don't worry, the family can learn better ways to cope with Jennie's disruptive tics. Scenarios like the two above are frequently uncovered in a Functional Analysis.

Functional Analysis

In a functional analysis, a therapist works to identify the situations or factors in the child's daily life that may serve to maintain or increase her tic frequency and severity. Often, the therapist uncovers processes that the child, family, and school were all unaware of. The most common forms of tic reinforcement tend to be:

1. Social Attention—getting a reaction from another person. This might be "good" attention, such as hugs and sympathy from Mom, or "bad" attention, such as getting yelled at. Getting a sibling annoyed might be fun, but for some kids, even getting yelled at by Mom is more reinforcing than getting no attention from her at all.

2. Escape from a Situation—a change in the demands on the child. If Jennie gets to skip homework or avoid sitting with the family at dinner because of her tics, the tics are being negatively reinforced. The behavior therapist will try to identify:

1. **Common Situations** when tics occur, e.g., mealtimes, TV time, and homework.
2. **Common Antecedents** (what happens before the tics start). Does the child tic more when her parents tell her to do something? When she's teased? When she's anxious or stressed?
3. **Common Consequences** (what happens after she starts ticcing). Is she comforted by a parent? Told to "Stop ticcing"? Teased or yelled at by siblings? Does she get to leave the table, classroom, or other situation? Is she allowed to skip homework or chores?

Once the therapist has identified all the different factors involved in reinforcement of the tics, he can design the interventions.

Functional Interventions

Functional interventions improve behaviors by eliminating the factors that reinforce those behaviors. Again, this is *not* meant to imply that the tics are caused by, say, teasing or sympathy. Tics are caused by chemical processes in the brain. But outside factors can make the tics worse, and the aim of FI is to get rid of those factors.

In a sense, FI teaches those around the child with TS to treat her as "normally" as possible. Tics should not dictate what the child does or does not do, and the child should not receive any special treatment for her tics. Whenever possible, family, friends, and teachers should ignore the tics completely. Of course, that may be easier said than done, especially if the tics are distracting to others or look painful.

A trained behavior therapist can prescribe specific ways to address problems with an individual child. But there are general rules that can be useful for many families:

1. **Give the child a 15-minute warning** and free time to calm down before you require her to begin specific tasks such as homework or chores. (This addresses antecedents.)
2. **Don't respond to tics *in the moment*** by teasing, telling the child to stop, comforting her, etc. This means parents, sibs, teachers, *everyone*. (This addresses social consequences.)

3. **Allow no escape from responsibilities** because of tics. (This addresses escape consequences.)
   - If tics interfere with a task, have the child leave the situation for fifteen minutes, then return.
   - If she leaves the dinner table because of tics, she must come back in fifteen minutes and finish eating the meal.
   - Homework must begin every day at a set time, regardless of tics. Allow the child to take brief breaks according to a set schedule.

Some of these rules may prove challenging to different parents. For example, if you were raised in a strict household where kids were expected to jump when parents told them to do something, fifteen-minute warnings may feel overly indulgent. On the other hand, if you've been giving your child a neck and shoulder massage whenever her head-rolling tic starts up, you may feel like you're being "cold" when you tell her to sit down and start her homework anyway.

Keep in mind, though, that it's not indulgent to give a child with TS fifteen minutes to calm her nervous system, any more than it would be indulgent to build a ramp for a child in a wheelchair.

And now that you know that the neck massage is probably reinforcing the head-rolling tic, is that really what a loving mother should do? You can always give your child a neck rub later in the day, when she isn't ticcing—just don't discuss the tics while you're doing it.

What do kids with TS say they want more than anything? They say they want to be "normal." Ironically—but happily—treating them as "normal" as possible can make their tics and related difficulties improve.

Back to Our Example

In our earlier example, Jennie came home stressed out from a tough day in middle school. She went to the den, where her sister was watching TV, and began ticcing loudly. Her sister got upset, screamed for Mom, and teased Jennie. Jennie's tics get even louder.

Since this was a frequent scenario in Jennie's family, her behavior therapist did a functional analysis, and made the following recommendations:

1. Jennie's sister is given a choice. She may: a) skip watching TV right after school; b) watch it on the little TV in her

room with her door closed; or c) watch it in the den, but she may not yell at or tease Jennie if she begins having tics.

2. At the same time, if Jennie's tics get loud enough that they'd interfere with her sister being able to hear the television program, Jennie will remove herself from the room for fifteen minutes. She may continue watching the program on a different TV if one is available.

3. No one may yell, including Mom. If either Jennie or her sister fails to abide by the rules, Mom will tell the offender to leave the room. If both break the rules, Mom will turn the TV off, and it will remain off for the rest of the afternoon.

Once Jennie and her sister see that Mom "means business" (i.e., turns the TV off when they began fighting), things settle down. Jennie removes herself from the den when her tics are particularly loud. And on days when Jennie's sister is feeling a little grouchy and knows that she's likely to get annoyed by even less volatile tics, she watches TV in her room. Now that the various reinforcements have been removed, Jennie tends to tic less during the after-school TV time.

:: How Well Do Behavioral Interventions Work?

Though HRT was first proposed for tic control in 1973, few controlled studies were undertaken until recently. Two studies funded by TSA in the late 1990s showed very promising results. At UCLA, a study with children showed an average 30 percent decrease in tic severity over the course of eight sessions over ten weeks. The second study, done with adults at Harvard University and Massachusetts General Hospital, resulted in a 35 percent decrease in tic severity over fourteen sessions. Even more significantly, in both studies, the degree to which tics actually impaired the participants' daily lives decreased by 55

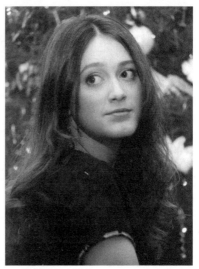

percent. Months later, study participants retained most of the improvements they'd gained through the HRT.

Recently, the National Institutes of Health provided funding for two four-year, large scale studies of behavioral interventions for Tourette syndrome and chronic tic disorders. The studies—one for children and adolescents (funded in 2004) and one for adults (funded in 2005)—are being carried out by the Tourette Syndrome Association Behavioral Sciences Consortium through a collaboration of some of the leading Tourette syndrome clinical research centers in the country, including UCLA, Harvard/Massachusetts General Hospital, Johns Hopkins School of Medicine, Yale University, University of Wisconsin-Milwaukee, and the University of Texas Health Science Center-San Antonio. These studies are examining the effectiveness of HRT in combination with a functional intervention. Individuals with other problems, such as ADHD, OCD, anxiety, or depression, are allowed to participate in the study, provided that these other problems are stable and that the tics are the primary problem. Although we're still in the early stages of these studies as this book is published, results look promising.

Before you begin any course of treatment for your child's Tourette syndrome, it's always wise to check into the most up-to-date research available. The Tourette Syndrome Association (www.tsa-usa.org) and the National Library of Medicine (www.medlineplus.com) are good places to start.

■■ Choosing a Therapist

There are some, but not a lot of, therapists out there who are familiar with Habit Reversal Training for tics. If you can find a local therapist who is—or if you can enroll your child in one of the NIH-funded studies listed above—great! But if that's not feasible, a well-trained and experienced cognitive-behavioral therapist or behavior therapist who is willing to learn about tics/HRT is an excellent second choice. Once the NIH studies are finished, assuming the treatment is shown to be effective, the research groups will work with TSA to launch a big training effort to teach as many doctors and therapists as possible how to do the treatment.

∷ Conclusion

Medication is still the most common and well-studied treatment for the symptoms of Tourette syndrome. But if you have an older child or teen whose tics cannot be sufficiently controlled by medication, or if you're concerned about the safety or side effects of the recommended medications, it's reasonable to look into behavior therapy.

Although tics are involuntary, there's a growing body of evidence to show that Habit Reversal Therapy can often reduce the intensity or frequency of tics. In HRT, the therapist targets one single problematic tic at a time, teaching the child a "competing response" to the urge to perform a tic. It takes consistent work over a period of several weeks for a child to master a CR, so this approach works best if your child is very motivated to be rid of a particular tic.

If you don't have a therapist experienced in HRT nearby, look for a cognitive behavioral therapist or behavior therapist who's willing to learn. Meanwhile, keep in mind the best response you can give to your child's tic is no response at all. Don't punish your child for her tics, but don't reward her for them (with sympathy or extra attention) either. What kids with Tourette syndrome most want is to be "normal." So, do your best to treat your child that way.

5

DAILY LIFE WITH YOUR CHILD

Marilynn Kaplan, M.Ed.

For most parents, good advice on childcare is easy to come by. When they have questions about development or behaviors, they have only to consult their own parents, their neighbors, or their child's pediatrician for suggestions. But when you have a child with Tourette syndrome, you may find that what works for other parents does not always work for you.

It's not that your child's daily care needs are any different from any other child's. It's just that his TS (or "TS Plus," which is the combination of TS together with any related conditions such as AD/HD, OCD, sensory integration problems, or developmental delays) sometimes makes daily care more challenging. For example, children with TS and AD/HD have trouble keeping their attention focused on one activity, so they may need more reminders or supervision when they are cleaning their room, setting the table, or completing some other chore. Children who also have obsessive-compulsive symptoms may have rituals or routines that interfere with their family's daily routine. If a child has a compulsion to wash his hands repeatedly before breakfast, his parents might have trouble getting him dressed and ready for school in time to catch the bus.

In addition, the need to keep your child's tics to a minimum by reducing stress can dictate the way the whole family's life is run. Each day, you may have to follow a set routine so that no unexpected events increase the stress your child feels. Since a child's TS symptoms wax and wane and frequently change, you must constantly reevaluate your child's needs and develop new strategies to meet them.

In the end, how you adapt your daily care routine to your child will depend on his personality, symptoms, and developmental abilities. Because children's personalities and TS symptoms vary so widely, there are no magic formulas and no absolute right or wrong answers. With attention, planning, and nurturing, however, you can learn what works with your child. And although your role as a parent may sometimes be more challenging, you can help ensure that your child develops the independence and self-esteem he needs to succeed as an adult. This chapter is designed to help you learn to analyze your child's unique needs and then develop ways to take care of them.

∷ Providing a Supportive Home Environment

From birth onward, most children are masters at making their physical needs known. They wail when they need to be fed, squawk when their diaper needs changing, and shiver when they need an extra blanket. Like any parent, you undoubtedly learned to interpret these signs early on and to take care of your child's physical well-being. But besides having physical needs, all children have a variety of emotional needs that may not be so obvious. Perhaps most importantly, they need to feel loved and accepted in order to feel good about themselves and their abilities.

For children with Tourette syndrome, the need to develop feelings of self-worth is just as acute as it is for other children. But because their TS often makes them feel different or "defective," it can be harder for them to develop good self-esteem. By providing a supportive home environment, you can help your child with Tourette syndrome conquer negative feelings about himself and feel like a valuable part of his family and community. The sections below describe some specific strategies that are often helpful.

Coping with Tics

One of the best things you can do for your child's emotional well-being is to make sure he feels comfortable having tics at home.

Children with TS may hold back their tics when they are in public because they don't want to seem different from other children. They need to know that there is at least one place where it is always acceptable for them to release their symptoms. Furthermore, helping your child feel comfortable with his tics lets him know that your family accepts him and his disability, which is crucial to the development of his self-esteem.

Constantly pointing out tics or blaming your child for having them only increases stress and usually makes tics get worse. Conversely, ignoring your child's tics usually helps relieve the stress he feels and therefore helps to reduce tics. Professionals usually advise parents to ignore their children's tics. There may, however, be times when you want to briefly acknowledge a tic to let your child know that you understand what he is going through and accept his disability. For example, if your child has a new shoulder tic, you could say, "I see that you are shrugging your shoulders. Let me know if you would like a massage tonight."

Ignoring tics is sometimes easier said than done. Phonic tics in particular can be very disruptive. Some parents wear earplugs or listen to a portable radio or CD player to help them ignore tics. In addition, having your child listen to music can sometimes have a calming and quieting effect on tics. Experiment with all styles of music. Music with a constant beat may be more soothing than relaxation tapes for some kids. Because many children with Tourette syndrome need to hear favorite songs over and over again, make sure your child's CD or MP3 player has a replay mechanism.

Listening to music may also help diminish your child's tics when riding in the car. Another strategy to use when traveling is to involve your child in activities that help him block out stressful stimuli and focus on something else. For example, you might give your child a tablet and crayons or play guessing games with the odometer, clock, or things you see outside.

If your child has a socially unacceptable tic or compulsion, such as spitting or licking others, it may be possible to substitute a more socially acceptable tic or compulsion for the less desirable one. For example, a child with a spitting tic may be able to change the tic to a swallowing tic or other mouth or tongue tic. A child with a compulsion to lick others might learn to lick his teeth instead. And a child with coprolalia might learn to substitute a word such as "fork" or "fu" for the swear word he might otherwise say.

Just as the ability to control tics varies with each individual with TS, so does the ability to successfully substitute symptoms. It may help to talk to your child about possible substitutions. Children can often describe what tics feel like or what movements or sounds they need to make to "satisfy" a tic. Trust your child if he says he cannot substitute a particular tic. As children grow older, tic substitution sometimes occurs more easily, and many adults with TS learn to use it as a coping strategy. A psychologist trained in "habit reversal" may be able to help a child who's not able to substitute a tic on his own (see Chapter 4).

If your child's tics cannot be reduced or controlled, then it is up to your family to accept that fact. Some people with uncontrolled disruptive tics say that keeping a sense of humor and allowing others to do the same works best in these situations. You and your child should also understand that there may be times when a family member needs to go into another room and shut the door to get away from the tics. For example, if your child's tics keep a sibling from focusing on a book report he is writing, he should leave the room, just as he would if a television were disrupting his concentration. As discussed later in this chapter, if there are times when you feel you simply must have a break from coping with tics, you may also benefit from respite care services.

Rarely, children with TS may have self-injurious tics such as head banging, eye poking, picking their gums, or burning themselves. These tics cannot be ignored, and you should seek professional help immediately from your child's physician or a mental health professional. They can advise you whether a change in medication or an attempt at symptom substitution may help.

Providing Structure, Consistency, and Routine

Structure, consistency, and routine are important for all children, but they are even more important for children with TS, especially those who also have AD/HD, Asperger syndrome, or OCD. Children with OC or Asperger tendencies often have a need to know what will be happening throughout the day. Surprises can be stressful for them, and may cause anxiety and increased symptoms. Children with AD/HD, on the other hand, can become anxious and hyperactive or withdrawn if they are not involved in directed activities. Many things in the environment, but especially unexpected events, can over-stimulate them. In order to stay calm and in control, children with these symptoms need daily events to be predictable.

The keys to providing your child with the predictability he craves are structure, routine, and consistency. Providing structure basically involves setting well-defined boundaries for behavior and activities. Your child needs to understand what he is expected to do, when, and how. When your child is at home, it is often up to you to tell him what he can or should be doing by planning after-school and evening activities. Outside the home, a structured school or daycare setting can help. During summer vacation, you can help to keep your child's day structured by enrolling him in a YMCA or community recreation center program.

Developing routines, or set ways of doing things, helps to reduce surprises that may be stressful to your child. Generally, the more "sameness" in your child's life, the better. If he can get up at the same time each morning, sit in the same spot at the breakfast table, even eat the same cereal every day if he so desires, he will feel more secure. Occasionally, of course, routines must be broken. For example, instead of coming straight home after school, your child may need to go to the dentist. When changes are necessary, keeping a family events calendar in a prominent location can help your child prepare ahead of time.

Being consistent in your parenting style is also important in providing predictability. Not only should you try to handle specific situations the same way each time, but you and your spouse should try to handle situations in the same way. If you have different ideas about parenting, work together to develop a system that combines both of your strengths. When you and your spouse present a united front, your child will be less likely to play one parent against the other, and will be less confused as to what is expected of him.

Keeping an Eye on Your Child

All babies and young children require close supervision to ensure their personal safety. As children grow up, they usually become more cautious and responsible for their own well-being. Children with TS and AD/HD, however, may continue to need a great deal of supervision as they get older. This is because they are often impulsive and have a tendency to wander beyond their boundaries. For parents, constantly supervising an active child can be very tiring. It may help to limit the amount of time your child spends on stressful activities that may worsen his symptoms. If he starts losing control, try to redirect his energies into another activity. For example, if he becomes overexcited while playing video games with friends, send them outside to swing or play tag.

Setting and enforcing physical boundaries inside and outside your home may also help. An enclosed backyard, a bedroom, or a special nook or cubby can give your child privacy, time to unwind, and relaxation. Let him pick the spots himself (with your approval), so they're sure to be places he feels safe and comfortable. The idea is to provide specific areas where your child will not be over-stimulated and where he will gain a clear understanding of where he fits into his environment.

If you take the time to let your child's siblings, friends, and neighbors know about your child's impulsivity, they can keep an eye out for him outside the house. Sitters can also help to relieve you of some of your supervising duties, especially if they know that you are not far away.

Occasionally, you may wish to make some alterations to your home to avoid persistent problems. For example, if your child always helps himself to snacks when you are not looking, you may want to lock up all the junk food in a separate cabinet and leave the healthy food readily accessible. If your child has a compulsion to climb out of windows, you might install bars on the upstairs windows that snap out in case of fire. If your child frequently gets into dangerous situations, talk to your physician or a mental health professional about ways of dealing with your child's behavior.

Providing a Physical Outlet

By providing your child with opportunities to take part in exercise and sports, you can help him reap both physical and emotional benefits. Many children with TS have fewer tics when they are actively involved in a physical activity. Some experts believe this is because exercise produces or increases certain brain chemicals that have a calming effect. If your child has AD/HD or sensory integration problems, he may find exercises such as climbing, jumping, spinning, or swinging very calming. This is because children with these problems often have a need for the increased stimulation of their movement (vestibular) sense that these activities provide.

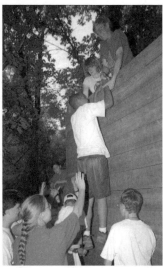

At home, there are many ways you can encourage your child to work off energy. A mini trampoline or an old mattress in a play area may work indoors. Outside, you may want to install a basketball hoop, swing set, climbing tower, or a soccer goal.

In the sports arena, there are numerous individual and group activities that can benefit your child. Swimming is one of many individual sports that works well for children with Tourette syndrome. It teaches a life skill, involves the whole body, and provides a physical outlet for excess energy. It can be enjoyed either competitively or recreationally. Your child may feel comfortable swimming in a public pool, but if he prefers warm water, check for area hospitals that have therapeutic pools or facilities for people with disabilities or chronic illnesses. Some recreation centers and YMCAs offer indoor heated pools as well. Other good choices of individual sports include skiing, ice skating, roller skating, dancing, biking, and jogging.

If group lessons make your child too anxious, consider arranging for a few private lessons. After he feels more secure in his ability and surroundings, he can be worked into small group lessons. Be sure to discuss your child's symptoms with all instructors before classes begin.

Some kids with Tourette syndrome do well in team sports, but don't push your child if he doesn't. There are many stress factors inherent in team sports, and stress is what many children with Tourette syndrome need to avoid. Of course, some children will insist on pursuing an activity even if it makes their symptoms worse. If this happens, you will have to weigh the pros and cons of him continuing, and perhaps discuss it with the professional who is treating your child's TS.

As with any activity, there is a chance that your child may become compulsive with his chosen sport. If so, encourage his interest and try to use it to enrich other facets of his life. For instance, if your child likes to play baseball, encourage him to explore books on baseball. Or if he loves ballet, try introducing him to classical music. If your child is so compulsive about a sport that he becomes overtired, you will need to limit the time he is actively participating and promote quieter, related activities such as score keeping, charting, or reading about the sport.

▪▪ Discipline and Behavior Management

Teaching appropriate behavior is an ongoing concern for parents. Indeed, it is one of the most important responsibilities of parenthood. All children need to learn how to get along with others and how to follow safety rules. They need to learn, for instance, not to dart out into traffic and to ask to borrow another child's toy.

When your child has TS, teaching appropriate behavior can be especially difficult. Your child may be unable to control certain socially unacceptable behaviors because of the nature of his disability. Although he may understand that some of his motor and verbal tics or obsessive-compulsive behaviors are unacceptable to many people, he may not be able to control them. He might also be impulsive, hyperactive, aggressive, disorganized, or socially and emotionally immature, making him even more prone to do things that others see as "misbehaving."

As a parent, you must decide which behaviors society will need to learn to accept and which behaviors your child will need to learn to control if he is going to live in the community. The behaviors that are referred to in this section as "inappropriate" are those that can cause physical or emotional harm to your child or to others, or destruction of property. Examples include hitting other children, slamming doors, hanging out windows, stealing, punching holes in walls, doing karate kicks on windows, and the like.

Once you have identified which behaviors you want to discourage and which you want to encourage, you must then find the combination of behavior management strategies and discipline that works for your child. "Behavior management" is a general term for techniques used to help children learn appropriate behavior. Some examples of behavior management include praising desired behavior, ignoring unacceptable behavior, and punishing inappropriate behavior. "Discipline" refers to the rules and standards for acceptable behavior that parents establish for their children. Discipline forms boundaries within which children learn to act and behave appropriately.

Sometimes, traditional behavior management strategies do not succeed with children with Tourette syndrome. Many parents of children with TS consistently follow the guidelines for good behavior management, yet their children still have persistent behavior problems. As the parent of a child with multiple motor and phonic tics, AD/HD, and OCD, I was perplexed for many years until I finally figured out why the usual methods didn't work. Most behavior management strategies suggested to parents don't address the problems that arise when a child does not have normal impulse control and may have very compulsive behavior as well. This realization made me start exploring ways to handle children with neuro-behavioral problems.

Another reason many traditional behavior management systems do not work well with many children with Tourette syndrome is that these systems are primarily "reactive." Parents respond or react to their child's actions by giving some kind of consequence that may or may not relate to the behavior they want to change. For example, two siblings might be playing a board game on the floor, when a third sibling runs into the room and slides into the game, scattering the game pieces all over the room. A reactive strategy might be to send the culprit to his room for a five-minute "time out." Professionals assure us that if these kinds of consequences are given repeatedly and consistently, behavior will change. But if the culprit in this instance has a compulsion to run in the house, a compulsion to slide into games, or often acts impulsively, a reactive strategy may never change his behavior.

If the typical *reactive* types of discipline are not right for your child, you may be more successful with a *proactive* approach. Rather than waiting for your child to do something wrong and then reacting, try setting up the environment to prevent undesirable behavior from occurring in the first place. In the example above, the siblings could be told to play their game on a table instead of on the floor. Meanwhile, their impulsive sibling could be redirected to an activity such as playing basketball outdoors that would not give him cause to run into the game board.

Over the years, I have found that such proactive strategies really work. For example, my son went through a period when he kept slamming the laundry chute door. At first, I tried reactive methods, punishing him every time he slammed the door by giving him "time outs." When that didn't stop the behavior, I tried taking away privileges, but that didn't work either. I finally decided that the behavior was very compulsive and resistant to change. Taking a proactive approach, I removed the laundry chute door for several months. By the time I replaced the chute door, my son's compulsion to slam it was gone.

Obviously, you cannot always change the environment to accommodate your child, but you may still be able to use a proactive approach. For example, for several weeks my son had a compulsion to throw chairs in his classroom. Two possible proactive approaches would have been to remove all the chairs from the room or to nail them to the floor, but that would have caused too much disruption for the other children. Instead, I used a less intrusive proactive approach and removed my son from the main classroom until he was able to control his compulsion. For a few weeks, he was educated in a smaller, less stimulating room where he was able to calm down and regain self-control more easily.

Aside from benefiting your child, a proactive approach can also help you. In deciding how and when to deal with your child's inappropriate behaviors, you will no longer need to ask yourself which behaviors are due to Tourette syndrome and which are not. Nor will you need to sort out which behaviors are caused by medications. As long as you use proactive strategies, you do not have to differentiate between causes of misbehavior. You simply try to prevent it before it occurs, regardless of cause. Instead of punishment, the emphasis is on setting up the environment for success, praising acceptable behavior, and redirecting unacceptable behavior.

Crucial to the proactive approach is cultivating the type of supportive environment described earlier in this chapter. If you can avoid stressful situations while providing structure, routine, and consistency, your child will have an easier time controlling his actions. It is especially important that discipline be clearly defined and consistent. If rules keep changing, your child will be confused. But if he knows what to expect, there will be fewer variables and unknowns, and he will feel less stress.

The sections that follow offer a number of proactive strategies for helping parents of children with TS manage challenging behavior.

Cues and Redirection

Redirection means changing your child's focus of attention when he has lost control of his behavior—or better yet, when you see that he's about to do something inappropriate. It can be accomplished by physically moving your child from one place or activity to another or by suggesting another activity for him to do.

For children with TS, redirection works best when used *before* they have begun to behave inappropriately. This makes it important for you to learn to recognize the *cues* or signs that your child is on the verge of losing control. Cues might include more frequent vocal or motor tics, an increase in hyperactivity, an angry facial expression, or uncontrolled giggling. Redirecting your child quickly and calmly will help him regain control before he loses it completely.

I often used redirection to help my son cool down when he was angry. For example, when he played team sports in grade school, my son frequently got angry if his performance was anything short of perfect. His anger usually started with yelling and accusing someone else of cheating.

Depending on the situation, I tried to redirect him, either by having him sit quietly for a while in a safe area, or by having him move over to the swings for a few minutes. If he remained angry, I wouldn't allow him to play the sport for the remainder of the afternoon and helped him select another activity, such as score keeping or playing a completely different game. Had I not redirected him at that point, his anger would have probably escalated to throwing equipment or rocks, or kicking something across the yard, without concern for anyone else's safety.

You might see signs of frustration while your child is trying to do his homework or work on a project. Encourage him to take a break, and suggest something he could do for a few minutes to calm down. For example, you could ask him to move the lawn sprinkler or taste the chili you are making. Be sure to praise your child for helping you afterwards. To help your child feel as if he is an active part of the plan, discuss with him, in advance, why he might need to be redirected and how you might redirect him.

Redirecting Obsessions and Compulsions

Learning to use redirection is especially important if your child has obsessive and compulsive symptoms. Children with OC symptoms might become frustrated if they are "obsessing" on something that it is too difficult for them to do. In these cases, it can be helpful to try to channel the obsession into something they can do more easily, but still feel satisfied. For example, if putting together model airplanes is too difficult for your child, suggest that he draw airplanes or do some library research on airplanes.

If your child has an Asperger-type "obsession" (i.e., all-encompassing interest), try to channel it into broader or more productive activities. For example, if your child is obsessed with horses, give him opportunities to play with toy horses, read about horses, draw horses, go to a farm and watch horses, and arrange for a horse ride.

Use compulsive behaviors to develop talents such as music, dance, or art. A child who is compulsive about practicing the piano, for example, might be encouraged to become an accomplished musician. There are several famous sports figures who have Tourette syndrome and acknowledge that their OC symptoms helped them achieve their success.

Redirection can make a significant difference between your child feeling out of control and feeling good about himself. Take the time to get to know your child's cues, and experiment with different types of redirection. Remember that redirection should only be used with relatively harmless OC behaviors. If your child's symptoms are socially unacceptable, self-injurious, or harmful to others, they should be dealt with by a neuropsychiatrist who specializes in working with OCD. As Chapter 3 explains, there are several medications that can often improve OC symptoms. Habit reversal training may be useful as well (see Chapter 4).

Time Outs

Another method of helping your child regain control is the "time out." To use "time out," you and your child agree upon a "safe place" where he can go when he is about to lose control or is already behaving inappropriately. Ideally, you can help your child learn to recognize his own cues that signify he is in danger of losing control of his behavior. He can then take responsibility for his own behavior and retreat to his "safe place" long enough to regain control. If he's already lost control, you may need to send (or take) him to his "safe place." If it's helpful, stay there with him, perhaps helping him to calm down by stroking his back or using soothing words. On the other hand, some children calm down faster if left alone—just be sure to stay within earshot.

"Time out" should be explained to your child as a positive way to calm down, rather than as a punishment for bad behavior. You may wish to re-label it "calm time" or "relax time" if your child already associates "time out" with punishment.

Handling Transitions

Children with TS+ may have trouble making transitions when they are physically or mentally involved in something else. That is, they may find it difficult to end one activity and move to another or start a new task. Parents are often frustrated at having to constantly nag at their children to get them to do something or go someplace.

If your child has trouble with transitions, it may be very helpful to provide visual reminders of what he needs to do and when it needs to be done. For younger children, charts with pictures work well. These can be done by hand or computer. For example, you might design a chart with pictures of each morning task: get dressed, eat breakfast, take pills, brush teeth, put on jacket. Then hang the chart in a visible location. As your child completes each task, he can check it off on the chart. Once your child knows his numbers, it is easy to use a digital clock for visual cues. Tell your child what time he should do specific tasks and, if necessary, write the time and task on a chart. Be sure to praise your child for each task completed.

Charts are particularly helpful when there is a change in routine. For example, when your child returns to school in the fall, it may be difficult for him to change from his leisurely summer schedule to a more organized, fast-paced, get-ready-for-school routine. Using a chart on which he can check off tasks as he completes them and/or visual cues such as pictures of a toothbrush and toothpaste may help him organize his morning more efficiently and get off to school with minimal fuss.

Older children can design their own lists of what they need to do, together with a time schedule that will help them get the tasks done within an appropriate amount of time. Using charts in this way can not only provide needed structure for your child, but also teach him to be responsible for himself. This self-reliance becomes extremely important when your child eventually moves out to live on his own.

At times, you may need to give verbal reminders about transitions. Allow enough time for your child to complete what he is doing or to put it aside in a way that is less stressful for him. For example, if you want your child to go shopping with you, you might tell him he must be ready to leave in thirty minutes. Ask him if he needs help getting ready or ending his activity. If he resists, let him know the consequence of not being ready in thirty minutes. In this scenario, you might tell him that for every additional minute you must wait for him, he will lose that amount of play time later. When fifteen minutes are up, remind your child again and tell him you will give him a reminder five minutes before you will leave. When the time is up, it's time to go. Insist that your child accompany you, even if—as my son does—he tells you that he "can't" stop what he's doing to go shopping. Understanding your child's special needs *is* important, but following through with consistent discipline will help your child learn his boundaries.

There are some tools that can help smooth transitions. Some parents use a timer that signals the stop time. One that many experts recommend is the "Time Timer" (available at www.timetimer.com), which uses a simple visual display to count down the remaining time. Older children may use alarms built into watches, cell phones, computers, or personal digital assistants (PDAs).

Modeling Appropriate Behavior

Children learn behavior from their parents, so, in essence, we are all teachers. If we want our children to behave in a certain way, then it is important for us to behave in the same way. For example, you cannot expect your children to be kind and cooperative with each other if you and your spouse constantly fight and criticize each other. If you use physical punishment such as spanking, then the chances are good that your child may hit others to try to get his way.

Because children with TS often have trouble controlling their impulses, it is especially important for parents to model non-violent behavior. You and your spouse should learn to discuss your differences using calm, non-threatening language, so that your child can hear and see how it is done every day. In addition, regularly praising family members and friends will encourage your child to be respectful of others.

Praising Your Child

Children with TS often hear so many negative comments about their symptoms and behavior that they start to believe that they are bad people. To counteract this misperception, catch your child being good and praise him whenever possible. Try to be specific when praising him; tell him exactly what it is that you like. If your child has cleaned up his room, you might say, "Marc, your room looks really nice. Cleaning your room shows that you care about your belongings. Also, it gives me more time to play with you." Be careful not to dilute your praise with subtle criticism. For example, if the way your child has made his bed isn't up to your adult standards, don't say, "That's a pretty good job even though the bedspread is crooked." Instead say, "I'm proud of you for making your bed without having to be reminded."

To encourage the least stressful sibling relationships, remember to praise all your children. Each needs to feel special and worthy. Praise your children for their kindness and cooperation, tasks completed or attempted, bravery in new situations, and other accomplishments. Sometimes I gave my children or their friends paper medallions with special inscriptions for doing something well. For example, I've made awards for "1st place room cleaner," "Best cooperative play for one hour," "1st place diver," or "Gold award for bravery for staying overnight at John's house."

Children like to hear that they are good. It makes them feel proud and accepted, and also makes it more likely they will repeat the behavior they have been praised for. You may want to keep a "Special Person" notebook in which you list the things your kids do well each day. This list can be reviewed with each child at night before bed. Likewise, your children can make "I'm Proud of Me" books and share their positive experiences and feelings with the family.

Reward Systems

Volumes have been written on using reward systems to shape children's behavior. But the basic principle behind reward systems can be stated quite simply: You can either reward your child for resisting something you don't want him to do, or you can reward him for doing something you do want him to do.

Before you try using a reward system, you must first decide which behavior you wish to reward, then decide how the system will ensure your child's success, and finally, pick a reward. Here is an example of how you might do this:

Let's say you want your child to stop teasing his sister. That means that you want to reward behaviors that *don't* involve teasing his sister. Don't expect him to immediately stop all teasing—that's an unrealistic goal. Instead, you need to reward incremental successes. You might have to start, for example, by giving your child a star for every thirty minutes that he does not tease. If he receives six stars in a day, then he may receive a sticker, balloon, or whatever reward you decide will inspire your child. (Ideas for rewards are endless, but some professionals advise against using money or food for rewards.) If your child easily earns six stars, you may want to gradually increase the number needed for a reward. If your child cannot earn six stars, you will need to back up as far as necessary for him to achieve success. As his behavior improves, you can increase the stakes for getting the reward, remembering to praise your child even if he has a more difficult day.

If your child is older, you might award him points that can be used to "purchase" something from your family store. The list of items available and number of points needed to buy them can be posted on the refrigerator. These rewards can be services that others will perform, such as Dad cleaning the child's room for one hour or Mom taking the child to a park to fly a kite. They may also be special privileges, such as being allowed to stay up one hour past bedtime or choosing a video to watch. My children often picked going to the car wash with me as a reward. Reward systems are only limited by your creativity and your child's desires.

While you are using a reward system, remember that it is only a temporary measure. Ultimately your child must perform the desired behavior without receiving any more reward than praise and self-satisfaction. Although some unacceptable behaviors may return when you discontinue your reward system, others will not. It is worth a try to experiment with reward systems to break the pattern of unacceptable behavior.

Handling Aggressiveness and Anger

If your child has trouble controlling aggressive behavior or he experiences prolonged anger and rages, safety can become a pressing problem. Seek professional help for your child immediately. Try to find a specialist who is knowledgeable about TS-associated behaviors (not just tics) and medications, and who does not blame your child for his behavior.

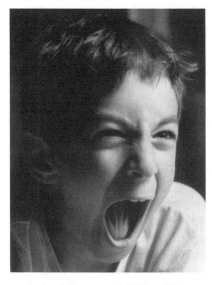

Your child's doctor will teach you specific ways to deal with his anger and frustration, but there are some general strategies that can help many children.

Prevent Behavior. Once again, it is easier to prevent an inappropriate behavior from occurring rather than react to it once it has begun. For example, if your child is aggressive with other children, limit the time he spends with friends. End the play period while your child is still in control. Let your child know that his play time with friends will increase as he shows you that he is able to play appropriately. Some professionals recommend that everyone in the family refrain from watching all television programs and movies that are violent and use abusive language, including most cartoon shows. They also recommend removing both real and toy guns and weapons from the home.

Teach Ways to Express Frustration. Because you cannot prevent all frustrating situations from occurring, teach your child a variety of ways to express himself and handle frustration. For example, you might set up a safe place for him to go to calm down. The area might have pillows, a mattress, stuffed animals, or other unbreakable objects. The area should be as free of visual and auditory distractions as possible. Let your child remain in his area for as long as necessary for him to feel that he is back in control.

Use Calming Techniques. Being held helps some children with Tourette syndrome regain control, but makes other children become more angry or aggressive. Some children want to be left alone, which is fine if you've provided a safe place to go. Other activities that may calm your child include having a back massage, swinging, rolling into blankets, crawling into a box, taking a shower, or soaking in a bathtub.

Redirect Anger. If you can, try to redirect your child's anger before he loses control. Have him draw a picture of his anger, write a couple sentences about appropriate behavior ("I will say kind things to my sister"), or say three nice things about the enemy ("Amy is good at drawing"). The first tries may end up crumpled and tossed, but eventually your child will settle down as his focus shifts from internal stress to external expression.

Whatever strategy you use, keep reassuring your child that he will calm down, and praise him when he does. Remember that using physical punishment to teach a child to use non-violent behavior does not work. Reversing aggressive behavior takes time, supervision, appropriate role models, and sometimes, professional help.

Teach to Make Amends. Once your child has regained control, allow him to make amends for his behavior. He may apologize, share a toy, color a picture, or do whatever makes him feel okay about himself again. Don't expect or demand immediate remorse. Although many children will do something to make amends quite naturally, others need to be taught how to do this. Your child may need to repeat the same mistake many times before he understands why it is wrong. But if you allow your child to learn from his behavior, ultimately he will learn to be responsible for his actions and their effect on other people.

Help Siblings Learn to Cope. Your other children also need to learn how to deal with their sibling's anger. Teach them to quietly move away from their brother or sister if they see he is losing control, and to notify you that this is happening. Going to another room or to a friend's house may provide them with safety and security until your child with Tourette syndrome has calmed down. If your child with TS is a threat to the safety of other family members, professional intervention is needed. Your child may need to be removed from your family until he is on medication that improves his symptoms or has learned to control his aggressive behavior. There are hospital and residential treatment programs that can help your child learn to cope with his symptoms in non-violent ways.

∷ Other Strategies for Daily Care

Building Self-Esteem

One of the most important goals of parenting is building self-esteem—feelings of self-worth and self-acceptance—in all of our children. High self-esteem is a vital component of good mental health. To a large extent, it determines how willing people are to set high

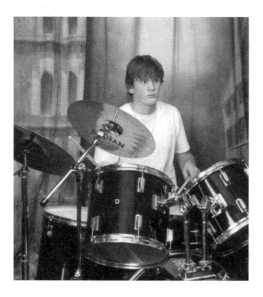

goals for themselves, as well as how hard they try to meet those goals. In fact, research shows that high self-esteem is more important to professional and personal success than high grades in school or a high I.Q.

Children with Tourette syndrome are often very intelligent and are quite aware of their inappropriate behaviors, tics, and noises. They are also very much aware of other people's reactions to them. As a result, they may feel different, unaccepted, and left out, and their self-esteem may suffer. Because you don't want to add to these feelings of "differentness," you should make sure that your daily care routine is aimed at building self-esteem and understanding.

Behavior Management and Self-Esteem

How you manage your child's behavior on a daily basis can have a major impact on your child's self-esteem. You must avoid making your child feel as if there is something wrong with him for not being able to control tics and other symptoms associated with his TS. By using the proactive, positive behavior management techniques described earlier, you can avoid punishing your child for behaviors that are out of his control. And as long as you use techniques that help him succeed in following through on family rules, his opinion of his own abilities will rise.

It also helps if you can let your child know that the purpose of discipline is not to punish him for unacceptable behavior but to help him learn to act appropriately and build self-control. In other words, be sure to convey the message that you want him to learn to make wise decisions about his behavior—and that you believe he is fully capable of doing so. This will help him understand that he is a loved and accepted part of the family, and will, in turn, boost his self-esteem.

Protection vs. Overprotection

It is natural for parents to want to protect their children with TS from negative reactions from people in the community and to rush to their defense when they are blamed for actions they cannot control. But sometimes it is better to let your child take care of himself rather than to intercede. Knowing where to draw the line between protection and overprotection is essential to building your child's self-esteem.

When your child is young, you will certainly want to protect him from harassment and inappropriate punishment for his symptoms. As he grows older, however, you must encourage your child to learn about TS, his own particular symptoms, and how to deal with other people. (See the section on "Handling Others' Reactions," on page 140.) As he becomes able to communicate about his disorder to others, you must allow him to make his own way in the community. Otherwise, if you try to shield your child from all undesirable situations he might encounter, you risk sending him the message that he can't make it on his own in the real world.

Recognize When Your Child Needs Help

Educators and parents often remark that some children with TS use their TS as an excuse not to do something that they are capable of doing. But if TS really does interfere with a child's abilities, it can be damaging to his self-esteem to be accused of not trying. If your child is having trouble doing something, it may be worthwhile to look for alternate ways to allow him to succeed. For example, a boy in third grade claimed he couldn't take spelling tests because he had TS. The teacher got angry at the boy, and blamed the parents for being overprotective of their son. In reality, the boy had great difficulty writing due to tics and sensory-motor problems. When the boy was allowed to dictate the answers to someone else, he was able to take spelling tests. The point is that the boy was correct in his initial statement, but he was not able to elaborate all the intricate details of his problem. Obviously, it is far better to make minor adaptations that allow your child to succeed than to let him wallow in feelings of failure.

Let Your Child Make Choices

Children with TS are always being reminded of what they cannot control—their tics and behaviors. Allowing your child to make choices for himself is a good way to focus instead on the control he has over many aspects of his life. Daily choices such as what to wear, what movie to attend, and what to buy for a birthday party should be encouraged. Asking your child's opinion on many topics from how to fix a broken appliance to what he thinks about current events can also help strengthen his sense of competency and control.

Focus on Your Child's Talents and Abilities

All children with TS have unique talents and abilities. One may excel in art, while another may be a computer whiz. It is vital to your child's self-esteem that you give him frequent and positive feedback about his areas of special talent and ability. This helps offset the feelings of failure he may have because of his symptoms and his inability to be like everybody else.

Mealtimes

Many children who have TS+ have trouble behaving at mealtimes as their parents would like them to. One reason is that children are often left to their own devices while Mom or Dad is busy in the kitchen. This may be fine for most kids, but some children with TS might start losing control while they are waiting for dinner if their time is too unstructured. Furthermore, if a child has hyperactivity, he will have trouble sitting still at meals. And if he has obsessions about certain foods, planning meals can be challenging. There may be no way to eliminate mealtime madness altogether, but a few tricks can make mealtimes more pleasant.

One technique that can help make mealtimes more manageable is to give all your children specific mealtime chores such as setting out napkins, plates, and glasses. You can remind your children who is responsible for doing each chore by listing the chores on a chart. You might also let your children prepare easy meals and serve them. If your child with Tourette syndrome is focused on his responsibilities, he is more likely to be in control of his behavior.

To avoid arguments and confusion about who will sit where during meals, have your children draw names for seat assignments or assign them on a rotating basis. Let your children know how long the assignments will last. Have them make place cards. If your child has an obsession about where he must sit, accept that this is not harming anyone, and, if possible, work around his need.

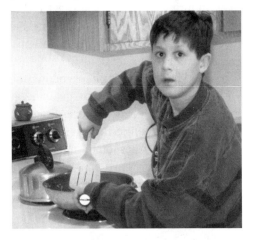

Wherever your child with Tourette syndrome is seated, don't expect him to sit for very long if he has AD/HD. Instead, establish basic rules of conduct during meals. For example, tell your children they may eat only when sitting down in their assigned places at the table, they must pass food instead of throwing it, and they must use utensils to eat. If your child feels he must move around during a meal, tell him specific things he may do, such as walking around the living room twice or standing by his chair, but don't allow him to eat unless he is sitting in his assigned spot.

Remember that the more structured and calmer the mealtime, the easier it will be for your child to stay in control. Some families find that if they defy the experts and watch TV during meals, their child has better control. This brings a little peace and sanity to their mealtimes. It does not, however, help the child learn to behave appropriately at meals served away from home. (For tips on eating out, refer to the section on "Restaurants" on page 141.)

Sometimes children with TS+ will only eat certain foods. This can be for a variety of reasons: some children have obsessions about particular foods; some kids with Asperger syndrome take comfort in the "sameness" of a consistent diet; some with sensory sensitivities intensely dislike certain food textures. Regardless of the reason, you should work with your child to develop nutritious menus. Often, if you provide the foods that he feels he *must* eat at each meal, he may eat other foods as well. And he may eat foods that are closely related to foods that he refuses to eat. For example, your child may not eat yellow vegetables, but he may eat green vegetables. In addition, your child may eat a greater variety of foods if they are served on a specific plate that he likes. Limiting between-meal snacks to fruits and vegetables may give your child the nutritional supplements that he isn't getting at mealtime. If you are unsure whether your child's nutritional needs are being met, enlist the help of a nutritionist.

In addition to having idiosyncratic food preferences, some children with Tourette syndrome also have allergies or sensitivities to certain foods, additives, or dyes. Experts disagree as to whether and to what extent allergies actually affect symptoms of Tourette syndrome. But some experts think allergies sometimes make symptoms worse. For example, some children may have an increase in tics, increased hyperactivity, persistent runny nose, skin irritations, or a general feeling of restlessness. Many people with TS say that their tics get worse if they consume caffeine. Others claim their symptoms increase after eating foods with certain dyes. Because of the waxing and waning of the disorder, it is often difficult to make determinations by observation alone.

Professional allergy testing by a pediatric allergist may be helpful if you suspect that your child is reacting adversely to certain foods or airborne substances. If your child is hyperactive, don't assume that sugar is the culprit and automatically switch to diet products. Artificial sweeteners may cause more problems for some children with Tourette syndrome than sugar does. In any case, if you are considering eliminating something from your child's diet, be sure to consult a nutritionist or your child's physician to see if a nutritional supplement is needed.

Finally, a word about special meals. Don't invite guests unless they are familiar with Tourette syndrome and associated behaviors. Adding another person to the table changes routine and adds stimulation. If guests are expected, let your child know ahead of time, review the family rules, discuss any changes in the normal meal routine, and remind him that he can go to another room if he feels he is losing control. Have holiday meals at noon, if possible. The longer everyone has to wait, the greater the anticipation and excitement. For a child with Tourette syndrome, that usually means more tics and other symptoms. If your child must wait, it may help to involve him in structured activities, such as making the table centerpiece, place cards, or window decorations. If your child is older, let him cut vegetables or prepare dessert.

Dressing and Clothes

Dressing can pose special problems for you and your child if he has Tourette syndrome Plus. Children who have difficulty with executive functions (the skills involved in planning, self-regulating, and completing tasks) often have trouble organizing themselves enough to select their own clothes and get dressed in a limited amount of time. Some with obsessive-compulsive or Asperger symptoms may become obsessed with wearing a specific item of clothing or a specific color of clothes. One way to ease these problems is to help your child set out his clothes before bedtime. It is usually easier to resolve the issue of what to wear at night rather than during the morning rush. This gives you time to wash your child's favorite shirt or mend the only pair of shorts that he will wear.

Your child may also have trouble accepting new clothes if he has OC, Asperger, or sensory processing symptoms. If so, try laying the clothes out in his room for several days before you ask him to put them on. Pre-wash the clothes so they feel softer and smell more familiar. Some kids are very sensitive to touch and need very soft fabrics. They are excellent recipients of "hand me down" clothes or consignment shop bargains. Remember to cut out all tags, and don't be surprised if your child can't stand the feel of synthetic fabrics, synthetic thread, wool, or lace. Sock seams are such a common complaint for children that some manufacturers now make seamless socks. (If you can't find them locally, there are numerous sources on the Internet.)

Some children with TS+ have difficulty making seasonal transitions in clothing. For example, as the weather grows cooler, your child may still insist on wearing summer clothes. One idea is to have him start the transition by wearing his summer clothes under warmer clothes. As he becomes accustomed to wearing the new seasonal clothes, he'll probably discontinue wearing the summer clothes underneath. When my son started first grade, he wore his bathing suit and a shirt to school for two weeks before he was able to change to shorts and jeans. His teacher said she never even noticed. We often have so many issues to deal with every day, it is important to play down those that are less significant.

Sleep

Most parents wish their children would sleep from 8 p.m. to 8 a.m. each day and wake up refreshed, clear-headed, and happy. When your child has Tourette syndrome, the reality is that this is very unlikely. To begin with, medications used to control tics or other symptoms may cause sleep problems. Some drugs make kids sleepy and others keep them aroused. Sleepiness may occur during the day, and arousal at night. In addition, some children get more hyperactive as they become fatigued. And children with OCD may have trouble getting to sleep until everything feels just right and all rituals have been performed. For example, a child might need to prepare for bed by doing certain things in a specific order. Toys may have to be lined up in a certain order, pillows may have to fluffed and re-fluffed, and sheets and blankets may have to be loosened or tightened.

You can't *make* your child fall asleep, but you can determine what time he must be in bed, ready for sleep. Most kids with TS are very active and need a good night's rest, and so do you, the parents! Besides, keeping to a consistent bedtime helps satisfies your child's need for routine.

Often a bath or a back massage before bed will help your child to relax. Be sure to tell him what he may do in bed and what he may not. Playing music softly or looking at books are usually calming activities. You may want to purchase a vibrating pad, carried by most discount stores, and let your child rest on it. (The vibration provides tactile stimulation which is relaxing for many children.) Jumping on the bed and shooting Nerf balls are examples of activities that should not be allowed. If you can ensure that your child's bedroom is quiet and remove distractions that are too stimulating, it will be easier for him to settle down.

To help your child get used to a calming bedtime routine and to get ready for bed independently, use a chart or reward board until the routine is well established. List each thing that your child should do to prepare for bed. For example:

Bedtime Routine
- Take a bath
- Brush teeth
- Put on pajamas
- Select clothes for tomorrow
- Read a story with Mom or Dad
- Listen to soft music
- Lights out

Give your child points that can be redeemed for rewards later when he completes each task on his chart. After your last hug and kiss, wish your child a good night and let him know that you'll be nearby, but it's now your private time.

If your child keeps leaving his room, redirect him back to his room and praise him when he settles down. Remember that many kids don't want to miss out on anything, and may challenge you for quite a while. Once you let your child know the rules and routine—and he realizes (probably through testing you) that you won't make exceptions—it will be easier for him to follow through.

Sometimes sleep problems may be caused by emotional stress. If you suspect this is the case, encourage your child to share his concerns and frustrations. A caring hug may ease his tension.

Finally, as mentioned above, sleep problems may be linked to your child's medication. Adjusting the dosage or time of ingestion may bring relief. Be sure to report significant sleep changes and difficulties to your child's physician, and don't make any adjustments in medication without his or her advice.

Aversion to Odors

Because many children with TS have sensory processing difficulties, some are very sensitive to certain odors. Smells that may be agreeable or only mildly offensive to you may be intolerable to your child. Listen to your child's complaints and eliminate the odors if possible. There are now many fragrance-free products that can make your life easier. When it is necessary to use something with an odor offensive to your child, try to use it when he is out of the house. For example, clean your oven when your child is at school and open windows and use a fan to remove the smell more quickly. If you plan to paint, it may be a good time for your child to visit Grandma. If you wear perfume or aftershave lotion, and the smell bothers your child, wait to put it on until you have left the house.

Some of these strategies may be a little inconvenient, but irritating your child's senses can increase stress and may cause an increase in symptoms. For example, one older child with TS told me that he gets a feeling of restlessness and general irritation when he is near someone wearing perfume.

Organization

Many children with TS+ have trouble with executive functions such as organizing their belongings and their time. Besides making it difficult for them to make transitions or get dressed in the morning, this lack of organizational skills can affect everything from how tidy your child keeps his room to how well prepared he arrives at school.

To help your child get organized and keep organized at home, try using masking tape or pictures to label where things are supposed to go. For example, label dresser drawers "underwear," "T-shirts," and "socks," and label shelves in his room or play area "books," "crayons," and "paper." If your child is supposed to help with kitchen chores such as putting away dishes or groceries, you could also label those shelves and cabinets. If there are certain activities you'd like to restrict to certain places in your house, it may help to mark off play areas on the floor. For example, use tape to mark off an area where building blocks are permissible. These visible boundaries and visual cues will usually help your child understand where things belong.

How you communicate with your child can also affect his ability to get organized. When you are giving directions to him, especially if he has AD/HD, make them simple and specific. For example, instead of saying, "Put your clothes away," you could say, "Put your socks in your sock drawer." When that task is completed, praise your child, and then say, "Put your underwear in the underwear drawer," and so on. Many children like to take care of their belongings and help with family chores, but are overwhelmed if the directions are too vague.

To help your child get organized for school, designate a specific place for him to assemble the things he needs to bring to school. You might make a checklist of items needed every day. Then make a note each day for additional things that your child must take. Whenever possible, have your child get his school things ready for the next day at night before he goes to bed. If he takes a lunch from home, make a menu for the week so the lunch can be ready to go without a fuss.

If homework is a problem, ask the school to provide an extra set of textbooks to be left at home. Work with your child to set a good time for homework. Some kids with Tourette syndrome need free time before homework to relax, let out tics, or run off energy. Others, particularly those with OCD, may feel a need to do homework right away. If you see that your child is overwhelmed with homework, work with him and the school to plan reasonable expectations. Chapter 8 provides more detail about how to make adjustments in your child's school program to accommodate his special needs.

Electronics

Video games, the Internet, MP3 players, cell phones, portable DVD players, and other electronics have become very popular forms of entertainment and recreation. Although they may have positive benefits, some children need very specific limits for their use.

Tics may subside while your child is playing a video game, but increase when the game is finished. Your child's mood may deteriorate after prolonged playing, as well. Some children with TS and OCD get "stuck" on video or computer games, isolating themselves from personal interactions with peers and family, and even becoming angry or aggressive if they can't advance in the game. Be sure to check the rating on any game your child plays—some games depict disturbing violence. Observe how your child behaves during and after a video game, and set appropriate time limits. Some kids with TS can handle a reasonable amount of game time daily or on weekends. Others might be better off without a video game system in the home.

The Internet can provide a wealth of useful information, and it's playing an increasingly large role in all our lives. Many children learn to type while sending emails or instant messages (IMs) to their friends. Many kids today—even in elementary school—need Internet access to complete their homework assignments. However, children and teens need to be protected when they're online, to prevent them from viewing inappropriate websites or "chatting" with strangers. Parental control software offers some protection, and some programs even allow you to set time limits to prevent compulsive use. These programs are far from perfect, however. Perfectly innocuous websites may get "blocked" (which can cause a lot of upset and frustration for the child), while some shocking sites manage to slip through. Many children learn to bypass parental control programs, as well.

Bottom line: you need to supervise your child's Internet use personally. Rather than letting him have Internet access in his room, limit it to a computer in the family room or den, where you can be nearby.

Cell phones are great for keeping in touch with your children. But children can also misuse cell phones by running up huge bills, cheating on tests by text messaging answers, inappropriate video-taping, etc. Now videos, games, and music can all be downloaded onto cell phones—for a fee. If you choose to provide your child with a cell phone, set rules on how it's to be used, and what the consequences will be if your child misuses it. You may want to consider a phone designed specifically for preteens, which only allows the child to call numbers that you've approved in advance

The world of electronics is advancing quickly. Keep up with what products are available to your child. Learn how they may affect his symptoms. And, most importantly, supervise when, where, and how they're used.

▪▪ Your Child in the Community

When you and your child are out in the community, you often confront problems that you don't need to deal with at home. Unlike at home, you cannot always set up the environment to make it easier for your child to control his symptoms. And particularly if your child has AD/HD, sensory sensitivities, or Asperger's syndrome, the stimulation from

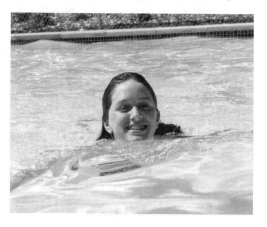

unfamiliar people and places may send him into a frenzy. At times, you and your child may feel as if everyone is staring at you—and you may be right.

Difficult as it can sometimes be to brave an outing into the community, it is important not to let Tourette syndrome take over the lives and activities of everyone in the family. Your child with TS needs to feel like an important, accepted part of the outside world, and so do your other children. All of your children need to learn how to get along as independently as possible in the community.

How your child adapts to life outside the home depends largely on you, the parent. If you appear to be at ease with your child in public, he is more likely to feel comfortable as well. By following your lead, he will learn to handle stares, comments, and potentially awkward situations. Friends and strangers will also take their cue from the respectful way you treat your child. Some strategies that may be useful in integrating your child into the community follow.

Educating Others

Many problems children with TS encounter in the community arise from others' ignorance about Tourette syndrome. Other children may tease or make fun of your child, while adults may scold him for misbehaving, because they don't realize he can't control his tics and other symptoms. Consequently, as your child's community gets larger, it becomes important to educate people about TS so they will understand your child's symptoms and behaviors.

Although the media often sensationalizes TS by focusing on coprolalia, public awareness of TS has dramatically increased over the last twenty years. It's up to you to educate and provide accurate information to the people who come in contact with your child. In the process of trying to answer other people's questions about TS, you will find yourself learning more about the disorder, your child's particular symptoms, and how best to deal with them.

Although you can wait for people to ask you questions, it is often preferable to educate others before your child gets into new situations. Again, this really depends on the severity of your child's symptoms and how they affect others in the community. Because my son's symptoms were so obvious during his school years, we held "inservice" sessions for all of his school classmates, teachers, friends, neighbors, relatives, and teammates. My son wanted others to know about his disorder, so that he didn't have to constantly answer questions about his tics and behaviors. On the other hand, some children don't want anyone to know about their TS. It is up to you to determine if it is in your child's best interests to tell people. Now that he is an adult, my son's symptoms are less obvious, and he picks and chooses when and with whom he discusses his TS.

If you decide to "inservice" and educate, the national Tourette Syndrome Association has many prepared pamphlets and videos about TS that you can purchase as well as materials for educators. (See the Resource Guide for the address of the national TSA.) Check with your local chapter to see if it has materials available for loan or purchase. You may even find a local group that will send an expert to your child's school to do a presentation. If you ask, your local newspaper may run an article on TS. Your local radio and cable TV stations may help you produce a talk show on TS. Educating the public about such a complex disorder is not easy, but it is necessary to ensure more understanding and acceptance of Tourette syndrome.

Handling Others' Reactions

Many parents feel anxious about doing things in public with their children because they worry about how others will react to their children's TS symptoms. Although you cannot predict how strangers will respond, you can rehearse a variety of strategies that can help you and your child through awkward or potentially embarrassing situations.

In general, there are three ways you and your child can deal with strangers' questions and comments:

1. Ignore the comment.
2. Acknowledge the tic without explaining the cause. For example: "I have a tic that makes me jerk my head; I don't do it on purpose."
3. Educate the person about Tourette syndrome. Your child could say, for example, "I have Tourette syndrome and licking my lips is a tic I can't control." Some people carry informational brochures about TS (available from the Tourette Syndrome Association) or hand out cards that they have had printed with a brief explanation of TS and a phone number to call to get more information.

It may help to "role play" different scenarios with your child. Act out many possible remarks people could make about your child's tics, and let your child practice different positive responses rather than reacting in a negative or aggressive way. For example, if your child gets a very red, chapped face from a rubbing tic, you might mimic, "Hey kid, did you fall into a vat of tomato sauce?" First, your child could try ignoring your comment. He could then try offering a general, neutral explanation such as "My face is chapped." Finally, he could attempt to explain a little bit about Tourette syndrome: "I have Tourette syndrome. Rubbing my face is a tic. It makes my face chapped."

Sometimes children with TS unintentionally insult or upset a stranger with inappropriate touching, name calling, or other behaviors. In these instances, it is often best to tell that person that your child has Tourette syndrome and give a very brief explanation of the disorder. Although your child should not have to apologize for having an impairment, most people will expect an apology. You and your child should discuss this possibility and do what is comfortable for you.

Planning Ahead

There are some places you can go where your child's symptoms will be more noticeable and disruptive than others. For example, your child's tics may go unnoticed at a baseball game, but attract quite a bit of attention at a library. This does not mean that you should avoid all potentially troublesome settings, but that you should minimize stressful situations by a little advance planning. Some strategies for handling specific situations are outlined below.

Movies and Concerts

In any kind of quiet social gathering, it is usually best to prearrange a place where your child can go if his symptoms become disruptive. For example, at movies or concerts, your child can go to the lobby or into the restroom if he feels he is losing control. Taking seats on the aisle, toward the back, is usually a good idea.

Use your best judgment when deciding on concerts and movies. If your child has AD/HD, he will be more likely to sit still if the movie holds his interest. Disruptive symptoms will probably not be noticed at a rock concert, but may cause problems at a symphony. Outdoor concerts are less stressful and less likely to exacerbate symptoms.

Rather than chance an embarrassing situation, some people with disruptive tics prefer to watch videotapes or listen to music at home with a few friends. Although you and your family understand coprolalia, most people do not, and a movie theater or concert hall is not always a good place to start educating them.

Restaurants

Eating out can be especially stressful if your child gets overstimulated or is hyperactive. You may be able to prevent some potential problems if you reduce waiting time by ordering ahead, picking a buffet or fast food restaurant, or selecting a restaurant with a video arcade or other form of kids' entertainment. It may also help if you bring crayons and paper or a puzzle book to use during the wait for service. Seat your child next to and across from people who will help him stay in control, rather than near a child who may over-stimulate him. Be sure to review the rules of eating out before you go and when you arrive at the restaurant. Again, many children with TS need to know very clearly what they can and cannot do in a given situation.

If your child starts to lose control, take him outside or into a quiet area for a few minutes, so he can settle down. If all else fails, be prepared to leave. On the rare occasions when our family went to a restaurant that was difficult for our son, my husband and I usually drove in separate cars. If our son had to leave, he went with one parent while the other remained at the restaurant with our daughter. Although it is hard not to blame your child for this inconvenience, you have to remember that over-stimulation makes the symptoms worse, your child is not deliberately trying to drive you crazy, and he usually feels worse than anyone else. Your child needs encouragement, not reproach.

Shopping

Tics and vocalizations often get worse at a shopping mall. Children with TS+ often become over-stimulated or find some obsession that will cause them to run ahead, bounce around the floor tiles, or hide in the clothes carousels. To minimize these problems, take your child shopping only when necessary and only when the stores are the least crowded. Be sure to call ahead to see if the desired items are in stock. If you haven't already, you might also want to look into catalog or online shopping.

If your child "needs" everything in sight, this can pose problems in grocery stores, drug stores, self-service shoe stores, and other types of establishments with a vast array of products to choose from. These large stores are also over-stimulating for many kids. Where you see aisles, they see racetracks—just inviting them to run! To reduce problems, tell your child ahead of time where you will shop and exactly what you intend to purchase. If your child will be picking out something to buy, try to decide on the exact item or reduce the possibilities to only a few before you leave home. Save your browsing for a shopping trip by yourself. When shoe shopping, try to find a store where shoes are kept in the back room and your child must sit in a chair to be waited on. Be sure to praise your child for what he does well, such as staying with you or calmly selecting his shoes, and tell him how much you enjoyed the shopping trip with him.

Libraries

You may feel especially reluctant to enter a library with your child. But all the public librarians with whom I've spoken insist that everyone is welcome in a library. They encourage anyone with any disability to use the facilities. Furthermore, they point out that public libraries are not really as quiet as many people think, because kids are often using computers and doing group projects. Still, if you or your child feel too conspicuous, librarians are usually willing to make accommodations. For example, they might allow your child to use a conference room if he feels he is bothering other people. You might also plan to visit the library during the hours when it is less crowded.

:: Changes in the Teen Years

The teen years for any child bring many changes to the family. When you have a child with Tourette syndrome, these changes can be especially dramatic. Depending upon the course of your child's symptoms, daily life for your family may become either more or less difficult.

In many children with Tourette syndrome, tics and AD/HD symptoms begin to decrease during adolescence. Children may become less hyperactive, and their ability to focus and stay on task improves.

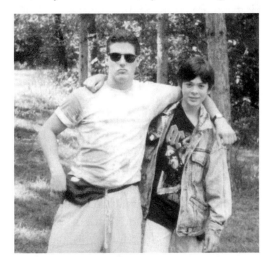

Many teenagers develop a much better capacity to understand Tourette syndrome and advocate for their own needs. These kids can also become positive role models for younger children with Tourette syndrome.

Other children, unfortunately, have increased symptoms in the teen years. It is important to understand that these changes can make your child feel different and lonely. Listen to your child and encourage him to talk about his feelings. If you can find a support group for teens with Tourette syndrome, your child may find it very helpful. You might contact your local chapter of the TSA to see if such a group exists in your area, or if they could help you set one up.

Because of changes in body hormones, your teen's medications may need to be adjusted or changed. Medication checks should be scheduled at regular intervals with your child's physician. Be sure to tell your physician about changes in your teen's emotions, sleep patterns, attitude toward school, family, and peers, in addition to reporting tics and other symptoms. Any of these can indicate that a change in medication is needed. School refusal and depression are not uncommon in teens with TS and should be treated by a professional. Sometimes a medication change or psychological or psychiatric counseling is needed. Chapter 3 provides more information on medications used to treat TS.

During the teen years, you should also alert your child to the hazards of recreational drugs. Because Tourette syndrome is a disorder involving brain chemicals, some street drugs can be more dangerous for people with Tourette syndrome. Since there are still so many unknowns about how drugs affect the brain, tell your child to say "no" to all street drugs. Remember, too, that substances such as caffeine and alcohol can also have undesirable effects on your child's symptoms, and their use should be discussed with your child's physician.

On the flip side, your teenager may read articles or online information about nicotine and/or marijuana (THC) being used to reduce TS symptoms (see Chapter 3). Some teens may even be tempted to "self-medicate." Educate yourself on this issue, and be prepared to discuss it with your child. You may want to be proactive and bring it up yourself. Definitely ask your teen's physician to discuss with him the pros and cons of these alternative therapies.

If your child has coprolalia or symptoms that could be misconstrued as intoxication, make sure he carries cards that give a brief explanation of Tourette syndrome and the phone number of your child's physician, the local Tourette syndrome organization, or the national Tourette Syndrome Association. You can also purchase a Medic Alert bracelet and have information about your child's disorder engraved on the tag. These cards and tags can come in handy if your child is ever stopped by a law enforcement official and has symptoms such as uncontrolled swearing, walking in unusual step patterns, punching, kicking, spinning around in circles, or falling to the ground.

You can ease some of the changes in the early teen years if you prepare your child for his progression from elementary to secondary school. Have him help you educate his new teachers about Tourette syndrome and his particular symptoms. If your child has difficulty organizing his time and belongings, the homework requirements—especially long-term projects—can become quite daunting in middle school and beyond. Continue to emphasize the good homework routines you started him on in grade school, and if he seems to be struggling (in school or at home), work with him and the school to make whatever adjustments are necessary. (See Chapter 8 for more information on schools and education.)

Most teenagers want to drive a car, and this usually causes anxiety for parents. How and when to approach this with your child with TS takes even more planning and decision-making. We included a driving assessment with our son's "transition programming" in high school. The assessment (which included tests for distractibility, coordination, reaction time, and impulsivity) was performed by specially trained professionals at Minneapolis' Courage Center (a not-for-profit resource center for people with disabilities). Courage Center also provided the driver's training program. If that type of program is not available where you live, it is very important to evaluate your child's readiness for driving as well as the cost factors. My son mastered all of the technical skills of driving long before he mastered the responsibilities that accompany operating a vehicle. It's vitally important that you don't let your child behind the wheel until he's mastered *both!*

One final issue that is extremely important to teenagers is friendships and dating. As your child's interest in the opposite sex increases, he may find that the interest isn't always returned. Many teenagers simply do not want to associate with anyone who seems different. Educating peers about Tourette syndrome may help, but for many, the need to conform outweighs compassion and sensibility. Reassure your child that as he gets older, he will meet many people of both sexes who are more understanding and accepting of people with disabilities. Acknowledge what Adam Seligman, a young man with Tourette syndrome, observed in an article written shortly after his graduation: "High school is not a place noted for the maturity of its inhabitants." In the meantime, encourage your child to pursue activities that interest him in school and in the community. People who share similar interests and talents may be more able to see beyond the symptoms of Tourette syndrome. Lastly, be prepared to accept friends that may seem "weird" to you at first. Kids who don't quite "fit in" often find each other, and very special friendships can develop.

∷ Transitioning to Adulthood

One of the primary goals of parenting is to prepare your child for adulthood. You want your child to eventually be able to live independently, find a suitable career, pay his bills on time, and take care of his physical, emotional, and spiritual needs.

Throughout his school years, your child can be acquiring various skills that will ease this transition to responsible adulthood. By the time he's in high school, your child should be starting to self-advocate. That means he needs to:

- learn about Tourette syndrome and be able to explain it to others,
- take an interest and an active role in his own medical care,
- understand his own strengths and challenges, and
- be able to identify and ask for what he needs.

If your child is on an IEP (Individualized Education Program) at school, the IEP team (including you *and your child*) should work together to set "transition" goals for after high school, and make a plan for how your child will achieve those goals. Depending on the child, goals could include post-secondary education, vocational training, employment, leisure and recreational activities, transportation, housing, and community involvement. You may want to invite individuals from your county social services, housing, or vocational rehabilitation programs to join the IEP team.

If your child plans to attend college, keep in mind that IEPs aren't used in college. However, if he had an IEP or 504 Plan in high school, he may be entitled to accommodations such as a modified means of getting notes, extended time for assignments, a separate space for testing, priority registration for classes, etc. These accommodations aren't automatic though—even if he did receive them in high school. Your child will need to find out what disability services are available at his chosen college and what is required to access the services—preferably before he hits the campus. If his accommodation needs are extensive, this should be taken into consideration when he chooses a college, since the available accommodations—and, in some cases, services—can vary tremendously among universities.

The transition years, leading up to and following high school graduation, is a period when your child can truly grow and blossom, if everyone works together to reach realistic, gratifying goals. For you, it is also a time to gradually step back and allow your child to take the reins. Easy? No. But necessary, and ultimately rewarding, when you see your adult child functioning as a happy, responsible member of the community.

▪▪ Taking a Break from Child Care

When you have a child with Tourette syndrome, spending quality time alone with your spouse or friends is very important. Parents have a tendency to get so involved in the welfare of their children, they forget about nurturing themselves. B.C. (before children), most parents had many interests and hobbies. Take time to pursue those activities and share your talents with others. Eat properly, get enough sleep and exercise, keep yourself healthy, and try to find something to laugh about every day. Keep your own stress level down. Treat yourself to a massage, a concert, or a movie. Don't feel guilty about taking time for yourself. You deserve it!

Finding competent sitters who are comfortable with your child can be a challenge, but don't give up. In some cases, simply explaining your child's symptoms to a mature teenager is sufficient. But if your child's behaviors pose too big a challenge, there are many other avenues. Students in special education, occupational therapy, or nursing programs at nearby colleges, as well as vocational school students, often make excellent sitters. Disability organizations in your area may also be able to recommend competent sitters with experience caring for children with special needs. And don't overlook other parents of children with Tourette syndrome as a source of names. You may even be able to trade off watching each others' children occasionally.

Some families of children with Tourette syndrome need more than an occasional evening away from their child. These families can often benefit from *respite care*. Respite care gives parents a respite, or break, from caring for their child. In the most common form of respite care, your child goes to the home of a qualified caregiver on a regular basis, usually for a weekend, but sometimes for longer or shorter periods. You may also be able to request respite care on an emergency basis, with little or no advance notice. Don't be surprised if your child behaves differently at the respite home. A change in environment can reduce behavioral difficulties on a short-term basis or increase them.

"In home" respite care or personal care attendant services are other options. If you qualify, a trained person comes into your home on a pre-set schedule to relieve you or to help you with child care.

To find out about respite care or personal care attendant services in your area, contact your county social service agency or local TSA chapter. Eligibility criteria vary, but in many counties you must qualify by showing a need for the service. Fees are usually on a sliding scale and based on family income. Some private social service agencies, such as those run by churches, may also have respite care programs.

Don't be afraid to ask for help. The daily stress of living with a child with Tourette syndrome can sometimes be overwhelming, even for the best of parents. In addition to out-of-home respite care arranged through our county, I got help from a wonderful woman who answered an ad that I ran in our local newspaper. For two years, she came to our home before school and helped restore order and sanity to our lives. During puberty, when my son's symptoms and behaviors intensified, we arranged for personal care attendant (PCA) services through our county. The PCAs came daily for a few hours to help supervise his play and daily activities. The PCAs were primarily young men who were great role models and physically up to the challenge of keeping up with a very active boy. Whether it is a friend, relative, respite worker, or PCA, you, too, may find that an experienced helper can make your daily life more enjoyable.

:: Conclusion

Several years ago, a newspaper reporter came to our house to write a story about my son. She had heard about his TS, AD/HD, OCD, and sensory motor problems. I don't know what she expected to see, but she said she was pleasantly surprised to meet a boy who was bright, creative, full of zest for life, and blessed with a great sense of humor. It was a wonderful reminder that our children with Tourette syndrome are kids like all other kids—they have special gifts and talents, and they must be nurtured and loved and given all the opportunities that life has to offer.

It is true that you must make special accommodations for your child with TS, and daily life may seem more complex. But by trying the strategies presented in this chapter as well as others that you discover, daily life certainly can be manageable, not to mention enjoyable. Take pride in yourself and your parenting skills. You're doing great if you can even find the time to read this book.

:: Parent Statements

The baby books can really throw you off. So can books on such things as the strong-willed child or on how to discipline. Usually these books do not acknowledge that other things such as neurological problems may be influencing behavior.

❧❀❧

When my daughter was younger I was so worried about how severe her symptoms would get. We tried our best to be good parents. I read the books available on behavior management. Now she is a young adult and I am so proud of how she turned out. Her tics are not noticeable to anyone but her now.

❧❀❧

One of my favorite people is the mother of a boy who was harassing my daughter in middle school. After the school had handed down its discipline, the mother said it wasn't enough. She had her son apologize to my daughter and wanted to hear from my daughter that it had happened.

❧❀❧

It takes so much involvement to stay on top of planning things for my son that I'm often "drained" in my free time.

❧❀❧

At a ball game, I take Tyler for a walk or to get refreshments a lot. He counts all the bathroom stalls and blow dryers in the men's and women's restrooms and compares the number of each.

❧❀❧

Punishment and time out don't work for Zach. He doesn't understand them, because he didn't get out of control on purpose. It's as if his computer is overloaded with stimuli. If we allow the computer to become overloaded, we know what will happen. Proactive behavior management techniques are so much more successful.

❧❀❧

Once when he was thrashing around on the kitchen floor, I held him— so he thrashed me around with him! But I told him I was there and wouldn't leave him, and that I loved him and he was a good little boy. That was what he needed then, and I had to stay with him for nearly an hour. It made me more determined than ever not to ever let him down, but to support and reassure him and "be there."

❧✿❧

The hyperactivity and compulsive behaviors are draining. But it helps when you understand why your kid is acting that way.

❧✿❧

Michelle's self-esteem greatly improved at TS Camp. She was impressed with the cool teenagers with TS. The acceptance she received there gave her quite a boost.

❧✿❧

There's no getting around the extra amount of energy needed to parent a child with TS, especially if he has complications such as LD or OCD.

❧✿❧

He's got the impulsiveness, the obsessive thinking, the anger from having been treated unkindly. I worry about how he will end up. I hope my best efforts will be enough to make things come out all right in the end.

❧✿❧

Every once in a while I feel like I should give him a damn good spanking and everything will be OK. But it doesn't work that way. We have to accept that we have a child with a disability, and we have to work with that.

❧✿❧

For my child with TS, Asperger's, OCD, AD/HD, and sensory issues, the childhood years were the hardest. After adolescence things calmed down and he is doing so much better.

❧✿❧

The single most important thing you can do for your child with TS is to build up his self-esteem.

❧✿❧

Remember the ABCs of Tourette syndrome. A: Accept the fact that your child has TS. Accept the tics and noises, the impulsivity, the immaturity. Your child may have little control over his symptoms, but you can have control over your reactions to them. B: Build your child's self-esteem. C: Choose your fights. Ignore the ignorable. Figure out ways to cope or get around the really disruptive tics and behaviors. Concentrate on those which are a danger to your child or others and ignore the rest.

❧❀❧

Tourette syndrome is an explanation for unacceptable behavior, not an excuse. Kids with TS have to have consequences for their behavior, but the consequences must be appropriate to the amount of control the child is able to exert over his symptoms and behavior.

❧❀❧

My son doesn't like to talk about TS. He doesn't think he'd have any friends if they knew.

❧❀❧

When asked whether his tics bother him, Nathan says that if he had his druthers, he'd like them to go away, but that generally, he's not too troubled by them. **We** are bothered by the tics, but are grateful for our son's attitude.

❧❀❧

Remember the 5 R's of Tourette syndrome. 1) Reduce stress—provide structure, no surprises, no timed tests. 2) Realistic expectations—when tics are at their worst, don't expect behavior or school performance to be on the same level as when tics are mild. 3) Reinforce good behavior—there's no such thing as too much praise or affirmation. 4) Redirect unacceptable behavior. 5) Remove your child from the scene—as a last resort, but without anger or blame.

❧❀❧

Punishment makes the person who punishes feel better. Discipline helps the person who committed a mistake realize what he did wrong and learn from his mistakes. Discipline involves teaching. Punishment is easier, but it usually doesn't do any good.

❧❀❧

In order to think proactively, you have to put away conformity and use common sense and creativity. Parenting then becomes more exciting and rewarding.

❧❀❧

Show your child by your own "self-praise" that it's OK to say to others that you did a good job. It's even OK to say that you're totally awesome!

6

CHILDREN WITH TOURETTE SYNDROME AND THEIR FAMILIES

Carl R. Hansen, Jr., M.D.

▓ Introduction

Parents often have no idea what they're getting themselves into when they decide to start a family. They may be caught off guard by the many responsibilities that parenting brings, as well as by changes in their routines and priorities. But although raising a family may be challenging at times, most parents feel that the rewards far outweigh the demands. In fact, most parents find that providing a safe and harmonious family life for their children is one of the most rewarding experiences of life.

Family life for parents of children with Tourette syndrome is not always more challenging than it is for other parents. Especially if your child has very mild symptoms of TS, you and your family may not run into any special problems. But for many parents, having a child with TS complicates the already complex job of raising a healthy, happy family. Stresses and strains within the family are different, if not greater, than they are for other families. Relationships can become strained, for example, if tics such as spitting or obscene gestures are directed at other family members, or if family members continually have to explain TS symptoms to people outside the family. And both parents and children may need to develop special coping strategies in order to live peaceably and productively with one another.

How well your family adjusts to having a child with Tourette syndrome depends primarily on you, the parent. Children, other family members, and friends will all follow your example. Indeed, how you treat all of your children will send them important messages about their own place in the family and in society.

Because the parent's role in family life is so crucial, this chapter begins with a discussion of some common problems that can make it harder for you to give your family the guidance it needs. It then reviews problems that other members of the family may encounter, and suggests ways you can help family life run more smoothly.

❚❚ Feeling Good about Yourself as a Parent

Having a child with TS does not change your ability to be a good parent, but it may change how you look at your ability. Because of the many ways TS and associated difficulties such as AD/HD and OCD affect

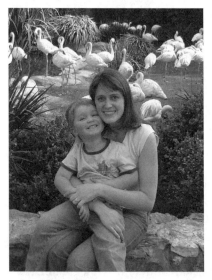

your child and your relationship with her, your self-confidence may plummet—even if you have successfully raised other children. You may, for example, feel as if it's your fault that your child's social skills lag behind other children's. You may blame yourself if your child cannot follow rules when playing a game with other children her age, or if other children in the neighborhood don't want to play with her. Then, too, repeated frustration at not being able to get your child to "behave" can make you feel like a failure. Even though *you* understand that your child's tics and other behaviors are out of her control, you may blame yourself in front of friends, family members, or teachers.

If feelings of failure persist too long, parents sometimes take it out on their child through inappropriate discipline and criticism. Or they may turn away from their child, immersing themselves in their work, outside activities, or even alcohol or drugs to escape the pain. At a minimum, they are likely to feel depressed and wonder why they should keep trying so hard.

Obviously, learning to cope effectively with the special challenges that confront your family is crucial. For this reason, the next section offers suggestions to help you recognize and begin to work around some problem areas you may encounter.

Altered Expectations

Parents tend to judge their success as parents by the success of their children. But when your child has Tourette syndrome, her accomplishments may seem to lag behind other children's. In the neighborhood, tics and associated conditions may lead to problems making friends and to delayed social development. In the classroom, tics, learning disabilities, or attention problems may make it harder for your child to make progress in some academic subjects. Your child stands out—but not for the reasons you would have hoped.

All parents must learn to reconcile reality with fantasy—to see that in place of the idealized, perfect child they dreamed of, they have a flesh-and-blood child with a unique set of strengths and weaknesses. For parents of children with TS, it's especially important to acknowledge your disappointment and frustration. You cannot accept your child's weaknesses and vulnerabilities unless you work through your feelings about them and acknowledge that the problems are part of your child's underlying condition. Denial of your feelings makes it harder to move ahead and cope with these problems. At the same time, you don't want to dwell too much on what your child *can't* do. Focusing only on your child's weaknesses and failures can lead to overwhelming disappointment and hopelessness. It can also prevent you from recognizing and appreciating your child's many successes—and there usually are far more things that children with TS *can* do than *can't* do.

Indeed, the key to dealing with your feelings about your child's failures is to work together on achieving success. Chapter 5 discusses why success is so important to your child's self-esteem. But helping your child achieve and celebrate successes can also give your self-esteem a boost. Consequently, when you help to reduce the stress that increases your child's symptoms, or steer her toward activities in which she is more likely to succeed, you are helping yourself while helping your child. For example, your child may find the beginning of school especially stressful. But if you anticipate the problems she typically has on the first day of school, you can take steps to minimize them—perhaps by taking her to visit her new classroom and teacher before school starts, so she'll be more comfortable with the new surroundings. Likewise, if your child wants to play sports but has a hard time taking turns, you might guide her toward individual sports such as swimming or running. The less frustration and failure your child experiences, the more successful everyone in the family will feel.

Most parents don't have to make a conscious choice about many decisions that will encourage their children to succeed. These values are passed from one generation to the next. But when you have a child with special needs, you have to make many conscious choices about the various details of daily life. Having to plan out so many details in advance can complicate your life in the short run, but in the long run, choosing to work with your child to help her succeed is one that you are not likely to regret. Consult Chapter 5 for specific strategies for building success into your child's daily life.

Concerns about Appearances

To outsiders, children with TS often look as if they are "misbehaving." For example, children with TS may have tics that cause them to spit or to make faces that others feel are rude or obscene. Or if they have OCD or impulsiveness associated with AD/HD, they may be unable to control the urge to touch things in a store. Although you may understand that your child cannot control his behavior, you may still feel inept as a parent when you see other children doing exactly as their parents say. Unsolicited comments and advice from others about what you are doing "wrong" and how you can "correct" the tics can further undermine your confidence in your parenting abilities.

As Chapter 5 discusses, there are many strategies you can try to help your child behave appropriately. But there also may be many behaviors your child simply cannot control. Once you are confident that you are managing your child's behavior properly, it may be necessary to ignore criticism in the confident knowledge that you are doing what is best for your family. Your family just may have to look different than the average family on the block. For example, you know that asking your child to suppress tics is asking for trouble. Even if she is able to hold the tics in for a time, the effort of doing so can dangerously increase stress and make it harder to concentrate on what is important. OCD behaviors, too, often cannot be controlled or resisted even with considerable effort. Consequently, your family may need to ignore swearing that other families would punish, or ignore compulsive behaviors such as poking

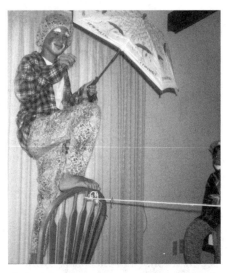

others, stomping, or opening and closing doors. Or you may need to do things in a way that looks a little odd to others. For example, if your child constantly pokes her brother when riding in the car, it may work better for a parent to sit in the backseat with the child having difficulty.

Your child's well-being must take precedence over your own concerns about appearances. In the end, what matters is not what onlookers think about your abilities as a parent, but the knowledge that you are doing what is right for your child.

Looking After Your Own Needs

Because of your child's TS, you may devote more time and energy to caring for her than you would have otherwise. For example, if your child has trouble making friends, you may spend a great deal of time arranging play opportunities or playing together with her yourself. Or if there is a danger to your child or others because of symptoms of impulsiveness or aggressiveness, you may need to provide additional guidance and supervision. If tics or other symptoms interfere with learning, you may also have to make numerous trips to school to help plan the educational program. And if your child has separation anxiety or cannot tolerate any change in routine, you may be a virtual hostage to your child's needs; even leaving her with a babysitter for just a few hours may seem out of the question.

Such demands have a way of sidetracking parents' personal goals. You may, for example, find yourself weighing career advancement and opportunities against your child's needs. You may even change or lose jobs because you feel you must be free to respond to crises at home or at school whenever they occur. You might also have to put plans for further education on hold, or say good-bye to parts of your social life.

Although there are many reasons why you might find your role limited to being the parent of a child with TS, this is not a healthy situation. If you feel as if your child is consuming all your time and energy, you may turn your anger, resentment, and frustration on your child—or on your spouse, if you feel you're getting stuck with more than your share of the childcare. Frustration with your child can get in the way of acceptance; frustration with other family members can lead to disharmony in the family and make it harder for everyone to support one another and work together as a team.

A social worker may be able to help you work out a compromise between your child's needs for care and supervision and your own needs for fulfillment. You should be able to locate a social worker through your county Human Services department, or through the special education program at school. Finding a respite care provider can also give you some breathing room. As Chapter 5 explains, respite care is skilled childcare provided by a worker trained in looking after children with special needs, and may be available for a day, weekend, or longer, if needed.

Most importantly, you and your spouse need to work together to make sure that each of you has some time to devote to your own needs for growth and independence. Often one parent (usually the mother, but sometimes the father) winds up shouldering the majority of childcare responsibilities—either because she doesn't work outside the house, or because her job has more flexibility, making it easier to look after the children's needs. In general, there's nothing wrong with this arrangement, unless the spouse with primary childcare responsibilities always gets stuck looking after the children, even when the other spouse is around to help. For example, if a wife quits her job to take care of her child with TS, but her husband keeps his job and continues moving up the career ladder, it is essential that the couple work out some way for the wife, too, to have a life outside the family. The husband might offer to stay home with the children in the evenings while his wife takes classes or joins a bowling league, or he might take over childcare responsibilities on the weekend so she can work on a novel. These are issues that you and your spouse must discuss openly and often, whenever one or both of you feels overwhelmed by the demands of raising a child with Tourette syndrome.

Being the parent of a child with Tourette syndrome takes more adaptation than usual. And the changes you will need to make likely won't come without anxiety and frustration. Accepting that your family life will be different from the idealized television or movie family is the first step in successful family management. If you don't change how you look at and work with your child, you will only meet greater frustration and failure. You may find it helps to remind yourself that you are doing things differently to increase your child's—and your own—success. And you will definitely discover that love for your child can help you weather seemingly unbearable difficulties and crises.

:: Parents with Tourette Syndrome

Parents who have TS themselves may encounter special problems in coping with the challenges of child care. When their child first begins showing symptoms of TS, they may feel as if they are reliving their own childhood. Especially if they were misunderstood as a child, painful memories they have long suppressed may be awakened. They may remember instances of emotional or physical abuse at the hands of teachers, parents, or other children, or times when they were laughed at or shunned. Some parents may have nightmares or flashbacks or become less able to cope with their own symptoms. They may also feel guilty or sad about passing TS on to their child. These feelings may make it harder for parents to see their child's situation objectively or as distinct from their own life.

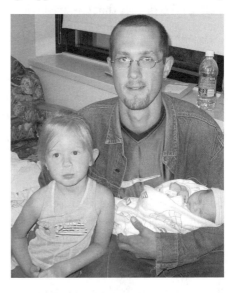

Your children's attitudes toward your Tourette syndrome can also affect your relationship with them. Just as parents wish for perfect children, children wish for perfect parents. They often idealize their parents, even in the face of extreme problems or illness. If you have TS, your children may deny the presence of the disorder or prevent their friends from meeting you to keep alive the fantasy-perfect parent they have described to others.

Often, frank and complete discussion of concerns with a mental health professional or members of TSA support groups can help allay anxiety and other painful emotions. Medications may also be helpful. Parents who have symptoms of severe depression—suicidal thinking, changes in appetite or sleep, loss of energy—should consult a psychiatrist. Coping may not be easy, but most parents with TS are eventually able to come to terms with their feelings and get on with their lives.

It's worth remembering that adults with TS often have a special talent as parents of children with TS. They have a special empathy and understanding of what it's like to have TS, and can offer their child tried and true methods of coping with TS symptoms. They often feel driven to see that their child does not have to go through the same negative experiences they faced as a child, and can become dedicated advocates for their child at school and elsewhere. Most importantly, they can serve as a positive role model for their child, demonstrating through their actions and attitudes that children with TS can grow up to be successful members of their community.

■■ Family Life

Although TS may sometimes dominate your time and attention, it should never be allowed to become the focus of your family life. If everyone is to feel like equal and contributing members of the family, they must be treated that way. Everyone deserves to have their needs and problems taken seriously *and* to have their talents and strengths nurtured. And everyone should share equally in family obligations and chores. Otherwise, their self-esteem will suffer and they may have trouble developing to their full potential.

For the sake of all members of the family, it is important to strive for as normal a family life as possible. Of course, you don't want to push your child with TS into situations that are too stressful for her. But you also don't want to keep your family cooped up in the house, thereby sending the message that there is something "wrong" with them. As a family, you need to go out to eat, to shop, to see a movie, to attend a concert, to visit an amusement park, to fly a kite in the park—to do all the normal activities that other families do. These normal activities help all family members develop social skills and expand their world. They also provide the good times that help everyone weather conflicts and crises when they arise.

How much your child's TS contributes to conflicts and crises within your family will depend to some extent on the severity of the tics and other problems. When tics are very mild, they may have little or no impact on family relationships. But symptoms such as loud vocal tics, compulsions to touch others, or impulsive behaviors can definitely affect the way family members interact. The empathy and compassion that members of your family have for one another can also make a tremendous difference in how everyone gets along. Because you, the parent, can have a profound effect on family relationships, the next section discusses how you can help keep friction to a minimum and foster the atmosphere of understanding and acceptance that everyone needs to grow.

Siblings

Brothers and sisters can grow up to be the best of friends or mortal enemies—or anything in between. Exactly what kind of relationship develops depends on many factors: common interests, differences in age, personalities, parental guidance. In other words, your child's TS alone is probably not going to make or break relationships with brothers or sisters. It may, however, present special challenges for your children to deal with in getting along with one another. Some of the most common problems are discussed below.

Embarrassment

Children often want others to believe that their family is perfect or at least just like any other family. But when a sibling has tics or other unusual behaviors it is impossible for a child to hide the fact that the family is different. Siblings may discourage their friends from coming over to the house for fear that their brother with TS will embarrass them. Or they may refuse to join in family activities if their sister's behavior often attracts unwanted attention. Embarrassment frequently becomes a major issue during early adolescence when children feel an acute need to conform and fit in. During these years, they are very self-conscious about *any* difference, including braces or eyeglasses, so having a sibling with TS can make them feel as if they really stand out.

There is probably no way to keep siblings from feeling embarrassed, but you can help them cope with their feelings. First of all, you need to teach your children that all people are different, and if someone makes fun of them or their sibling, it is not their problem, but the problem of the person who is doing the ridiculing or harassing. Second, help your children understand that it's their sibling's TS symptoms that are embarrassing them, not their brother or sister with TS. Remember, a child with TS is not deliberately behaving this way to draw attention to your family, and in fact, would give anything to be able to stop.

It's also important to help your children realize that embarrassment is perfectly natural, but also survivable. You can do this by being honest about your feelings and creating an atmosphere of open communication. For example, after an awkward incident, you might say, "Boy, was that embarrassing. Did you see that man's face when Maddie poked him?" Encourage everyone, including your child with TS, to share their feelings, and to see the humor, if any, in the situation. Finally, encourage your children to educate their friends about TS. If friends accept your child with TS and understand that tics are not done on purpose, siblings are less likely to be embarrassed when your child discharges tics in front of their friends.

Fighting and Aggression

Because of your child's tics and other behaviors, sibling relationships may sometimes be strained to the breaking point. Away from home, your other children may witness "inappropriate" behavior from your child with TS and may feel real or imagined pressure to make their sibling straighten up. Of course, since the tics are involuntary, your child *can't* shape up. But especially if your child persists in coprolalia or violent or aggressive talk, increasing frustration may lead siblings to try to beat a child with TS "out of the tics." Likewise, if your child has a tic that causes him to poke, kick, pinch, or slap siblings, tension is guaranteed to mount and may lead to fighting. The daily tension can lead to longstanding resentments and scapegoating. Whenever something goes wrong, siblings may blame your child with TS, even if it has nothing to do with TS. For instance, a sibling may blame the child with TS for not being invited to a birthday party, when he may just have been overlooked. In addition, some children have long memories and bear grudges over their sibling's inappropriate behavior. Eventually, they may take steps to "pay back the wrong" they think was done to them by fighting with or picking on their sibling with TS.

To help your other children handle the urge to fight with their sibling with TS, it helps once again to let them know that you understand their feelings. Let them know that you, too, think it is unfair that they have to deal with unusual behaviors on a daily basis, and that it's understandable that they would sometimes lose their temper. Talking about problems as they occur can help to diffuse rising anger. For example, if your child's tics are disrupting family TV time, talk openly about the problem and try to work out a solution. And giving your other children plenty of individual time and attention when they are *not* fighting makes it less likely that they will become angry because their sibling seems to get all the attention. A sibling might also benefit from talking to a counselor about how he feels about living with a brother or sister with TS.

Children with TS can be on the giving as well as on the receiving end of fighting. If a child with TS has difficulty controlling anger, she may be more apt to take out aggressive impulses on siblings. A child may push siblings around or lose her temper easily. Although your child may not be able to control these impulses, Tourette syndrome should not be considered an excuse to victimize family members. If family members must continually fend off impulsive or aggressive behavior of a child with TS, their psychological well-being can suffer.

Whenever necessary, you must take swift and protective action to prevent siblings from being injured. When your child with TS is younger, you should step in and divert her to some other activity, such as running or bike riding. As your child grows older, help her learn to recognize signs that she is losing control and take action to extricate herself from the situation. As Chapter 5 discusses in more detail, you can plan safe activities to release pent-up emotions. If aggression is a significant problem, you may need to work with a psychologist or other specialist who is knowledgeable about the neurological nature of TS and associated behavioral difficulties.

Disruptive Symptoms

As earlier chapters discuss, it's important to ignore your child's tics and other symptoms as much as possible in order to keep stress to a minimum. But sometimes this can be easier said than done. Your child's tics will change over time and some may be difficult to ignore. Your child may kick the furniture, make loud noises while siblings are trying to watch TV, or insist on having all the cabinet doors open all the time. In some cases, symptoms may seem to be directed toward a particular member of the family. For example, your child may spit at her sister or poke her shoulder. Teaching your other children to simply leave the room if they cannot ignore a symptom may work in some, but not all cases. Many children with Tourette syndrome have delays in social skills or sensory integration problems that make it difficult for them to observe boundaries. Consequently, they may follow their siblings around the house or into their rooms.

Your child has a "right" to have his tics, but your other children also have a "right" to concentrate on their homework, a game of chess, or a favorite book without being constantly distracted. When tics and other TS behaviors are too overwhelming to ignore, siblings must have a place where they can get away from it all (and lock the door, if necessary). Everyone needs privacy occasionally. You must also teach your child with TS to respect her sibling's right to solitude. Keep explaining why she must leave her brothers or sisters alone and keep enforcing boundaries—as often and as long as it takes. During periods when tics are especially severe, you may want to arrange for respite care for your child with TS or for time away for siblings to give everyone a break.

Handling Siblings' Needs

Your other children need to be treated as children in their own right—not just as siblings of your child with Tourette syndrome. Unless they are appreciated for who they are, their confidence in themselves

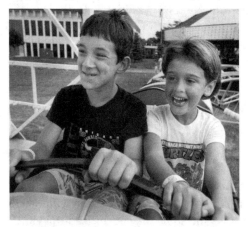 and their abilities will suffer and they may have difficulty reaching their own potential. True, their needs may not seem quite so dramatic as those of their sibling with TS, but they still deserve your serious attention.

Because having a child with TS can reduce the amount of time you have to devote to your other children, being able to recognize siblings' needs as they arise is especially important. Many of these needs will be no different than other children's, but others will be directly related to having a brother or sister with Tourette syndrome. For the sake of your children's emotional well-being, none of them should be neglected.

Information

In order to cope effectively with the challenges of living with a sibling with Tourette syndrome, your children will need regular doses of information about TS. Information can be the best antidote to fears and frustrations. It also gives siblings the background they need to deal with questions from classmates and friends. Furthermore, understanding how and why their sibling with TS behaves the way she does can help brothers and sisters respond more appropriately. For example, if they understand that their sibling cannot control coprolalia or aggression, they may be able to ignore this behavior instead of starting a fight.

Your children's need for information and ability to absorb it will change as they grow older. Depending on the severity of their sibling's symptoms, preschool children may not even notice that their sibling is different. If they do notice symptoms, they may wonder if TS is a disease that their sibling will die from, or if they can "catch" TS by drinking out of the same cup. At this stage, what they need most is calm reassurance and the chance to see that their sibling is more like them than different.

As children reach school age, they become ready and able to understand a great deal about TS. They can be told that Tourette syndrome is caused by a problem in the nervous system, that their sibling does not do these tics on purpose, and that they should ignore symptoms as much as possible. They can also benefit from watching children's videos from the national TSA. *I Have Tourette's but Tourette's Doesn't Have Me* is a good one for this age group

In the teenage years, siblings may become preoccupied with the genetics of Tourette syndrome. They may wonder if they carry the TS genes, and what the chances are that they will pass TS on to their own children. They may benefit from reading literature from the TSA on genetics, teen issues, or any other aspect of TS. The TSA also has a variety of videos targeted at teenagers and adults.

Communication

Even when children understand in theory what TS is and how it affects their sibling, they may still have trouble handling TS on an emotional level. They may feel resentful because their sibling is allowed to get away with behavior that they are not, sad because she is different, and jealous because she seems to get more attention. Often, children keep these emotions bottled up because they think their feelings are "bad" or that their parents already have their hands full dealing with their sibling with TS.

Obviously, you can't do something about a problem if you don't know about it. This means that if your children don't come to you with their problems, you will have to be alert to clues that something may be troubling them—for example, fighting at school, worsening grades, or depression. In the beginning, you may have to do a little probing to find out what is at the root of these outward signs of emotional difficulties. The key is to help your children understand that you care about their feelings and will consider and respect them. As they begin to open up, you can let them know that their emotions are normal and understandable. You can help them understand that it is vital for all family members to talk about their feelings, as well as about any conflicts that are developing.

If your family was not in the habit of communicating openly before your child was diagnosed with Tourette syndrome, the lines of communication are not going to automatically open afterwards. Many families have great difficulty dealing directly with one another. If you and your family simply cannot seem to discuss your feelings, it may help to get family counseling from a mental health professional with expertise in Tourette syndrome.

Balance

Sometimes parents think it's OK to focus exclusively on their child with TS for a while, just until things "settle down" and they have more time to spend with their other children. This kind of thinking, although understandable, is wrong. Tourette syndrome is a chronic condition that cannot be cured. True, because of the waxing and waning, symptoms will sometimes be milder than they are at other times. But your other children's needs most likely do *not* wax and wane, and can't be conveniently scheduled for the times when tics are least disruptive.

In order to feel as if they are worthwhile and important, each of your children needs individual parental attention. When parents spend much more time with their child with TS, other children may feel jealous or unloved. These feelings fuel sibling rivalry. Your other children may misbehave to get your attention, consciously or unconsciously believing that negative attention from you is better than no attention at all.

To keep your other children from feeling neglected, try scheduling time each week to do something special with each child. It doesn't have to be anything elaborate—you might take turns taking your children out to lunch, or to the library, or out shopping. Be sure also to ask *all* of your children how their day went.

As part of your balancing act, make sure that each of your children is given his or her fair share of responsibility around the house. Each child needs to experience the satisfaction of a job well done and feel like a contributing member of the family. Perhaps your child with TS has difficulty focusing her attention on a chore long enough to complete it. But if you avoid giving her chores because of this problem, she will not learn responsibility, and siblings will resent her special treatment. Each child in your family should be given jobs corresponding to their age and ability levels, and they should be expected to do their best at their jobs.

Finally, keep in mind that while children want to be given equal treatment, they also want to be treated as individuals. Sometimes special needs and talents *will* need to be taken into account when meting out privileges and responsibilities. Ideally, all your children would be given the same privileges and responsibilities once they reached a given age. For example, at age eight, they would be allowed to stay up until nine o'clock, ride their bike to school, and use the microwave oven to make popcorn. But because children's talents and weaknesses vary widely, it is not always possible to treat each child exactly the same. Your child with TS, for instance, may not be able to be left at home without adult supervision at the same age as her siblings, or may not be able to handle full responsibility for a pet. In deciding what your children can and cannot do, be sure to consider their talents, disabilities, judgment, and maturity.

Organization

Chapter 5 discusses how important organization is for children with Tourette syndrome. Having a predictable, settled routine can help reduce tics and problems such as over-stimulation arising from attention problems. But organization is also important for your other children. *All* children (and adults) become frustrated, angry, and confused if their home routine is chaotic. Consequently, your family should try to follow a daily routine that is fairly constant on both weekdays and weekends. Meals, bedtime, play time, and homework time should basically come at the same time every day. When changes in routine are necessary, you should anticipate them and plan for them in advance. If you can anticipate a particular problem before it arises, you can take steps to deal with that problem. For example, if your child has an exciting birthday party to attend, and you know she may become over-stimulated, make sure that the rest of the day will be relaxed and on schedule.

Individuality

One of the constant refrains in this book is that your child with TS is a child first, and only secondarily a child with Tourette syndrome. Your other children, too, are children first—not just the brothers or sisters of your child with Tourette syndrome. Each child in your family needs

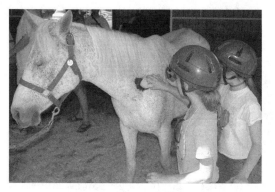

the opportunity to develop as an individual—to discover her own interests outside of the family and to pursue them with friends who share those interests. In other words, your other children need to be allowed to make their own friends. They should not always be forced to act as a playmate for their sibling with TS, whether or not she has friends outside the family. Experiencing social acceptance and success within the community is vital to your children's self-esteem.

In developing a sense of individuality, your children will also develop a sense of their own "specialness"—or what sets them apart from others. Your children may learn they have distinctive talents and abilities that make them special, but also distinctive problems and disabilities. For example, your child with TS may be gifted in academic subjects such as math, science, and reading, but have substantial delays in social and emotional development. Her brother may be unusually articulate and persuasive when speaking to a group, but have great difficulty putting her thoughts on paper. It's important that you help each of your children understand and accept that everyone has both strengths and weaknesses and encourage them to pursue their special interests and talents. But it's also important not to let special talents in one area blind you to serious problems in another that need to be worked on. This goes for all your children—not just your child with Tourette syndrome.

Although the main purpose of this chapter is to focus on potential family problems and their solutions, it would be unfair to imply that sibling relationships are always more challenging when one or more children has TS. In fact, having a brother or sister with TS can have many positive effects on siblings. For instance, having a sibling with Tourette syndrome helps many children grow up to be more tolerant of all people who are different. They learn that aggressive behavior need not always be answered with aggressive behavior, and that they can walk away from potentially dangerous situations. By working out compromises with their brother or sister with TS, many siblings also hone their problem-solving skills. Most importantly, however, when siblings learn to see their brother or sister as a person first, rather than someone whose major characteristic is TS, they learn invaluable lessons about the essence of humanity.

:: Your Marriage

When you have a child with TS, it's important not to let your marriage take a back seat to your responsibilities as a parent. Your child's well-being, after all, depends on the survival of your family, and the survival of your family depends on the survival of your marriage. Fortunately, many couples find that having a child with TS strengthens their relationship in the long-run. Jointly facing the challenges that TS brings and working together to meet their child's needs can bring them closer together than ever before. Other couples, however, find that their relationship suffers when a child with TS joins the family.

Having a child with TS *does* put some unusual stresses on a marriage. Dealing with tics and associated problems for months and years on end can wear patience thin and fuel intolerance. And constantly struggling to gain acceptance for your child in the community can leave you feeling too burned out to give your marriage the attention it needs to flourish. But too often TS is blamed for marital problems that have their roots elsewhere. The fact is, the presence of any chronic disorder in a family tends to bring out and intensify *existing* problems—not to create new ones.

Marital discord and breakup can usually be traced to core problems with communication, parental roles, or intimacy.

Communication

Chapter 2 discusses common emotions parents have when a child is diagnosed with Tourette syndrome. Because these feelings are often painful or are perceived as being shameful, many parents have trouble sharing them with their spouse. Other parents may think that if they ignore their feelings, they will go away. Unfortunately, denying or hiding these feelings can drive you and your spouse apart.

Honest communication is at least as important for you and your spouse as it is for siblings. It's crucial that both partners feel free to express all of their feelings, including feelings about their needs, their family life, or raising a child with TS. It's just as vital that these feelings be validated or supported by a caring spouse.

Active listening is the key to good communication. This involves setting aside time to listen to each other without making value judgments or blaming or criticizing your spouse. You don't have to agree with your spouse; but you do have to respect each other's feelings. It may help to remember that feelings are only feelings, and neither good nor bad. There are many popular self-help books on communication in marriage you may find helpful.

Parental Roles

Having a child with TS may bring added family pressures. Parents often have to spend time and energy taking their child to doctors

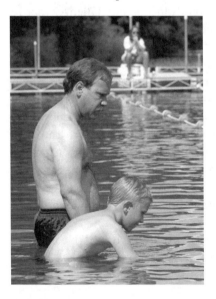

or counselors, attending meetings at school, or supervising their child at home and in the community. Consequently, as mentioned earlier in the chapter, parents need to put some thought into decisions about family roles. One spouse or the other should not have to bear *all* the pressures related to having a child with TS. You and your spouse need to recognize that you may not be able to rely on traditional roles or do things the way your parents did. The husband, for example, needs to be more than breadwinner and disciplinarian, while the wife often must be more than homemaker and nurturer. Sometimes spouses naturally gravitate to the parenting tasks they do best. More often, however, they need to formally figure out an equitable division of the responsibilities involved in keeping their family running smoothly. This is another area where being able to communicate openly is a godsend.

Intimacy

An intimate relationship is one that is based on trust, sharing, and closeness. Intimacy in marriage strengthens parents for the emotionally draining task of nurturing and supporting a family. It helps you feel that you aren't alone in the struggle to raise a healthy family. Intimacy is especially important in families with children with TS, as you may need extra energy to keep up with their children's day-to-day needs.

When you have a child with TS, time is often the biggest roadblock to increased intimacy. Because you may need to spend a disproportionate amount of time taking care of your child's medical, educational, and social needs, you may have less time available to spend with your spouse. It can be a vicious circle. The less time you have for intimacy with your spouse, the more isolated and exhausted you feel; the less energy you have, the harder it is to cope with the demands of parenthood. You must therefore make it a top priority to schedule some regular, unpressured time to work on your relationship with your spouse. Although this will reduce the *quantity* of time you are able to spend with your child, it will increase the *quality* of time you devote to her as you and your spouse recharge your emotional and physical batteries through intimacy.

Some couples are able to work out their problems on their own. Others may find it helpful to consult a mental health professional, especially someone who is knowledgeable about the effects of TS or other chronic disorders on emotions and relationships. All couples benefit from developing an outside support network. It can help take away some of the feeling that "we're doing it all alone." This support can come both through formal arrangements—from babysitters, respite workers, or support groups—or more informally, from neighbors, friends, and extended family. Chapters 2 and 5 provide more information on developing support networks.

∷ Single Parents

Divorce is never something to be entered into lightly. When a child with TS is involved, it can make day-to-day life considerably more difficult for both parent and child. A single parent has limited relief without a spouse to step in and help out with child care. Financial concerns, too, can be overwhelming. Parents may find their jobs in jeopardy because of the amount of time they need to spend on doctor visits, school conferences, and therapy sessions, and the cost of medications can be considerable. Then, too, the changes in routine that divorce brings can cause a child's tics and other symptoms to worsen.

Still, divorce sometimes is in the best interests of the family. For example, if one parent has significant problems with alcoholism or drug addiction or is abusive to the children, then the other parent alone could likely provide a more supportive home environment.

When working out a divorce settlement, it is essential you keep the financial, practical, and emotional costs in mind. For example, if the child with TS currently receives medical benefits under the terms of one parent's insurance, provisions should be made for that coverage to continue, or for the child to be switched to the other parent's policy at the time of the divorce. If your child goes uninsured for even a few weeks, it may be very difficult to get a new policy that doesn't exclude TS as a "pre-existing condition." Likewise, if one spouse has been abusive, legal action may be necessary to protect the children from harm after the divorce.

During the divorce process, counseling for spouses and children is often helpful. Most children become depressed and angry when their parents divorce. This can be even more of a problem for children with TS who have problems controlling aggression and anger. Children with TS may also worry that it was their tics and other behaviors that drove their parents to divorce, and they may therefore be consumed with guilt and remorse. A divorce can be especially hard on children with TS if it results in changes in routine. For example, if they are shuttled from one parent's house to another, they may find their daily life too confusing to handle. Often, professional counseling is essential to help children with TS through this period. Chapter 3 offers tips on finding a mental health professional with expertise in counseling children with TS. Your child's school might also have a children's divorce group.

Parents, too, often need help coping with emotions after a divorce. Some may need to seek counseling from a mental health professional in order to cope with the day-to-day demands of their family life and jobs. Respite care and a support system of family and friends can also help parents cope with the extra demands of single parenthood. In addition, some find it worthwhile to attend a support group for single parents.

Often, remarriage may appear to be the logical solution to the problems of single parenthood. But dating and marriage are like a double-edged sword for most single parents of children with Tourette syndrome. On the one hand, there is the hope that a new spouse will be able to provide the emotional and financial support everyone in the family so desperately needs. On the other hand, there are the internal conflicts and self-doubts that can arise. For example, parents may feel that they are undesirable because they have children, or because they themselves have a tic disorder. Some worry that after marriage, the romance may fade and that antagonism toward their child or themselves may develop as in their previous marriage.

The effects of dating and remarriage on the child with TS must also be considered. Dating and marriage produce major changes in a family's life. These changes can make the child with TS anxious, and as a result, tics may become worse. Problems may also result if a parent's new spouse or boyfriend or girlfriend does not understand Tourette syndrome. He or she may try to discipline the child with TS for tics or other behaviors that seem disrespectful or abusive, but are really out of the child's control. Obviously, no one should be allowed to discipline a child with TS until he or she understands the condition and has learned what management strategies are effective. Remember, no child or adult deserves to be mistreated, and it is up to the parent to take steps to ensure the safety of the family.

If you decide to remarry, professional counseling is often helpful. Family counseling with a psychologist or social worker can speed the adjustment period by helping everyone in the family develop better channels of communication. A counselor can also help spouses develop more systematic parenting—helping them decide in advance what behavior management strategies they will both use. It's also helpful to keep the medical and educational professionals involved with your child with TS informed about any changes the family is going through. They can provide support and help develop a treatment plan if it becomes necessary. For example, if your child has difficulty adapting to a new step-brother after your remarriage, they can devise strategies to help her adjust.

❖ Conclusion

Having a child with Tourette syndrome adds a new dimension to family life. All family members need to learn coping strategies and confront challenges that they would not otherwise encounter. But family life need not—in fact, *should* not—revolve around your child with TS. True, your family may need to make many adaptations, both individually and together, to accommodate your child's special needs. Remember, however, that other family members also have needs that are equally important. And just as your family pulls together to solve the problems that Tourette syndrome brings, they should also pull together to solve all the problems that face your family. As a parent, you call the plays. It's up to you to see that everyone feels like a welcome, valued member of the team.

∷ Parent Statements

Our daughter, Kelsey, who has Tourette syndrome, is nine and her little sister is five. While she knows that her big sister has TS and tics, all she really understands is that "big sis" sees the doctor and gets the attention for these "eye tics" and when the appointment is over, she gets stickers. So, on the way home from out last appointment, our five-year-old says, "Mom, I think I need to go to the doctor—my eye <u>pics</u> are sick." It was too funny and it really brightened our day and it made Mom feel a lot better.

❧

We had to let go a bit on our attachment for "things." Things get broken. Clothes are damaged. Walls are dented. What is more important, our daughter or "things"?

❧

Over the years my daughter's tics have included hitting, pinching, and tickling and when she was younger, she would sometimes "fake" her tics to get away with hitting, pinching, or tickling a family member. Though this was usually done in fun, we all got wise to it!

❧

In our family, I'm the one who tends to do all the research into treatments or educational approaches, and my husband is the one with the gumption to try to get the professionals to provide what we want for our son. For us, it's a good division of roles.

❧

Model the behavior you want your child to someday exhibit. I hold my child's hand, look people in the eye, and smile, then perhaps tell them a bit about TS. I am not embarrassed by her movements or noises. Today, my daughter is not embarrassed—she will smile at the clerk or fellow shopper, tell them she has TS and just makes these funny sounds. The other people are put at ease, they have learned something today, and may feel more comfortable the next time they meet a person with TS.

❧

Most recreational activities that people like are unstructured and loud. For my son, these things are extremely challenging. Ball games, family birthdays, state fairs are all a challenge. He is at such a high emotional state and seems to be at odds with his body. People talk to him and he answers with an unrelated comment or says nothing. So, we tend to do quieter family activities than most. Swimming is a good one for our family.

❧

A lot of people don't understand. When we're all in a restaurant or store and he gets hyper or throws temper tantrums, they really give us the looks.

❧

It's easier for me and my husband to ignore Dave's vocal tics than it is for his sister. She can get very annoyed by his ticking and it causes a lot of fights between them.

❧

We insisted that my daughter have personal responsibility regarding her tics/compulsions. If her tics "made" her hit or tickle her sister while they were watching TV, then it was her responsibility to move out of arm's reach, not her sister's.

❧

At different times over the years, one of the pastors has reintroduced our daughter to the church because there are always new people attending. This lets them see who it is who comes and makes those noises. The congregation has always been supportive as they have gotten to know her and learned about TS. A few years ago, a new pastor was hired whose son has TS. He talked about the congregation's easy acceptance of his son!

❦

Our daughter found achievement and acceptance outside of school that really helped keep her confidence and ego intact during the tough teen years. She got involved in theater, modeling, managing a football team (I wouldn't let her play), the humane society, even a job, to name just a few.

7
YOUR CHILD'S DEVELOPMENT

Gary A. Shady, Ph.D., C. Psych.
Robin Jewers, B.M.R., O.T.M.
Patricia Furer, Ph.D., C. Psych.
Rox Wand, M.D., FRCPC
Rosanne B. Papadopoulos, B.M.R., O.T.M.

Doctor, professional athlete, teacher, parent . . . You can find adults with Tourette syndrome in just about every profession. Their stories remind us that Tourette syndrome doesn't necessarily limit an individual's potential. Nonetheless, when your child has been diagnosed with TS, it is understandable that you would worry about how this disorder might affect his life. You may wonder whether your child will develop "normally" or master skills as well or as quickly as other children do.

Unfortunately, it is impossible to predict exactly how Tourette syndrome will affect any one particular child's development. Every child is unique. Some children with TS acquire skills at the same rate or even faster than other children do, while others may lag somewhat behind. Usually, however, Tourette syndrome is associated with some common strengths and weaknesses in development. Exactly how Tourette syndrome will affect your child's development may depend on many factors, including: the severity and type of tics he has; what kind of support he receives at home and at school; and whether he has any associated conditions such as attention-deficit/hyperactivity disorder

(AD/HD), obsessive-compulsive disorder (OCD), or Asperger syndrome (also known as Asperger's disorder). Individuals with TS who also have one or more such associated conditions are now frequently described as having "Tourette Syndrome Plus" or "TS+."

This chapter will provide a framework to help you understand your child's development and how it may be affected by Tourette syndrome. It also provides suggestions on how you can help your child overcome developmental difficulties and reach his full potential. Many of these suggestions have come from parents of children with Tourette syndrome and you will undoubtedly be able to add to the list.

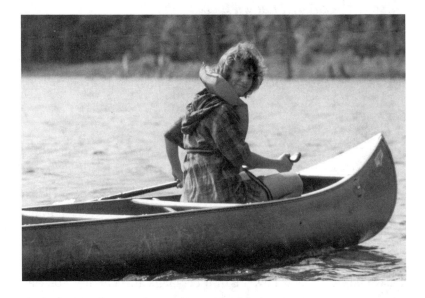

▪▪ What Is Development?

Most children grow and acquire skills, or *develop,* according to pretty much the same timetable. That is, there are certain skills that most children acquire by a certain age. For example, most babies sit briefly without support at around six months of age and can say a few words by around eighteen months. Most children also develop new skills in generally the same order—they crawl before they walk, and they understand much spoken language before they can speak themselves.

Nevertheless, there is a tremendous variety in rates and styles of development. This is because all development depends a great deal on biological programming. In other words, a child's genetic makeup sets the foundation for growth and acquisition of skills. For example, inheriting quick reflexes may make it easier to learn to catch a ball. Other factors such as environment, culture, and psychological makeup are also important. A child's temperament, as well as the availability of his caregiver, playmates, toys, or books can all affect early development. Because so many combinations of factors can occur, no child's development is exactly the same as another child's development. One child, for instance, may move carefully through each step of learning to talk, while another child may seem to pick up language skills in a rapid learning spurt later on.

TS may be considered a neurodevelopmental disorder. A neurodevelopmental disorder can cause some aspects of a child's development to vary from the norm. For example, a child with TS who has hand tics may read far above grade level, but lag behind his classmates in handwriting. In this example, not only does the TS cause a delay in the acquisition of a specific skill (handwriting,) but it also affects the order in which the child develops certain skills (with advanced reading coming before, say, legible printing). Ultimately, whether a child has a neurodevelopmental disorder or not, how quickly he learns to do something is not as important as how well he can eventually do it. If he needs to do it a little differently, that's OK, too.

The extent to which Tourette syndrome will affect your child's development can depend on the frequency and severity of his symptoms. For example, a child with only mild tics and no associated conditions may adapt easily and have few developmental difficulties, while a child with severe tics, OCD, and AD/HD may have more obstacles to overcome in many areas of development.

** Typical Course of Tourette Syndrome

The onset and development of TS can vary quite substantially. However, we can look at some typical stages that may occur during a child's growing years and into adulthood. We find it helpful to look at three very broad phases of development: ages birth to 9, 10 to 15, and 16 and up.

Stage One: Birth to Age 9

Most children with TS are born following a normal pregnancy and delivery. However, in the preschool years (often before the tics appear), parents sometimes notice mild, subtle differences in their child's behavior compared to that of other children the same age. Parents may worry that their preschooler seems hyperactive or too aggressive with other kids. Perhaps he has more temper tantrums than the other kids have at daycare, or "loses it" when Mom and Dad try to leave him with a babysitter. Maybe he can't go to sleep at night unless his stuffed animals are lined up "just right." These may just be passing phases of development that your child will quickly outgrow, but they may be cause for concern should they be extreme or persistent. The wide spectrum of "normal" behavior and development can be a challenge for both families and physicians.

The average age at which tics begin is seven, but this can vary considerably. Even after tics appear, it can take a while for TS to be diagnosed. Unusual eye blinking may look, at first, like the child needs glasses or is being bothered by allergies. If the child is "always on the move," his motor tics might be masked by all the running, jumping, and playing. Until very obvious tics emerge, parents and even the pediatrician may assume the child is just very active or perhaps has AD/HD.

Stage Two: Ages 10 to 15

If a child is not diagnosed with Tourette syndrome when his tics first appear, he probably will be diagnosed in preadolescence. Tics often peak when the child is between the ages of ten and twelve. Scientists believe that the biochemical, hormonal, and other changes the body goes through during puberty are probably to blame for the worsened symptoms (not that that's much consolation to a self-conscious twelve-year-old who just wants his tics to go away).

Stage 3: Late Teens through Adulthood

Fortunately, most people with Tourette syndrome find that their symptoms lessen in their late teen years or early twenties. In fact, an international research team (including professors Burd and Kerbeshian, who wrote chapters for this book) has followed thousands of people with TS for more than twenty years. They found that, once children with TS reach adulthood, 75 percent have few tics and feel that TS has only a very modest impact on their lives. Another 15 percent have moderate, but manageable, symptoms through adulthood, while only 10 percent have severe symptoms as adults. At this point, though, we are not yet able to predict *which* individuals will be fortunate enough to have their tics lessen or remit totally.

"How Bad Is It Going to Get?"

Once your child has been diagnosed with Tourette syndrome, you (and he) will want to know "how bad is it going to get?" But medical specialists may be reluctant to predict exactly how the disorder will affect your child's development and functioning. This is, first of all, because the range of symptoms in children with TS can vary so widely. In some children with TS, the only symptoms are motor and vocal tics. Other children may have obsessions, compulsions, hyperactivity, learning problems, frequent mood swings, or aggressive or self-injurious behaviors.

If your child does develop other symptoms, they will wax and wane, just as motor and vocal tics do. How severe a particular symptom becomes can vary tremendously from child to child. And the extent to which Tourette syndrome will affect your child's development can depend on the frequency and severity of his symptoms. For example, a child with only mild tics and no associated conditions may adapt easily and have few developmental difficulties, while a child with severe tics, OCD, and AD/HD may have more obstacles to overcome in many areas of development.

As a parent, the best approach is to educate yourself on the ways TS could affect your child's development, so you will recognize problems quickly if they should arise. At the same time, keep in mind that most children's Tourette symptoms remain mild, and a diagnosis of TS is no reason to panic.

∷ Areas of Development

Although every child with Tourette syndrome *is* unique, the disorder generally has at least some effect on social, emotional, or academic development. It may also impede development of sensory processing, cognition, fine and gross motor coordination, and language skills. The sections below review some of the ways TS *may* affect a child's development. But, as you read, keep in mind that not all children have the same developmental concerns. Very few children with TS have *all* these difficulties. Your child may have many of these problems, but then again, he may develop few or none of them.

Motor Development

A child's *motor skills* are his abilities to use his muscles appropriately to perform tasks. Of course, motor skills are dependent not just on the

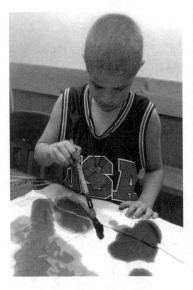

muscles, but on the brain, skeleton, nerves, and joints as well. In *gross motor development*, children learn to control their bodies through the use of large muscles such as those in the legs, arms, and abdomen. Rolling, sitting, crawling, and walking are examples of basic gross motor skills, which later develop into more advanced skills such as running and climbing. Because these types of skills enable the child to master the environment and explore the world, they play a crucial role in development in other areas. In *fine motor development*, children learn to use smaller muscles such as those in their hands to make precise, detailed movements. Pinching, holding, and touching things with the hands are all examples of fine motor tasks. Fine motor skills lay the foundation for later development of academic skills such as handwriting, as well as self-help skills such as tying shoelaces.

Some children with TS have motor development problems and others do not. Children with TS+, with an associated disorder such as AD/HD or Asperger syndrome, are the ones most likely to have motor difficulties. These children may be sloppy eaters or have difficulty in learning how to ride a bike. Typically, they don't have any significant delays in reaching motor milestones—they lift their heads by around four months, walk around twelve months, etc. But they may have what professionals refer to as *soft signs* that suggest subtle neurological problems. Some of these signs are:

- Awkward body posture during physical activities;
- Poor balance;
- Floppiness or stiffness in the body and limbs during movement;
- Difficulty identifying right and left;
- Difficulty with activities such as bowling or basketball in which both sides of the body must be used in a coordinated way;
- Difficulties with activities that involve coordinating the eyes and hands, such as catching a ball;

- Over-responsiveness or under-responsiveness to sensory experiences such as smells, bright lights, and loud noises.

On a day-to-day basis, gross motor development problems can make it difficult for a child to keep up in gym class. He may be reluctant to join intramural or team sports, and feel left out of playground or neighborhood games. A child who is not comfortable with athletic activities will often opt for more stationary pastimes such as computer games and TV. Of course, that can create a difficult cycle: the less active he is, the farther behind he will fall in athletic skills. The consequences can be far-reaching: Exercise is essential for good physical health, and sedentary children grow up to be sedentary adults. Moreover, the child who stays home to watch TV is missing out on the friendships that often develop through sports, as well as the stress relief that comes through physical activity.

Children and adolescents with either TS or TS+ may have poor fine motor control. This can result in difficulty in handwriting, dressing, grooming, eating, and arts and crafts. There are many possible reasons why a child may have poor fine motor control. The difficulties may be related to differences in how touch sensations are processed. For example, a child who is over-sensitive to touch might avoid working with papier-mâché, finger painting, or taking part in other activities that require touching gooey or slimy materials. This, in turn, may provide the child with fewer opportunities to develop fine motor skills. Other factors contributing to poor fine motor control can include: poor muscle tone, particularly in the shoulder, arm, and hand; difficulties understanding spatial information; and problems coordinating the eyes and hands. Tics, or the child's attempt to physically hold back an arm or hand tic, can also contribute to fine motor problems.

Symptoms of AD/HD can add to motor problems. Hyperactivity and impulsivity may prevent a child from focusing and can contribute to messy work or an inability to stay focused on an activity such as handwriting. Some studies also show that children with AD/HD have below average gross motor and fine motor skills, but it isn't clear whether these are difficulties they were born with or whether they are related to inattention.

OCD may also interfere with a child's motor performance. For example, excessive erasing, trying to get things "just right," or rituals such as counting certain letters can all get in the way of completing written work.

Children with Asperger syndrome frequently have motor delays and coordination problems. These may include an awkward gait (walking or running very rigidly), poor fine motor skills, and poor visual-motor coordination.

When a child's motor impairment interferes with his activities of daily living and academic achievement—and it cannot be attributed to an autism spectrum disorder or a medical problem—he may be diagnosed with *developmental coordination disorder (also known as DCD)*.

Strategies for Motor Difficulties

Depending upon the nature of your child's motor problems, he may benefit from occupational or physical therapy.

Occupational therapy (OT) is designed to help a child develop his motor and other skills so he can better cope with his day-to-day activities. For instance, an occupational therapist might help a child with TS improve his handwriting skills by having him use a special pencil grip, hold the pencil differently, play fine motor games, and perform exercises that develop arm and hand strength.

Physical therapy (PT) focuses more specifically on identifying and treating problems with movement and posture. If a child with TS has poor balance, a physical therapist might have him sit on a tilt board, bounce on a large therapy ball, and work up to jumping, hopping, and running.

One great thing about both OT and PT is that therapists can often combine treatment with play. That makes the sessions more fun for the kids and allows the therapists to work on several areas at once. A therapy session concentrating on gross motor skills might include a trip through an obstacle course that consists of a balance beam, a scooter board (for postural control), and bowling pins and balls (for visual aiming and motor accuracy), as well as floor mats for working on rolling or crawling. A therapy session focusing on fine motor skills and eye-hand coordination might include maze-drawing, playing with clay, and lacing. An OT might also work at decreasing a child's over-sensitivity to touch by playing with messy materials such as shaving cream and pudding.

As a parent, you can help your child's skill development by encouraging him to attempt a variety of fine motor and gross motor activities. Choose activities to fit your child's strengths and limitations and be sure to include him in the decision-making. After all, children are more likely to succeed if they are motivated to try an activity. For example, if your child enjoys playing in the water at the beach, then consider enrolling him in swimming lessons at the local pool; if he loves doing art projects, have him join a craft club at a nearby community club; if he adores music, he might want to learn to play the guitar, piano, or drums.

Where sports are concerned, keep in mind that although team sports can be a good opportunity to develop cooperative play skills, some children with TS or TS+ gain more satisfaction from individual sports. Team sports, such as soccer, may have motor (and social) demands that can be overwhelming. Individual sports such as karate, dance, gymnastics, archery, and swimming may be better choices. These sports help develop physical strength, endurance, and coordination, and promote individual versus team progress. They also help to develop self-confidence, which may be sorely needed for children with TS.

Cognitive Development in Children with Tourette Syndrome

Cognition refers to a person's ability to think, reason, problem-solve, and understand the environment. Cognitive development is influenced by many things, including genetics and an individual's interactions with the environment.

When a child is diagnosed as having Tourette syndrome, parents often worry that his intelligence will be impaired. Although TS can be very challenging for children and families to cope with, it does at least have the saving grace of *not* affecting overall cognitive or intellectual development.

Your child's cognitive abilities can be measured one of two ways: informally, by evaluating how he copes with daily life; or formally, through an IQ test, which compares your child's abilities with those of other children of the same age. Most children and adolescents with Tourette syndrome have average IQs. As in the general population, some children with Tourette syndrome are above average in intelligence, and some are below. Only a very small percentage of children with TS also have mental retardation—that is, cognitive capabilities that test far below average and affect their skill acquisition and performance in all areas of development. The percentage of children with Tourette syndrome who have mental retardation is the same as for the population as a whole—roughly 3 percent. Tourette syndrome *does not* cause mental retardation.

Although Tourette syndrome is not associated with low overall intelligence, it does appear to be associated with difficulties in some specific cognitive skills, since many children with TS share the same challenges. We have yet to figure out exactly *why* children with TS tend to have these problems. Nonetheless, you may find it helpful to learn about the kinds of challenges your child may encounter. Research suggests that areas of difficulty for some children with TS include:

- *Cognitive flexibility*, or the ability to shift ideas or thoughts easily (talking about something in social studies one minute and science the next);
- *Concept formation*, or the ability to understand or form ideas by taking in new information and mentally categorizing it with other relevant information (e.g., a child who already knows how to add will use that information, plus new input from his teacher, to grasp the new concept of "multiplication").

These cognitive difficulties relate to *executive functions* or the factors that help us plan, organize, and problem-solve in our daily lives.

Children with TS, and particularly those with TS+, may also find written arithmetic very challenging and often do better on oral arithmetic word problems. This may be related to carelessness, impulsivity, or disorganized written work. As a result, your child may have difficulty with mathematics at school, where these skills are typically taught and tested in a written format.

Another area that often is difficult for children with Tourette syndrome is taking timed tests. This may be painfully obvious in a classroom where students are given in-class tests or assignments to complete in, say, twenty minutes. If a child has difficulties with executive functions, he may have trouble allotting the appropriate amount of time to each portion of a test. Difficulties with *verbal fluency* can make it hard for him to come up with the "right" words to express his thoughts, especially under time pressure. If the test covers a broad range of topics, and the child has trouble with cognitive flexibility, it may take him extra time to make the "leap" between subjects. If concept formation is a problem, applying the math facts he knows to a word problem he's never seen before can slow him down. Add to any of these difficulties the fact that he may be having tics or engaging in compulsive behaviors at the same time, and you can see why timed tests can be so rough.

Children with TS+, especially those with AD/HD or Asperger syndrome, may have particular difficulty with some of the executive functioning skills outlined above. Additional challenges for these children may include a poor sense of time and timing, difficulty delaying gratification, poor judgment, a low "boiling point" for frustration, and difficulty working toward long-term goals. These children may also struggle to sustain attention in play activities and to listen to instructions on how to perform the activities. Organizing the various steps necessary to complete a task may be particularly challenging. Your child may, for example, have great difficulty following a set of instructions such as "Wash your face, brush your teeth, and comb your hair." Children with TS+ frequently forget one or two steps or seem to get distracted before the task is completed. Similarly, your child may have trouble remembering to do his homework assignments or to bring home the necessary textbooks. These types of problems can cause endless frustration for parents.

Besides interfering with the development of specific cognitive skills, the problems described above may also cause the intellectual potential of children with TS to be underestimated. People, including teachers and school officials, simply may not recognize how intelligent your child is. This can occur for several reasons. First of all, some motor and vocal tics directly interfere with *performance* in various activities at home and at school. For example, if your child has a vocal tic that makes him repeat his own words, an otherwise excellent speech can become virtually unintelligible. Your child's public speaking skills may thus be hidden by a tic. Secondly, your child's intelligence and abilities may be underestimated if any of the medications he takes for TS have a cognitive dulling effect and teachers or testers do not recognize that.

So, TS can create some specific cognitive challenges for your child. But it is important to remember that few people have equally developed cognitive abilities across all areas. We each have relative strengths and weaknesses. For example, you may be great with numbers but be less comfortable writing business reports. Your spouse, on the other hand, may write reports and creative essays with ease but find balancing a checkbook very difficult. Thus, we each have more difficulty with certain cognitive skills than with others. The same holds true for children with TS.

Strategies for Cognitive Difficulties

These potential problems underline the importance of having your child's intellectual potential assessed by a psychologist who is familiar with Tourette syndrome and the medications used to treat it. It is also essential that all professionals, teachers, and parents understand that a child's poor performance on a given task may be due to interference from tics or medication, rather than to a lack of ability or intelligence.

If your child has any of the cognitive difficulties described above, it's important that he learn to compensate for them. For example, if your child has difficulty with verbal fluency, he may be more successful using rehearsal strategies, reading from cue cards, or using other visual cues. If he has difficulties with written mathematics, the teacher could permit him to do at least part of the required work orally. Relaxing or eliminating the time restrictions on tests can be helpful for many children with TS.

If your child has problems with cognitive flexibility, you may find that playing word games—such as guessing alternate endings to a story—is helpful for him.

If he struggles with concept formation, try breaking words down or giving actual examples or scenarios. For instance, for the word "justice," you could show him scenes from a courtroom setting in a movie or television series. This type of exercise is helpful as a way to redefine and reframe abstract concepts into more concrete terms that your child can capture or understand more clearly.

Finally, if you have a child who seems to constantly forget things, he would probably benefit from predictable daily routines and good organizational strategies. And you, as the parent, may have to impose those strategies upon him until he's able to do it for himself. A child with organizational challenges needs a systematic approach for everything from getting ready to school to completing household chores. Together, you and your child might make "to do" lists on calendars, planners, or dry erase boards. Older children or teens might like using a computer program or an electronic organizer. (If you, the parent, have any tendencies toward AD/HD, you may benefit from these strategies as much as your child does. It's hard to organize your child if you aren't organized yourself.)

Use your own creativity and the teacher's expertise to brainstorm strategies to help compensate for your child's difficulties. Here are some ideas to get you started:

- provide as much one-to-one instruction as possible
- lecture less
- design tasks of low to moderate frustration levels
- use computers in instruction
- pair the student with a study buddy
- structure tasks
- maintain frequent communication between home and school

- allow time during the school day for locker and backpack organization
- have daily and weekly organization and clean-up routines
- prepare for transitions and change
- display rules
- have clear consequences
- use favorite activities as rewards
- highlight or color-code directions
- divide larger tasks into smaller segments
- repeat directions

See Chapter 8 in this book for more ideas on coping with TS in the classroom.

Development of Language and Communication in Children with Tourette Syndrome

Through language development, children gradually learn one of the most vital skills in modern society: communication. Usually, comprehension of language, including words or gestures, comes first. Later, the child develops the ability to communicate through use of appropriate gestures, words, or written symbols. For example, a child generally understands the word *milk* long before he can verbally request it. This ability to understand words and gestures is called *receptive language;* the ability to use language to communicate is *expressive language.*

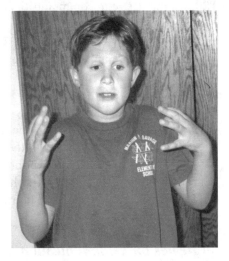

Parents sometimes wonder whether their child's vocal tics can be traced to abnormal language development in the early years. In general, that does not seem to be true. Most children with Tourette syndrome have normal speech patterns. Their verbal tics fit in with normal speech rhythm and often occur at the same point where a speaker would normally hesitate or pause, such as at the beginning or ending of a sentence. Speakers often hesitate while talking, making sounds such as *um* and *uh.* These sounds are produced by unnecessary, nonverbal movements of the lips, tongue, and vocal cords. So, as you can see, many verbal tics found in TS originate in normal behavior.

Once verbal tics develop, they are more likely to interfere with language expression, rather than comprehension. Research has shown that children and adolescents with Tourette syndrome often have good receptive language ability: they can repeat sounds they hear, remember what someone has said (except when long sentences are involved), and, in general, understand what they hear. At the same time, it is common for children with TS to stutter, or to have trouble elaborating on a story or finding the right word. Often these difficulties arise because the child is making a concentrated effort to hold back a vocal tic.

Interpersonal communication can also be disrupted if tics are expressed, rather than suppressed. This happens if tics involve word repetition or echolalia, or if the vocal tics are explosive, loud, or distracting. Listeners may lose track of the conversation, as may the speaker. This can be frustrating for both. It's easy to imagine the social and emotional anxiety that may result from being unable to verbally express your thoughts. Occasionally, an exasperated child or adolescent with TS loses the desire to communicate at all, which can lead to further language or social problems.

If a child with TS+ has Asperger syndrome, he may have different, or additional, communication difficulties. Unlike children with other autism spectrum disorders, those with AS don't have speech delays. In fact, many have very advanced vocabularies, even at a young age. However, children with Asperger syndrome tend to have difficulties with the *pragmatics* of speech—the ability to carry on appropriate back-and-forth conversations with their peers. Instead, they may tend to lecture on their special topics of interest. They also may have difficulties with receptive language (both oral and written), because they tend to interpret language very literally, and have trouble "reading between the lines."

Strategies for Communication Difficulties

To minimize the effects your child's verbal tics have on his language development, be prepared to be very supportive. To help him get used to communicating with others, encourage him to play with peers—first on a one-to-one basis, and then in small groups. Allow him to speak for himself in conversations, rather than answering for him.

A speech therapist may be helpful with stuttering or delays in speech and language development. Some speech therapists, as well as some psychologists, guidance counselors, and occupational therapists, provide *social skills groups* for children who have difficulty picking up the basic unwritten rules of society, such as knowing how far away to stand from someone when talking. A social skills group might, for example, look at a complex skill such as "starting a conversation," and break it up into a number of steps, then work on one step at a time. Giving a child opportunities to watch others complete these steps and then copy them is very helpful. It is also important to provide opportunities for your child to practice his newly learned skills in the real world. Parents, teachers, or other helping professionals may want to set up phone or play dates to encourage and develop social communication skills.

If your child has a verbal tic that is offensive to others and leads to social isolation, you might consider teaching him ways to turn or *shape* the tic into a more acceptable word or phrase (for example, turning "damn" into "darn.") Other strategies might include encouraging him to whisper the tic, placing his hands over his mouth when expressing the tic, or going somewhere private (like a bathroom) to express his tic.

Habit reversal training (HRT), a kind of behavior therapy designed to reduce tics, may also be helpful. Psychologists, or others trained in HRT, can assist your child to become more aware of a tic and the urge that may precede it, to use relaxation strategies, and to replace the tic with a *competing response*. A competing response for a vocal tic from his throat might be to breathe deeply through his nose with his mouth closed. (See Chapter 4 for more information on HRT.)

Social and Emotional Development in Children with Tourette Syndrome

As children develop socially, they learn to get along with others, as well as to respond with appropriate emotions. Usually, even very young infants take an intense interest in others around them. As early as two months of age, they may smile and watch others' movements. By about six months, they can recognize family members and are often frightened by strangers, especially when left alone with them. During the preschool years, children learn the difference between genders, begin to recognize feelings in others, and react to others with varied emotions such as shyness or anger. Also during these years, children progress from playing by themselves, to playing beside other children,

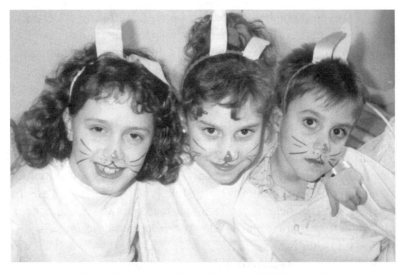

and eventually to playing together with other children in the same activity. By five or six, most children are able to form special friendships and show increased independence. All of these social skills help children to fit in and become functioning members of society.

Years before your child developed tics, you may have noticed problems with his social and emotional development. This is common. Although tics may begin as early as age one or two, they usually do not appear until after age five. Other problems, however, often start in the preschool years. These include temper tantrums, hyperactivity, aggressive behavior, difficulty sharing, and separation anxiety. Often these types of difficulties run in families, and siblings may also have similar problems, although only one child actually develops TS.

When a preschooler has problems with emotional or social skills, his behavior may disrupt family life. Parents may believe that their child intentionally misbehaves at home and in the community. Parents' frustration may turn to anger, and they are likely to repeatedly, but unsuccessfully, correct and discipline their child. The child, in turn, is likely to resent the criticism and may feel isolated from other family members. Children who have little control over their behavior may feel intense frustration, which can interfere with various aspects of social and emotional development. Family relationships can become strained even before the onset of a child's first tics.

After the motor and vocal tics develop, your child and the whole family will face additional challenges. For example, you may initially think that your child's tics are a way of expressing anger toward you, other family members, or playmates. As a result of this misunderstanding, you may discipline or correct your child, and siblings or playmates may ridicule him for behaviors he cannot control. This, of course, will only add to the child's frustration, and he may begin to isolate himself from people and activities. The child with TS may even begin to believe that he's "bad," and that he is deliberately misbehaving.

Once you know that your child has TS, some of these misunderstandings may be cleared up. Most families, however, find that the motor and vocal tics, especially when complicated by AD/HD or obsessions and compulsions, continue to disrupt the family and the child's social and emotional development in many ways. For example, your child may often try to hold back his tics to appease you, his teachers, and his peers. But tics can only be held in for so long. If your child succeeds in controlling the tics and associated conditions while in school or other public places, he will have to release many tics once he gets home. This often creates disharmony in the family, particularly when brothers and sisters demand equal leniency for their own disruptive behavior.

To make matters more difficult, it is often hard, as a parent, to tell whether a given behavior is an involuntary symptom (which is best ignored) or a willful behavior for which your child should be held accountable. This uncertainty puts additional pressure on family relationships. Mom and Dad may feel guilty and frustrated, while siblings resent the child who gets "special treatment." The child with TS may feel angry, guilty, hurt, and frustrated.

All these factors may add up to reduced opportunities for socializing and for developing social skills. For example, if members of your family are embarrassed by the TS symptoms or your inability to make the child with TS "behave," you may forgo outings to restaurants and theaters or withdraw from other social and recreational activities.

As children enter adolescence, their "different" behaviors often increase. Tics may become more frequent or severe. Obsessive-compulsive symptoms may worsen and AD/HD frequently continues unabated. Ongoing academic difficulties may also cause worry.

Poorly developed social skills become much more obvious when children reach their "tweens" or teens, and some adolescents with TS seem to have more difficulty understanding and changing their behaviors than their peers do. Families and classmates often see them as immature or lacking in social skills. Just at the stage in life when the need for peer acceptance is greatest, your child may feel captive to a condition that appears bizarre to his friends. He may hesitate to participate in important social activities such as dances, parties, dating, or part-time employment. As a result, he may feel isolated and lonely. The lower his self-esteem gets, the harder it becomes for him to seek out new opportunities in social relationships.

If you are the parent of an adolescent with TS, you may frequently find yourself acting as your child's best friend, nurturing the development of social skills, social relationships, and self-acceptance. Children with TS who have the additional diagnosis of Asperger syndrome may experience particularly severe struggles in the social realm.

Strategies for Social or Emotional Difficulties

As a parent, you play a vital role every day in helping your child learn appropriate social skills. This is true whether or not your children have TS, of course, but may be particularly important for those who do. You can best help your child by concentrating on *gradually* improving social skills. First reinforce bits and pieces of skills that are close to being right, then work up to more complete skills. For example, your child might have trouble understanding others' reactions to his behavior. He might not realize how frustrated other children get when he refuses to share his toys. If he does consent to share a less favored toy—even with a reminder from you—praise him enthusiastically. He can gradually work up to sharing a variety of toys and doing so without parental prompts.

You may find it helpful to prepare your child for common challenging social situations. Try role-playing or rehearsing ways to respond to, for example, unkind comments from classmates. That can increase your child's ability to handle such situations effectively and may also decrease his social anxiety.

Because social development can frequently be interrupted or delayed if your child is ridiculed or unfairly disciplined, you also have an advocacy role. Make information about TS available to your child's teachers and classmates (see Chapter 8). Providing this information may help demystify the unusual behaviors which baffle children and adults unfamiliar with the syndrome.

In addition to increasing understanding of TS among teachers and friends, you can also enhance your child's social development by enrolling him in group therapy or recreation programs at facilities that treat children or adolescents with TS. Summer camp programs for kids with TS can also boost your child's sense of well-being and social skills. By sharing information and feedback with other children with TS, your child can learn new coping styles that may ultimately lead to better relationships at home and in school. The National Tourette Syndrome Association or a local chapter can help you find programs that may give your child a boost in social development.

If your child is struggling with depression, OCD, or other anxiety problems in addition to the TS, consider consulting with a professional who is familiar with effective treatments for these problems. Both psychological and medication treatments are helpful for depression and anxiety-related concerns. Cognitive-behavioral therapies may be particularly suitable for children with these problems. This approach to treatment emphasizes the interaction between feelings, behavior, thoughts, and physical symptoms, and involves learning strategies to reduce and cope more effectively with anxiety, depression, and other problems.

Self-Help Development in Children with Tourette Syndrome

At birth, babies are totally dependent on others for their survival and well-being. Through the development of self-help skills such as feeding, grooming, and dressing, they gradually learn to do things for themselves and become more and more independent. Self-help skills can develop early in life, particularly when children are given opportunities to act independently. For example, when physically able, a child can learn to use a spoon instead of being spoon-fed, as long as others at the table don't mind the mess. Not only does tolerating this type of independence help a child reach developmental milestones, but it also helps parents boost the child's confidence, which can make learning new skills in all areas easier.

For children with TS, many of the problems in other areas described above (such as executive function, motor skills, and language) can add up to poor self-help or daily living skills. For example, if your child cannot remember a simple series of instructions, he may have difficulty learning how to make breakfast, use the washing machine, or learn any number of self-help skills. If tics or speech and language problems delay his social development, this may hamper his ability to get along independently. For example, he may be unable to deal well enough with strangers to make a purchase in a store, ask for directions when he is lost, or place an order in a restaurant. As mentioned earlier, poor fine motor control can also lead to problems with eating, dressing, and grooming.

Children with TS may also have sleep problems. While sleep habits are not a "self-help" skill per se, a child who has difficulty falling asleep at night and getting up in the morning is definitely going to find his everyday activities more challenging. Lack of sleep can make it more difficult to pay attention at school, "hang in there" when problems with peers or schoolwork become frustrating, or slow down and resist solving problems impulsively. This list could go on and on. Just think how *you* feel and behave on days when you haven't had enough sleep! Chapter 5 discusses strategies for dealing with sleep problems.

Strategies for Self-help Difficulties

As with all children, if your child has delays in self-help skills, an OT should be able to offer helpful ideas and suggestions. To help your child with problems related to fine motor control, an OT might, for example, recommend pull-on and pullover clothing, sneakers with Velcro fasteners or elastic shoelaces, or special eating utensils. A therapist, or you as a parent, can also help your child break down daunting tasks into smaller, more manageable pieces. For instance, create a set of simple step-by-step instructions to post by the washing machine.

Checklists outlining morning routines or daily expectations may also be helpful for your child (for any child for that matter!). To be most effective, checklists should be as specific as possible (for example, "Set alarm for 7:30 a.m." rather than "Get up in the morning") and might even include some pictures or visual cues. Encouraging your child to participate in simple household chores, such as setting the table, at an early age will also help him develop some basic skills and feel good about himself. A key point to remember is to establish as much predictability and routine in your day as possible. This allows your child more sense of control over his day and promotes independence.

Sensory Processing Issues in Children with Tourette Syndrome

Another developmental issue that may affect your child's growth and learning is *sensory processing* (or *sensory integration*). Sensory processing has to do with how your brain takes in, interprets, and uses the sensory information it receives from inside and outside the body. There are seven senses that send information to your brain. The five senses most of us are familiar with are touch, sight, hearing, taste, and smell. They send your brain information from outside of your body. There are two more senses that send your brain information about what is happening *inside* your body. These senses are called the *vestibular* and *proprioceptive senses*. The vestibular sense (regulated by your inner ear) responds to changes in your head position and helps you maintain your balance. The proprioceptive sense, also known as the *position sense* or *muscle sense*,

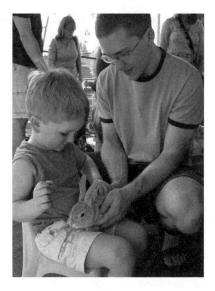

sends your brain information about where different parts of your body, such as your hands and legs, are when you can't see them.

When there is a problem with how a child's brain handles sensory information, he may have a *sensory processing disorder* (or *sensory integration dysfunction*). Sensory processing disorder can take three forms.

Sensory Modulation Disorder. One form is commonly referred to as *sensory modulation disorder*. Children and adults with sensory modulation disorder can be over-responsive or under-responsive to sensations or they may need to seek out sensory experiences. For example, if your child is over-responsive, he may perceive a gentle tap on the shoulder as a hard hit. His automatic reaction might be a "fight, flight, or freeze" reaction: he may slug the person back. On the other hand, if your child is under-responsive, he might not notice a gentle tap on the shoulder. You might need to give him a deep squeeze at the top of his arm for him to notice that you are touching him. Finally, if he is a "sensory seeker," he may be the one touching you on the shoulder!

Sensory Discrimination Disorder. The second form of sensory processing disorder is *sensory discrimination disorder*. This is when there is a problem noticing differences in how things look, sound, taste, etc. For example, your child might not notice that you have added a different spice to your chili. Or he might not notice when you make a change to your hairstyle.

Sensory-Based Motor Disorder. The third form of sensory processing disorder is *sensory-based motor disorder.* A child with this kind of disorder may have difficulties with movement and coordination because of underlying sensory processing problems. He may have a particularly tough time learning a new movement or set of movements—for example, learning how to swim the crawl or tie shoelaces. He might also appear clumsy or accident-prone.

Sensory processing issues may affect how your child learns and may become more apparent when he enters school. If he has trouble dealing with the many sensations bombarding his brain, he may find it difficult to concentrate, sit still, and focus on a math lesson without being distracted by sounds coming from the school hallway. Standing in line, eating in the cafeteria, or taking part in gym or music class might also be overwhelming to him because of the many sounds, lights, and unpredictable activity around him. These feelings and his consequent actions—for example, having a "melt-down" in gym class--may further contribute to delays in his gross motor skills and social development because they are taking him away from valuable motor and social learning experiences. It is easy to see how sensory problems—added to the tics of TS—can very easily lead to low self-esteem and poor relationships with family and friends.

Strategies for Sensory Difficulties

There are a number of strategies that you can try to help with sensory processing disorders. Simply becoming aware of your child's sensory processing differences is the first step. An OT or someone else trained in sensory processing/sensory integration can complete a formal assessment This assessment might involve having you or your child's teacher complete some checklists related to how your child responds to different experiences at home and in the classroom. The therapist might also observe your child as he completes a series of motor exercises.

Once your child's unique sensory pattern or "profile" is established or a particular sensory processing disorder is identified, a plan can be put into place. Often the first step is to make environmental adaptations (i.e., find "fixes" for the things that bother him). The bumpy seams of his socks irritate your child? Replace them with seamless ones. Unwanted sounds distract him? Arrange with his teacher for him to wear noise-filtering headphones when he's doing quiet work at his desk.

A second approach might be for an OT to prescribe a *sensory diet* for your child. This is a "menu" of sensory activities designed to help your child maintain an optimal level of alertness and behave in a more organized manner throughout the day. Sample menu items might include chewing on gum or a plastic "chewy tube" to stimulate the facial muscles and satisfy oral needs, bouncing on a mini trampoline, or wearing a weighted vest (a vest with beanbag weights in the pockets) to provide deep stimulation to the sensory receptors in the skin, muscles, and joints.

A third method of helping a child with sensory difficulties is to have him participate in a specific program of activities that help "train his brain" to respond to sensory experiences in a more typical way. Each program needs to be carefully designed by a therapist with sensory processing expertise, so that the activities are not distressing or overwhelming for the child. These therapeutic activities often involve lots of movement, and might include riding across the floor while your child lies on his tummy on a scooter, moving through an obstacle course, or swinging on special swings.

Finally, there are many things that you can do at home to develop your child's sensory processing skills. For example, if your child is sensitive to touch, encourage him to rub his skin with different kinds of textures. Start with something soft (fur, silk, or cotton) and progress to something coarser or harder (terry facecloth, loofa sponge, or plastic kitchen scrubber). If your child has a hard time maintaining his balance, encourage him to walk on unstable surfaces (like a sandy beach or snow-covered sidewalk) or sit on a large therapy ball. The trick to home activities is to balance fun and success with a challenging experience for your child.

▪▪ Development in Adolescence and Adulthood

The end of childhood does not mean the end of development. All people, including those with Tourette syndrome, continue to grow and learn throughout their lives. Early milestones do lay the foundation for most major skills, but there are also important developmental goals in adolescence and young adulthood.

In adolescence, teens continue to tackle challenges in cognitive, physical, and social development. For example, they master increasingly complex academic subjects, become more skilled in athletic pursuits, and learn to maintain long-term friendships. These are all steps toward becoming independent adults. It's not surprising, therefore, that adolescents may feel anxious when development doesn't go as expected. By the same token, their confidence seems to grow more rapidly than in childhood,

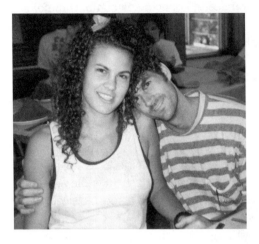

because when they succeed, they truly feel that they have reached their goals on their own.

In reaching independence, adolescents with Tourette syndrome may need to overcome more than the usual number of obstacles. Some typical social problems at school were touched on earlier. Teenagers with Tourette syndrome may also have problems with dating, fitting in with peers, or being accepted on the job. Each individual needs to make his own choices about whether, when, and how to talk about his TS with employers, coworkers, and friends. There is no single strategy that will work perfectly for all individuals in all situations.

Strategies for Adolescence and Adulthood

These barriers to full independence can be surmounted. Three factors are especially important in helping teenagers with Tourette syndrome make the final step to independence. First, your teen must strike a reasonable balance between early successes and failures. For example, it's not necessarily a bad thing to start learning a musical instrument and then lose interest. Everyone has interests that change over time. However, your teenager will likely feel better about giving up on music if he then takes up a sport or other leisure-time activity that he enjoys and sticks with it for a reasonable length of time. Second, your child needs a real sense of support and encouragement from others, both inside and outside the home. Much of this support will come from you, the parent. But remember, teachers can also be strong advocates for your adolescent and help out by teaching others about this disorder. Often, you need only give teachers the opportunity to learn about Tourette syndrome to enlist their support. And finally, your teen must have access to a reasonable flow of accurate information about Tourette syndrome and its real or fictitious limitations. This kind of self-education helps your teen gain some control over a disorder that, by its nature, causes considerable difficulties in controlling movements and vocalizations.

Given this kind of head start, the chances are that your adolescent will either conquer most developmental differences or learn to compensate for them satisfactorily. Your teen will have every reason to hope for optimal employment, good relationships with friends and family, and good self-esteem. Most importantly, your adolescent can grow up to be a healthy adult, capable of reaching his full potential.

:: Helping Your Child Overcome Developmental Problems: Summary

At this point, you may feel overwhelmed by the developmental challenges your child may face, and also by the importance of your role in helping him deal with them. If you don't know where to begin, start with the following guidelines. They may help you focus on the areas that will most help your child.

Understand Your Child's Tourette Syndrome or TS+. Both you and your child should understand all aspects of your child's disorder so that you can make informed decisions when solving problems.

Treat Your Child as a Normal Child. As much as possible, treat your child as you would any other child. Consider his personal strengths and weaknesses where appropriate, but give him all the responsibilities and limits he needs to develop into a responsible adult.

Have Realistic Expectations and Set Realistic Goals. This is an inherent part of good parenting. Expectations and goals need to be reasonable according to your child's age, strengths, and limitations to allow for challenge and success. Success in reaching early goals creates the energy and motivation needed for future goals.

Let Your Child Make Choices. Allowing a child to solve problems and make choices is essential to his self-esteem. By making his own choices—even ones you may know won't turn out well—your child will learn to take responsibility for himself and will gain confidence in his ability to control his own life.

Make Learning a Part of Daily Life. Try to teach social skills and life skills on a day-to-day basis, as situations occur. Whether you are showing your three-year-old how to dump a pebble out of his shoe or your fifteen-year-old how to plunge the toilet, "on the spot" lessons will teach your child to face problems, not avoid them. If something goes wrong, teach him to figure out a more successful way to deal with the situation in the future. You might want to try role-playing the situation over again with your child so he can "try on" the new behavior.

Boost Your Child's Organization and Independence. Make use of any strategies and devices that will help your child become more organized or independent on a day-to-day basis. For example, use reminder charts, Velcro sneakers, or special grips on utensils—whatever fits his particular needs.

Seek Help. Perhaps you are beginning to feel frustrated after reading some of the guidelines above. You may already have tried some of these strategies, but found that they haven't worked for you. If so, that may signal that you need some help in establishing a parenting

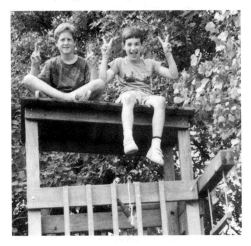

style that works for your child with TS and for your family as a whole. Or, it may signal that your child has additional challenges that need to be addressed. Either way, don't be afraid to seek help, not only for your child with TS, but also for your family. Your family doctor or your child's specialist can assist you in finding a psychologist or counselor, preferably one knowledgeable about TS, to help all of you deal with the stress of coping with TS. The doctor may also refer you to other developmental specialists if your child needs additional evaluations. Local TS support groups may also be helpful.

Obtain Needed Therapy Services. Occupational, physical, and speech therapists, as well as educational psychologists, can help your child overcome a variety of motor, self-help, and sensory problems. As explained in Chapter 8, these services are available free of charge through the school system if your child qualifies for special education. You may also want to consult private therapists, especially if your medical or life insurance will cover the costs. Other organizations that may help you find needed therapy services are listed in the Resource Guide at the back of this book.

▪▪ Conclusion

No two children develop in exactly the same way. Inborn strengths and weaknesses, as well as outside influences, all affect the speed and pattern of a child's development. Children with TS, too, will follow their own paths to maturity. Most likely, these paths will not be vastly different from other children's, although the TS and related disorders may make the journey more challenging. As a parent, there are many steps you can take to minimize the effects of TS and associated disorders on your child's development. You can seek help from professionals with expertise in treating developmental difficulties. You can work with teachers to develop the educational program and classroom atmosphere best suited to your child's learning needs. And you can support your child's efforts with information and understanding. Remember, if you view your child as an individual whose TS is only one aspect of his total being, he will be more likely to view himself as someone with abilities, rather than disabilities.

▪▪ Parent Statements

Children with TS seem to learn in big jumps, not in gradual, sustained progression. If your child is given the right kind of help, by the time he reaches high school, his behavior and ability to learn could be at an acceptable level.

❧

*Kids with TS and associated disorders often seem to be two or three years behind their peers socially and emotionally. They prefer to play with younger children rather than children their own age. **Accept** this symptom of TS. By the time your child is an adult, he'll have developed his own way of fitting in. Love him and build up his self-esteem. He'll catch up in his own time.*

❧

Concentrate on the abilities of your child with Tourette syndrome, not the disabilities.

❧

The hardest thing is that we have a child who doesn't look like he has a disability. But he acts extremely immature at times, trying to hide his tics by acting like a five-year-old. It's difficult, but we have to keep moving forward. We want to keep our son on the right track and work with his disability.

❧

TS can be compared to an electrical system that "shorts out" when it is overloaded, or to a computer that shuts down when it is overused. Kids with TS tend to shut down when they are bombarded by too many stimuli, too many directions, or too much activity. Anything that can be done to simplify your child's day, structure his activities, or help him to focus on only the most important skills or concepts to be learned will be helpful.

❧

Kathy's handwriting is so messy that she has to take a lot of her tests orally.

❧

My son is so good at echolalia; I think it could lead to a career in international translation.

❧

My son has incredible muscle tone from all his motor tics. That plus his high energy level makes him an asset on any sports team.

❧

Give value to special interest areas in children with Asperger syndrome and channel your child's interests into positive endeavors.

❧

I've recently been reading quite a bit about AD/HD and have learned about the role that executive function plays in getting yourself organized, prioritizing, following through on tasks. And it seems to me that a lot of my child's learning problems are actually related more to executive function deficits than to anything else.

❧

For me, it has always been difficult to know whether my daughter's developmental problems are related to any of her diagnoses, or are really more related to some developmental stage. I do think that just being an adolescent has a lot to do with some of the changes we're seeing in her these days.

◆✿❧

After six months of Sensory Integration therapy, my nine-year-old son is learning how to write, and his overall coordination has improved dramatically. He is learning how to stop and plan his actions rather than just acting impulsively.

◆✿❧

She used to lash out at anyone who touched her. After Sensory Integration therapy, she is much more tolerant of touch and has learned what kind of sensations and touch calm her down.

◆✿❧

I never thought Dave would be able or willing to play a team sport. We were thrilled when he joined a soccer team in fourth grade. He's always enjoyed individual sports, but participating on a team was really an achievement for him.

◆✿❧

Although many children who have TS Plus seem to have developmental delays, the same kids also have incredible talents in certain aspects of their development. It is up to parents and educators to nurture these special gifts and help each child reach his academic, social, and creative potential.

8

EDUCATIONAL NEEDS OF CHILDREN WITH TOURETTE SYNDROME

Larry Burd, Ph.D.

For some children, Tourette syndrome (TS) poses no special problem in the classroom. They keep up with the class in most, if not all, subjects. They discover special talents and interests, get along with most of their teachers and classmates, and eventually graduate with the academic, social, and vocational skills they need to fit into the adult world. But many children with TS do not progress through school quite so easily. Tics and other symptoms related to TS often produce academic or behavioral problems that require extra help if a child is to achieve her full potential in school.

The amount and type of help your child may need will depend on a variety of factors. First, your child may face special challenges in school, depending upon the severity of her tics and her attitude toward them. For example, if your child has loud, disruptive vocal tics or unusual motor tics such as touching or licking others, classmates may avoid or tease her. This can interfere with the development of age appropriate social skills. Regardless of how disruptive your child's tics are, she may have trouble learning if she expends a great deal of energy suppressing them. She may focus so much effort on not making sounds and movements that she has no energy left to accomplish her schoolwork.

Other conditions that often co-occur with Tourette syndrome can also lead to problems in school. For instance, nearly 60 percent of children with TS also have attention-deficit/hyperactivity disorder (AD/HD). If your child has trouble concentrating her attention, sitting still, shutting out distractions, or following instructions, that will obviously affect her learning. Learning disabilities related to reading, handwriting, spelling, and math are also very common. These problems are present in 23 percent (nearly one out of four) of children with TS.

Obsessive-compulsive disorder (OCD) is another problem often associated with TS that can cause difficulties in the classroom. Problems with obsessive and compulsive behaviors affect over 40 percent of children with TS. If your child must deal with obsessions in school, she may have trouble concentrating. Compulsions may also interrupt her work. For example, if your child has to silently count to 13 each time she thinks about the number 7, she will have difficulty completing her math assignments. If the teacher makes her keep working when she feels she has germs on her hands and wants to wash them for the twentieth time that day, she may not be able to work as rapidly as either of them would like.

Many children with TS plus OCD or Asperger syndrome have problems switching quickly from one task to another. They often feel they haven't finished the first task completely or that their work isn't perfect enough. As a result, they may become frustrated or irritable when they are asked to move on to the next activity, or when their regular routine is changed.

Despite the long list of possible problems, few children with Tourette syndrome have all of them. In fact, about 50 percent of children with Tourette syndrome have no educational problems or just have problems that require only minor adaptations to allow them to make satisfactory progress in school. Some may only require these modifications periodically when their symptoms are peaking, while others may need them more regularly. The other half can be helped through special educational programs tailored specifically to their needs. In time, the educational problems of many children in both groups become less severe. For about 60 percent of children with Tourette syndrome, educational difficulties peak between the ages of eight and thirteen, then gradually begin to decrease. By adulthood, the majority of people with TS have far fewer tics and related difficulties. The associated problems such as AD/HD and OCD typically get better in adulthood as well. But, in the mean time, you need to ensure that your child gets the best education possible, however severe or mild her symptoms might be.

To help you ensure that your child's school experience is as positive as possible, this chapter discusses how TS can cause problems for your child both inside and outside the regular classroom. It explains the concept of special education as well as why this may sometimes be the best route for children with Tourette syndrome. Finally, the chapter offers some specific solutions to common educational problems, and describes ways you can work with the school to help your child make the most of her school years.

∷ The Right Educational Program for Your Child

Because Tourette syndrome and related disorders can affect learning in so many different ways, there is no one "right" educational program for children with TS. Discovering what is best for *your* child may take some trial and error. Most often, children with TS start out in a regular classroom with their classmates of the same age. Extra help is usually needed only if they fail to achieve at the level of their ability in social, emotional, or academic areas.

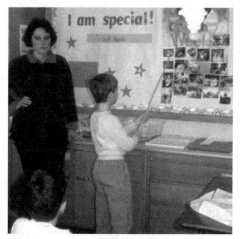

Even if your child's grades are good and her teachers do not report any special difficulties, it's wise to monitor her academic progress for problem areas once a diagnosis of Tourette syndrome is made. If your child *is* having academic, social, or emotional problems, in school or at home, she should be evaluated to determine the extent of the problem and to develop an appropriate intervention plan. This evaluation should be conducted by a "TS team" made up of you and your spouse, your child's physician, school personnel, and a resource person with expertise in developing management strategies for Tourette syndrome and the associated behaviors. Request that your school form a TS team if one is not already available.

From an academic standpoint, the TS team needs to evaluate reading, spelling, math, and handwriting skills, as well as your child's ability to pay attention and concentrate. From an emotional standpoint, the team should look at how well your child accepts her disorder and how it affects her self-image and her relationships with her teachers. Finally, the team needs to evaluate your child's social abilities: how well she gets along with others in her class, on the playground, at lunch, and home. For an adolescent, the team needs to monitor her progress with social peers. Does your child date? Does she have a peer group she "hangs out" with? Does she talk to friends on the phone or over the Internet?

One important concept that the TS team must keep in mind during the evaluation process is that many children with TS also have significant other impairments *that may not meet formal diagnostic criteria.* Yet these multiple *sub-threshold impairments* still need to be identified and addressed. For example, let's take a child with TS who has an all-encompassing interest in a collectible card game, gets very upset at any breaks in her daily routine, and erases her handwriting until she wears holes in the paper, because she wants it to be "perfect." She's also easily distracted, highly disorganized, and quite fidgety. This child may not meet the full DSM-IV-TR criteria for Asperger's disorder, obsessive-compulsive disorder, or attention-deficit/hyperactivity disorder—but she has some symptoms of each, all of which could interfere with her learning, behavior, or socialization. Sometimes even professionals forget that diagnostic criteria are just artificial frameworks that doctors designed to help understand and treat people with similar symptoms. If a child only meets, say, four out of six "required criteria" for a diagnosis, that doesn't mean she doesn't need help. It means the educational team needs to find interventions to address the symptoms, even if she isn't "coded" with the specific disorder.

Unfortunately, even though *cumulative impairment* from several sub-threshold disorders often causes academic difficulties, that fact is frequently missed in the assessment of children with TS. Three or more of these sub-threshold disorders can produce substantial impairments. Make sure that the person doing your child's assessment notes *all* relative weaknesses uncovered in the diagnostic evaluation, and describes their cumulative impact on your child's behavior, learning, and socialization.

Once the evaluation is completed, the TS team should meet and make recommendations. If the team agrees that your child's disorders are having a negative effect on her school performance, they will either recommend that she continue in the regular classroom with adaptations (this may be described as a "504 plan"), or they will recommend that your child be considered for special education services inside or outside of the classroom (usually only part-time). As a member of the team, it is your responsibility to help decide whether these recommendations or parts of them are appropriate for your child. Each of these options is discussed below.

Accommodations in The Regular Classroom

Within the regular classroom, your child may have academic or social problems that keep her from reaching her full potential. The TS team should work together to develop strategies to help her overcome these problems while remaining in her regular class. This should be the first option for children with problems in school.

Of course, before the teacher can understand how Tourette syndrome is affecting your child educationally, he or she needs a basic understanding of what TS is and is not. Too many adults misinterpret motor and vocal tics as nervous mannerisms or deliberate misbehavior. They often believe a child can control her tics—an impression that seems to be borne out when they ask the child to "quit it," and she is temporarily able to suppress his tics. Because attention problems may also wax and wane, the teacher may also incorrectly assume that because a child worked for twenty minutes on Tuesday, she should be able to do so every day. Most teachers see only a few children with Tourette syndrome during their entire teaching career and, therefore, misconceptions about TS are common.

To make sure all school staff involved with your child understand her specific symptoms and needs, the school should have a yearly inservice program on TS for all school personnel involved with your child. This session should be conducted by a knowledgeable professional from the nearest TS clinic, a representative from your local Tourette Syndrome Association (TSA) branch, or a teacher experienced in working with children with TS. You should also be present so that you can answer specific questions about how TS affects your child. The presenter should explain not only the symptoms that your child has now, but also the full range of symptoms and behaviors that may appear in the future and the waxing and waning nature of TS. This is important because symptoms often change—many symptoms that were present in September may have been replaced by others by June.

In addition to discussing your child's problems, the inservice program should include an opportunity for you and school personnel to discuss with the expert some proposed interventions, or ways of handling TS behaviors in class and of helping your child adjust and learn. These inservice sessions should be repeated on a yearly basis, since teaching the second grade teacher about Tourette syndrome does not inform the third grade teacher. In some cases, more frequent inservices may be necessary. A video on TS may not be sufficient for an inservice program, although videos and pamphlets can be used to supplement the program and provide examples of TS symptoms. The cost of inservice training *should* be a school responsibility. If your school doesn't readily agree to pay the costs, contact the TSA or other parents for help convincing the school district of its obligation.

Handling Symptoms in the Classroom

Educating the teacher about Tourette syndrome not only makes her more sensitive to your child's educational needs, but also to her emotional needs. Most importantly, it can help the teacher understand that by ignoring your child's tics, she can help reduce stress and, as a result, decrease the number and intensity of your child's tics. And because of the teacher's unique position as a role model, it is important for her to set an appropriate example. If the teacher ignores your child's tics, your child's classmates are much more likely to be able to ignore them as well.

Even if everyone in the class successfully ignores your child's tics, your child may still be quite aware of her own sounds and movements. This self-consciousness may lead your child to try to suppress her tics. This generally isn't a successful tactic. Suppressing multiple motor and phonic tics requires considerable attention and effort. If your child is working to hold back tics, she may not be able to concentrate and work up to her full ability in school. A better approach is for you and the teacher to develop ways for your child to release her tics in relative privacy. For example, your child could be seated near the classroom door so that whenever she feels the need, she can get up, walk down the hall for a drink of water, and discharge her motor tics. Or the teacher might allow her to go out to a private setting to discharge vocal tics. But remember, as important as these strategies are, it is just as important to have the teacher set an example by ignoring the tics and concentrating on getting the class's assignments completed.

If your child's tics are quite disruptive, embarrassing, or uncomfortable, her doctor may prescribe medication. This may or may not enable her to control her tics—or you may decide the side-effects of some medications outweigh the benefits. (It's important to note that the school does not have the right to demand your child be medicated.) If the medication isn't sufficient, or if you're hesitant about using it, a trained therapist may be able to help your child substitute a positive behavior that is incompatible with the tic. (See Chapter 4.)

Social and Behavioral Problems

Sometimes a child's symptoms may interfere with the development of normal social relationships. A child who has AD/HD in addition to TS may often be "in trouble" because of her behavior. If she is walking around when she is supposed to be sitting down doing her work, or she is talking when she should be listening, the other children quickly figure out that doing things with her will often get them into trouble too. As a result, many children may avoid the child with TS to avoid getting into trouble. Other children may also avoid or tease your child if she has tics that attract attention, such as sniffing, barking, or snorting, or tics that involve kicking, touching, or patting others.

Social skills training/therapy for a child who seems to have poor empathy or poor impulse control (e.g., blurting out whatever comes into her head—which can have a very negative social effect) may be an important component of her educational plan.

If your child's symptoms result in significant social difficulties, you, the teacher, and the TS team will need to develop ways to help her manage this problem. The first goal should be to design a positive and reward-oriented program that focuses on the behaviors you would like to see *increase* in frequency. All too often, schools begin with a list of problem behaviors and concentrate on eliminating them. They count how many times Crystal gets up out of her seat, how many spelling problems she doesn't finish, how often she talks out of turn. But they do not keep track of how often she's sitting in her seat, how many spelling problems she gets done, or how often she holds up her hand or waits her turn before she talks. Clearly, a focus on positive behaviors is often the preferred initial strategy. The more attention is paid to a particular behavior, the more likely a child is to repeat it.

An important key in improving behavior is to determine what your child finds rewarding and link that reward with a behavior you would like to see more often. For some children, praise may be rewarding; others need more tangible rewards such as smiley faces or gold stars on their papers or permission to do something fun. For adolescents, increased privileges or money may work. Generally, school personnel should link one particular reward with each different behavior they want to improve. For example, rather than using tokens that can be exchanged for treats to reinforce four or five different behaviors, it may be better to reward one behavior with time playing computer games, another behavior with a special visit to the library, and a third behavior with tokens.

Rewarding behaviors can be quite time-consuming for teachers. First, because rewards are only effective if they are given consistently, the teacher has to make sure he or she rewards your child nearly every time she demonstrates the target behavior. Second, to determine whether rewards are actually working, the teacher must count the frequency of your child's behaviors both before and after beginning the reward program. Therefore, it's often best if a teacher begins by concentrating on one or two behaviors. It is unlikely that a classroom teacher by herself could deal with more than three behaviors at a time. After all, if she has too much to do, she may not be able to accurately record the behaviors or give rewards consistently—let alone teach the other members of the class.

Academic Problems

If your child is having academic difficulties, you first need to find out why. For example, if she has trouble finishing work on time, is it because she's using all her energy to suppress tics? Does she have a compulsion to erase the words over and over until they are perfect? Is it because her medications make her feel dull and slow her thinking? The TS team needs this information in order to understand the problem and develop an appropriate intervention strategy.

Many children with Tourette syndrome have academic difficulties not because they cannot *do* the work, but because they cannot *complete* it. As noted above, this could be due to tics, attention problems, or obsessions or compulsions. Often it is helpful to break the work up into shorter segments. For example, instead of giving a child twenty math problems to solve, give her seven, five, or three at a time, several times a day. Then, as her work habits improve, the teacher can increase the number of problems she gives her each time.

Stress is another factor that can affect academic performance. The stress of taking a test, for example, may increase your child's tics and make it harder for her to concentrate. Time limits may be a problem for children with obsessions or compulsive behaviors, especially at the start of the behavior plan. If so, it may help if the teacher gives her more time to finish or allows her to take the test in a separate room.

A peer tutor—a classmate or older child who is doing well in school—may also be able to help your child. The peer tutor can work with your child side by side during school, or help her after school. For example, a peer might help your child do her work by reminding her to finish her last two problems or by setting a good example and not talking with your child when she is doing her own seat work. A sensitive, accepting older tutor can also be very helpful in improving your child's socialization skills and expanding opportunities for social activities. Selecting popular peer tutors can have many benefits socially, as well as educationally.

This section has provided only a brief summary of strategies to handle common problems within the regular classroom. For additional strategies that can be helpful both in the regular classroom and in the special education classroom, see the section at the end of this chapter on "Common Problems and Solutions."

:: Special Education

If your child has significant academic, behavioral, or social problems despite in-class modifications, she may be considered for special education. It's important to understand that "special education" means something very different today than it did a generation ago. Today, special education means instruction that is individually tailored to meet the unique learning needs of a child with disabilities. The goal of special education services is to enable children to learn as efficiently as possible so that they are eventually able to live the most independent lives possible. Consequently, special education does not just focus on helping children overcome difficulties in academic subjects such as reading, math, and history. It also includes special therapeutic or other services designed to help children overcome difficulties in all areas of development.

By law, a child's special education program must include all special services, or "related services," necessary for her to benefit from her educational program. These services are provided by one or more professionals trained in working with children with special needs. For chil-

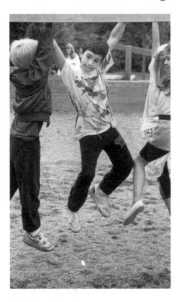

dren with Tourette syndrome, related services may include speech therapy, physical or occupational therapy, nursing services, inservice training, and a wide range of adaptations in a child's regular school program.

Special education is not an all-or-nothing proposition. Receiving special education services doesn't necessarily mean that your child will be sent to a different room all day. In fact, she will probably take most or all of her subjects in the regular classroom. For instance, if your child has a reading disorder, she may receive special assistance from a learning disabilities teacher who comes to her classroom several times per week, or she may receive "pull out" services in a special resource room. Or, the plan could simply have the mainstream classroom teacher modify his or her teaching methods or your child's materials in a way that will make it easier for your child to learn. If your child has wide fluctuations in her problem areas, she may benefit from having extra flexibility built into her program, allowing her to receive additional support and services when she needs them. Remember, the key is an individualized program to meet your child's unique needs.

The Assessment Process

Before your child can receive special education services, she must first be declared "eligible." As Chapter 9 explains, federal laws govern who can qualify for special education. Only a child with a disability that prevents her from making appropriate progress in school can receive special educational services at public expense. Your child may qualify for services if she's been diagnosed with a learning disability or if her tics or related disorders (OCD, AD/HD, etc.) interfere with her progress in school. Typically, the school will use the designation "other health impaired" to qualify your child for services. (TS is a neurological disorder, so it should usually *not* be coded as "emotionally behaviorally disturbed," as has been known to happen.) Once qualified, your child will be eligible for programming for the full range of her educational needs.

To determine whether your child needs and qualifies for special education, you or a school staff member must first make a written request for a special education assessment. This assessment cannot be conducted unless you give your permission. Once you give the go-ahead, your child's learning needs will be assessed, or evaluated, by a *multidisciplinary assessment team*. As the name implies, this team will be made up of specialists with different areas of expertise, as well as you, the parents. Usually, the same professionals who are on the TS team are a part of the multidisciplinary team.

To evaluate your child's abilities in each developmental area, members of the team will observe your child, collect data on her performance in the classroom, interview you and your child's teachers about her strengths and needs, and give her formal tests. The goal of this testing is two-fold: first, to identify problem areas, and second, to identify areas of strength that could potentially be used to compensate for the difficulties. For example, if your child has difficulty with handwriting, but is interested in computers, the team might suggest she be given keyboarding instruction.

In identifying problem areas, the team members will also try to determine whether a learning disability or some other underlying problem is interfering with your child's progress. For this reason, the multidisciplinary team should request input from your child's physician about the diagnosis, other associated difficulties such as AD/HD or obsessive-compulsive disorder, and side effects of any medication your child might be taking. It is also important that the physician provide information on the benefits of medications your child is taking so that the school is not misled by any apparent lack of symptoms. After all, the purpose of the medication is to suppress symptoms. But if school personnel don't observe the symptoms, they may doubt the diagnosis. This information is essential in planning a program for your child. With your consent, the physician can send his report to the school, or he can provide the TS team with the essential information through a phone conversation or letter.

After all team members have gathered information in their areas of expertise, the team will meet to share their findings. Then together you will develop a comprehensive summary report of your child's strengths and needs in all areas. At this meeting, the team members will discuss with you what they have discovered about your child's learning abilities and disabilities. The team will also decide whether your child is recommended for special education services. If you disagree with their recommendation, you may request a second assessment. Chapter 9 explains this process.

▪▪ Tourette Syndrome, Learning Disabilities, and Related Difficulties

Children with Tourette syndrome frequently have additional symptoms that negatively affect their school work. These difficulties occur even more frequently in children who have both Tourette syndrome and a specific learning disability, as illustrated in the table below....

Incidence of Symptoms and/or Disorders that May Affect School Performance

	Among Children with Tourette Syndrome but *No* Learning Disability	Among Children with Tourette Syndrome *and* a Comorbid Learning Disability
AD/HD	51%	80%
Anger/Rage Attacks	34%	46%
Sleep Disorders	24%	30%
Mood Disorders	18%	22%
Social Skills Difficulties	15%	33%
Anxiety Disorder	16%	20%

Developing an Educational Plan

If your child qualifies for special education, the next step is to develop a plan to meet her unique learning needs. This plan, known in the U.S. as an Individualized Education Program (IEP), will be designed jointly by you and school staff (as well as anyone else you want to bring) at one or more IEP meetings. Depending on your child's age and maturity level, she may participate on the IEP team as well.

Setting Goals

Your child's IEP will describe each of the areas in which your child has learning problems, as well as how the school plans to help her overcome these problems. For each area, precise, measurable, long-term goals will be set. For example, if your son has trouble spelling, a goal might be for her to pass the semester test. This overall goal would be broken down into smaller, short-term goals. For example, she might be expected to learn seven spelling words a week, or perhaps, two spelling words a day. If your child has difficulty concentrating because of AD/HD, a long-term goal might be to complete ten math problems in fifteen minutes. As a short-term goal, she might be expected to do five in fifteen minutes, then gradually work up to six, seven, or eight in fifteen minutes. Short- and long-term goals could likewise be set for a child with the OCD symptoms of writing, erasing, and rewriting until the work is perfect. If the ultimate goal is to have her write all her spelling sentences

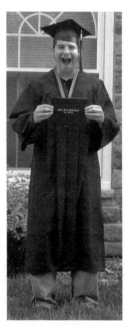

without erasing, a short-term goal might be to limit her to eight erasures, then seven, then six, and so on. Use of a computer might also help her make her letters "perfect," and therefore limit erasures.

When choosing goals, it's also important to choose rewards that will help motivate your child to work towards those goals. For example, it may be helpful to reward a child with *less* work when she does what she is supposed to do. For example, if your child has fifteen math problems and does ten in twelve minutes, the teacher could reward her by telling her she doesn't have to do the other five. That makes her more inclined to concentrate and work quickly next time. (As opposed to giving her additional work if she finishes a task quickly—a common mistake both teachers and parents sometimes make.)

If the TS team members determine your child needs assistance in nonacademic areas as well, they will write goals for additional services. For example, if she is having difficulty making or keeping friends, her IEP might include social skills goals. Her IEP might call for her to select one classmate each week to invite over to her house to play after school. She would then practice the required social skills—calling someone on the phone, inviting them over, suggesting games they could play, etc.—with the plan implemented by the school psychologist, counselor, speech therapist, or perhaps special education teachers. When the child is comfortable using the skills on her own, then a new social skill would be targeted.

Developing social skills is extremely important for children with Tourette syndrome. It may also be more difficult for them because they have a wide range of behaviors that are not completely under their control. These behaviors may drive potential friends away. After all, most children quickly learn that if you hang around with Dara and Dara gets in trouble, you will also probably get in trouble at the same time. That's why it is so important that teachers focus on increasing positive behaviors and try to ignore negative behaviors when possible.

Who Will Teach Your Child in What Setting

Your child's IEP will specify who is to work with her on each goal. This might be the regular classroom teacher, the classroom teacher and a peer tutor, a therapist, or a school aide. Or your child might need to work with a special education teacher or tutor specially trained in teaching children with special learning needs.

The IEP will also specify where your child is to receive this instruction—within the regular classroom or in a learning resources room. Generally, children receive services outside of the regular classroom only if they cannot work up to their level of ability with modifications or extra assistance given in the regular classroom. If your child does need to leave the regular classroom, it may just be to work on one particular subject or one skill. For example, your child might see the learning disabilities teacher once a day for special help in reading, but receive all her other lessons with the rest of the class. If her symptoms are so severe that they cannot be managed in the regular classroom with adaptations, she may require longer periods out of the classroom. In some cases, teachers (who are human and have all the limitations that trouble the rest of us) simply cannot deal appropriately with a child's behavior. If another teacher is not available, and support and training do not help the teacher deal with the child's behavior, then some out-of-class placement may be the only practical option.

Tips on Designing an Effective IEP

The following basic principles may help you or school personnel in designing an effective IEP for your child:

> **1. Focus on positive behavior.** Try to build on your child's
> strengths. If she has good attention but poor handwriting,

for example, it may help to have her use a computer or calculator for more of her work.

2. **Set goals based on what your child *usually* can do,** not on what she can do on her best days. This is especially important because of the waxing and waning of TS symptoms. When your child's tics (head turning, eye squinting) are at low levels, she will naturally be able to concentrate on her work better than when she turns her head thirty times an hour or squints twenty times every eight minutes.

3. **Provide support and motivation to increase skills.** Pay attention to positive behaviors and use positive reinforcement whenever possible. Be flexible—adjust the workload on more difficult days.

4. **Expect your child's school performance to vary.** As her tics and associated behaviors vary, so will her performance in school.

In developing an educational program, it is essential that you carefully weigh the pros and cons of each decision. Every member of the TS team should explain their recommendations and what short- and long-term effects they expect them to have on your child. As a parent, you should weigh the risks and benefits of each recommended objective before signing off on a program for your child. For example, are the benefits of special education greater than the problems? Is the benefit of a medication greater than its side effects? This balancing process is difficult because each child is unique and each situation is different. Often it comes down to deciding to try a given strategy or program briefly and then evaluate the results.

Monitoring Progress

In the United States, children are entitled to receive special education until the age of twenty-one, if they need it. But once your child begins receiving special education services, that doesn't necessarily mean she will continue receiving them for the rest of her school years. Depending on your child's needs, the duration of her special education services may vary. You and the school personnel will review her progress at a meeting called an *annual review*. Together, you will discuss whether she is learning faster or slower than expected, and whether the goals set in her IEP were too high or too low. Your conclusions will be incorporated into a new IEP for the coming year.

Every three years, at a minimum, your child will receive a *triennial evaluation*—a complete reassessment conducted by the multidisciplinary team (unless all members of the team agree that a new assessment is not needed). After reevaluating your child, the team will decide whether she still requires special education. If she doesn't, they will recommend that she no longer receive special education services. You and your child's teachers may also request that she be reevaluated after less than three years if you think a special education placement is no longer appropriate for her. On the other hand, if you feel the team is not recommending sufficient services, you can also request a reevaluation.

To Label or Not to Label?

Often when parents are asked to consider special education for their child, they worry about the possibility of the twin "stigmas" of having their child labeled "disabled" and "special ed." Clearly, in the best of all worlds, children would not have problems like TS or AD/HD. This, however, is simply not the world we live in, and many children *do* require additional help in school.

Unfortunately, there is some stigma attached to anyone who is different or requires extra help. Even in the first grade, children can quickly recognize the top reading group—whether it's called the Bluebirds or the Beavers—and they can also recognize the "lower" reading groups. Differences are not something we should try to hide. Instead, we should try to equip children to see these differences *and* the inherent value in each person as an individual—whether they have difficulty with handwriting, reading, or sitting still.

It's true that requiring children to fit into a disability category to be eligible for special education can be construed as labeling the child. But you could also view this as giving the child every opportunity to do her best and live up to her potential. Depriving your child of these services because you fear how she may react to a label may not be in her best interests. This is particularly true if your child will have significant academic and social problems if she tries to manage on her own, but could conquer these problems with additional help in school. Your child may even feel relieved to be doing something about a problem that she knows sets her apart from other children.

The "stigma" of special education services has changed over the last twenty to thirty years. With so many children diagnosed with AD/HD, learning disabilities, and Asperger syndrome nowadays, many parents are more concerned that their child isn't being given *enough* services, rather than being reluctant to have their child "labeled."

▪▪ Common Problems and Solutions

There are no foolproof methods for dealing with the educational problems related to TS. But there *are* many methods that are often effective, whether your child is taught in a regular or special education setting. To help you and your child's teacher handle potential difficulties, some of these common problems and possible solutions are described below.

Tics

Tics and Stress

It's important for teachers to understand that stress often makes tics become more frequent or pronounced. For example, taking a test, giving a speech, or being teased or punished may cause tics to intensify. Increasing your child's involvement in activities that she enjoys such as sports or music can help reduce stress. Often children with TS don't have as much time to play as other kids do. As a parent, you should keep track of your child's free time and encourage her to participate in fun activities with other children.

Waxing and Waning of Tics

There are several things teachers need to understand about the tendency of tics to wax and wane. First, they should know that even though symptoms will change over time and appear milder at some times than at others, that doesn't mean the tics are under your child's control. Furthermore, if they ask your child to suppress her tics, she may feel increased stress and have less energy to devote to her schoolwork. Second, if your child has severe TS, they should realize that it may be necessary to have two educational plans—a fallback plan for days when her symptoms are at their most disruptive, and another program for her average or better days. For example, on the most difficult days, your child could be given more breaks, more activities outside the classroom, and shorter assignments.

In setting overall educational goals for your child, you and the school staff need to consider how she does on an *average* day. Explain it to them this way: If you go to a junior high basketball game, you might occasionally see a child make nine shots in a row. But it wouldn't be reasonable for the coach to expect the child to perform that well at every subsequent basketball game. Rather, the coach should recognize that making nine baskets in a row was an unusually good performance—far beyond what the child could be expected to do every time. Likewise, on an exceptional day, a child with AD/HD and TS might get her math done in class and stay seated during the entire class period. But on an average day, she may complete only ten out of fifteen math problems (with four reminders from the teacher) and get out of her desk three times. Expectations should be based on her average performance, rather than on what she can do on an exceptional day.

Motor and Vocal Tics

The general rule for motor and vocal tics is to ignore them. Teachers should not encourage or reward your child for not having tics, as this may encourage her to suppress them. Instead, teachers should provide a place for your child to go to release her tics when necessary. Asking the teacher to explain Tourette syndrome and the difficulties your child faces (or letting you or a local expert on TS come in to explain) may also help foster an accepting atmosphere in the classroom. Rarely, your child's motor tics may raise a safety consideration—for example, in shop class or chemistry. In this case, the TS team may recommend an alternate activity for your child. Finally, if your child has tics that are particularly distracting to other children, there are several strategies to try. You may want to consult with your physician about the use of medication (see Chapter 3), or with a psychologist who's trained in the latest behavioral techniques for reversing specific tics or compulsive behaviors (see Chapter 4). Of course, before starting any treatment program, make sure the specialist fully describes any possible side effects, so you can make an educated decision.

Mental Tics

Some children with Tourette syndrome need to repeat words, numbers, or phrases to themselves. Children with these kinds of mental tics should be given extra time to respond to questions, to complete assignments, and to refocus their attention from one activity to another. In addition, it often helps to break assignments into shorter segments. Making it easier for your child to predict what is going to be next may also increase her ability to complete her work. For this reason, the teacher and the TS team may need to work together to develop a schedule for the child that can be followed consistently.

Obsessive-Compulsive Behaviors

The treatment of obsessions and compulsions is complex. Nearly always, both a clinical psychologist and a physician will need to be involved, since medication can be very helpful. Chapter 3 discusses medical treatments for OCD symptoms.

The first step in managing OCD behaviors at school is generally to develop an understanding of the symptom and its frequency. For example, writing, erasing, and rewriting letters until they are perfect is a common symptom. To manage this symptom, the teacher needs to begin by counting how often the child erases her work, and then gradually limit the number of times she is allowed to erase, using a reward each time she finishes her work without going over the limit. Suddenly imposing a "no erasing" rule or taking the child's eraser away would only create more stress for the child and likely cause other symptoms to increase.

In treating obsessions, it may be helpful to set time limits for certain tasks. For example, if it takes your child eight minutes to write two sentences, the time allowed should gradually be reduced by ten- or fifteen-second intervals. Although many children with OCD are very slow workers, they can often learn to work more quickly if their time to finish a task is limited and linked to a positive reward.

Teachers also need to understand that, like tics, obsessions and compulsions can wax and wane. Just because your child didn't insist on washing her hands repeatedly last week, that doesn't mean she's "being difficult" when she insists on doing it this week.

Challenging Behavior

Anger or Aggression

If your child has difficulty controlling anger or aggression in the classroom, it may help if teachers allow her to channel her aggression into physical movement. For example, she might be permitted to walk down the hall for a drink of water or to lie down and pedal in the air. Relaxation techniques may also be helpful. If appropriate, a clinical psychologist can provide your child with a tape of relaxation exercises to keep in class and listen to on headphones when she needs to calm down.

It is also important to provide explanations for those likely to be the target of aggression. The TS team or teacher should lead the discussion with the other students, emphasizing that the child with TS has difficulty controlling her behavior, and that other children should not take her actions or aggression personally. The TS team should be sure to let the other students know how to react and what to do if they witness aggressive behavior.

Restlessness

If your child is unable to sit still or fidgets constantly, she should be allowed to move about safely and freely (within reason) as needed. The TS team may consider "fidget toys," special seat cushions, etc. as options for your child. Restlessness should be reported to your physician, as it may be a symptom of AD/HD and is sometimes a side effect of medications used to control tics. As discussed earlier, a positive reward program can also be very helpful in encouraging your child to do her work and complete her assignments.

Difficulty Disciplining Your Child

If your child's behavior causes problems in the classroom, teachers should first try to control it with positive behavior management. That is, rather than punishing your child for inappropriate behavior, they should focus on the behavior they would like to increase in frequency. In particular, they need to understand that they should never punish your child for tics, because the stress of punishment may increase her tics.

For a program to be successful, it is helpful if behavior is managed the same way at home as it is at school. Otherwise, your child will get mixed messages about which behavior is acceptable and which is not. For example, if both parents and teachers ignore a child when she has a tantrum, the child is less likely to use tantrums as a way of getting attention. But if parents give in to their child's wishes when she has a tantrum at home, then she is more likely to resort to tantrums at school, too, even if teachers try to ignore her behavior.

Attention Problems

Many children with Tourette syndrome also have attention-deficit/hyperactivity disorder. As a result, they may have poor concentration, be quite distractible, and have trouble finishing their work. In general, AD/HD in children with TS can be handled the same ways it would be in children without TS. However, the first line of treatment of AD/HD today is often stimulants. And while some kids with TS can handle the stimulants, others can't. As with behavior problems, the initial strategy for symptoms of AD/HD is posi-tive behavior management. Teachers should focus on the behaviors that they would like to increase in frequency. For example, rather than count-ing how many times your child does not finish her work, they should count how many problems she completed and how many reminders were necessary to get it done.

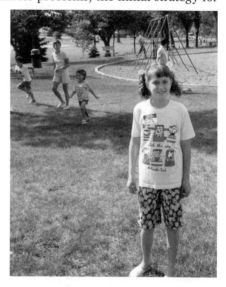

Keeping frustration at manageable levels also helps. Your child should not be given more work than she can han-dle comfortably, and assignments should be shortened if she cannot complete them. Rather than guessing, the teacher should make sure the length of the assignment is within your child's capability. No child can be expected to develop appropriate work habits if she is overloaded with work and then punished when she cannot do the work.

As your child grows older, she will probably need extra help devel-oping individual work and study skills. Using study guides or outlines provided by the teacher may help her stay focused while studying. Posi-tive reinforcement will also continue to be important. Your child should be encouraged to complete tasks before being given any rewards (e.g., she can get on the Internet *after* she's completed her homework).

Some children with AD/HD and TS may learn better outside of the regular classroom. It may be easier for them to concentrate and learn in a resource room where there are fewer distractions and where they can receive more individualized attention from teachers. This step may be recommended if your child fails to work up to the level of her ability and if modifications within the regular classroom do not improve her performance.

Learning Disabilities

As mentioned earlier, about 22 percent of children with TS also have learning disabilities. That is, there is a discrepancy between their level of intelligence and their achievement in reading, writing, or math that is not due to poor hearing or vision, poor school attendance, or limited proficiency in English. Learning disabilities affect three times as many boys as girls. The most common learning disabilities are in reading, spelling, handwriting, and math. Reading problems account for more than half of all learning disabilities and may make it difficult for a child to say the words she reads (decoding difficulties), or understand what she has read (reading comprehension disorders) or both. Spelling and handwriting problems are also very common and often occur together with reading problems or language disorders. Children with learning disabilities in math may only have difficulty with calculations, or they may have additional problems with mathematical reasoning, visual-spatial concepts, word problems, or following directions for assignments.

If learning disabilities are suspected, an evaluation by the multidisciplinary team described earlier is essential. This is because handwriting and math difficulties can also be the result of AD/HD, and if so, need to be addressed differently. For learning disabilities, the first step is usually to modify a child's regular curriculum. Your child may be able to make satisfactory progress with a tutor, reduced amounts of work, and use of positive reinforcement. With the emphasis on how much she is able to do, rather than on how much she can't do, your child's motivation may increase. Other in-class modifications might include oral tests and taped notes from the teacher for children with reading difficulties or the use of calculators for children with calculation difficulties. Likewise, computers can help children with handwriting problems improve their ability to express themselves in writing. A word processing program with spelling and grammar checkers allows the child to use any word she wants without having to worry about spelling it correctly or substituting easier words. Some children with learning disabilities may require educational interventions for the LD as well as the TS.

If in-class modifications are not enough to enable a child with learning disabilities to progress, she may receive special education services in her regular classroom or attend classes in a special resource room for part of the day. That way, she can benefit from instructional methods and materials specifically designed to help children with learning disabilities. The Reading List at the back of the book lists several publications that describe these teaching methods in detail.

The education program for each child with learning disabilities must be individually tailored to her unique needs. It must also be reviewed at least once a year so that any changes necessary can be made. This is particularly important for a child with TS plus learning disabilities, because her symptoms will likely change over time, peaking in early adolescence and lessening as she moves into her later teens. If a child's motivation and desire to do well are nurtured when she is young, her academic abilities will usually improve during adolescence and into adulthood.

Medications

As a parent, you need to ask your child's physician for detailed, current information about any medications prescribed for your child. If school personnel are to administer your child's drugs, make sure they understand how and when to do so. Be sure also to educate the teacher(s) about the side effects and effectiveness of these drugs. Ask him or her to report side effects to you and to let you know if the drugs are having the desired result. Teachers should be especially watchful for signs of cognitive dulling, lethargy, seeming lack of interest, irritability, tearfulness, or decrease in coordination. If these side effects appear, have your child reevaluated by her physician and find out whether the medication can be adjusted or given in the evening. If necessary, ask the teacher to allow your child extra time for studying and test-taking, extra breaks, or request a tutor if appropriate and not in the IEP already.

School Phobia

A small number of children with TS develop a school phobia—a strong avoidance of school (not wanting to leave home and go to school). Children wake up in the morning complaining of headaches, stomach problems, or other vague symptoms that they hope will keep them home from school. Attempts by parents to get the child to school may result in clinging and loud, tearful complaints. The child may also voice a wide range of fears about going to school—for example, "I'm afraid of the teacher" or "The other kids tease me." In severe cases, children may miss months of school if this problem is not successfully treated. Even in milder cases, frequent absences can result in serious disagreements between parents and school personnel.

School phobias sometimes emerge when neuroleptic medications such as haloperidol (Haldol™) or Pimozide (Orap™) are used to treat Tourette syndrome. If so, a change of medication may help. Often, however, school phobias require treatment by a team made up of the physician, a psychologist, school personnel, and family. See Chapter 3 for information on drug side effects, as well as on choosing and working with physicians and psychologists.

Social and Emotional Problems

Because of their differences, some children with Tourette syndrome feel isolated from their classmates. To help your child cope with loneliness or depression, the TS team should develop a plan to increase her self-esteem. For example, teachers might praise her for minor accomplishments and help her to recognize her special talents. All members of the team also need to encourage your child to participate in group and social activities.

Adults both at home and at school must make a concerted effort to prevent your child from being teased by other children. Teasing is tolerated far too often in the schools and is devastating to a child's self-esteem. When teasing occurs, it is not your child's fault. Rather, it results from the inability of teachers and other adults to control other children's behavior. Your child shouldn't have to "learn to ignore it" or "work it out with the other kids herself." Teachers and principals must explain to other children that TS symptoms are not under your child's control, and that teasing will not be tolerated. Educational films about Tourette syndrome can be helpful in opening up discussions about Tourette syndrome in the classroom. All school staff must be aware of your child's TS so that when she is teased on the playground or in the lunchroom, they will know how to intervene.

As a parent, be prepared to counter arguments from school personnel who may claim it isn't possible or reasonable for them to limit teasing. That type of thinking is outdated and hypocritical. Many schools today have implemented successful anti-teasing and anti-bullying programs. Ask the teacher how he would like it if his peers harassed him so much that he couldn't use a school bathroom without the principal accompanying him. Ask the principal how she'd feel if her peers pursued her every night after school, mocking her and threatening her. School personnel must teach acceptance of differences, and it's their duty to make school a safe place for every child.

If persistent teasing occurs outside the school, it is a more complex matter. You may be able to help by contacting the parent of the child who is teasing your child and politely explaining the situation to him or her. It often helps if you emphasize that you do not think the other child is deliberately being cruel, but that he or she just doesn't understand that the TS symptoms are really out of your child's control.

Because your child may have a variety of social and emotional problems related to school, it is important to encourage her to talk about her feelings on a one-to-one basis with you. You might also encourage her to join a peer group in which she can discuss her experiences with other children with Tourette syndrome (or other disabilities). The Tourette Syndrome Association can help you locate a group for your child.

Handwriting

Some children with Tourette syndrome have great difficulty with handwriting. These problems may be due to motor tics or related to the AD/HD that many children with TS have. Occupational therapy may help with her fine motor skills. Common classroom accommodations for handwriting problems include allowing your child to use a tape recorder rather than requiring her to take written notes; permitting her to use a classmate's notes or the teacher's lecture notes; assigning her oral, rather than written reports; providing her with a computer or access to a computer.

Teachers should be especially flexible in designing alternate ways for your child to take tests. Most states have specific rules about testing accommodations for the mandated assessments, and any testing accommodations should be stated in the IEP. They might, for example, allow her to dictate answers on essay tests. Or on standardized tests, they might allow her to circle the answers

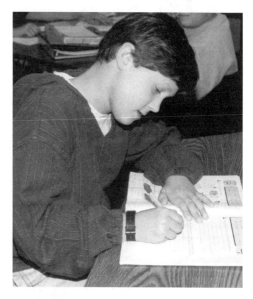

in the test booklet, rather than make her fill in small circles on an answer sheet. Being allowed extra time to take the test is another common testing accommodation.

Homework

For children with Tourette syndrome, homework often includes work they weren't able to finish in school because of AD/HD, mental tics, or handwriting problems. If your child routinely has trouble completing her schoolwork, work with her teacher to set a level where work can be finished in a timely fashion. For example, instead of expecting your child to do twenty math problems in a row, have her do three, then take a break, do three more, and then take another break.

Not surprisingly, the same problems that make it difficult for children with TS to complete their work at school also make it difficult for them to complete their homework. They often have trouble getting organized, getting started, and staying on task. On top of that, they are now working after a full day of school, when they may be tired. Thus, for some children homework may need to be limited.

You can help your child with organizational problems by setting aside a special place for her to do homework and making sure the area is kept stocked with pencils, paper, dictionaries, and other school supplies. It may also be helpful to set aside a specific time every day for homework. You might even want to establish a quiet hour for the whole family to spend reading or doing homework.

You may want to ask the school to provide a second set of textbooks for your child to keep at home. This can have two advantages: 1) She doesn't have to remember which ones to bring home each afternoon, and 2) If your child's symptoms cause her to miss parts of lectures, having the book at home will allow her to catch up (or allow you to understand her homework assignment)!

Although you may need to be more directly involved in your child's homework than you would if she did not have Tourette syndrome, it is important not to do too much for her. Don't let her take advantage of your extra help. Your aim should be to work with her to develop her skills so that eventually she can do the work independently. If homework becomes a source of increasing conflict, this problem may require a change in your child's IEP.

Parent-School Relationships

Parents of children with Tourette syndrome often start out on the wrong foot with their child's school. Frequently, problems develop before a diagnosis of Tourette syndrome is reached. Even though parents insist that their child cannot control her behavior, schools may attempt to punish the child for her tics. Or schools may punish children who cannot complete their work due to AD/HD or learning disabilities. Then, once Tourette syndrome is diagnosed, parents may feel the diagnosis gives a sense of legitimacy to problems the school has previously seen as willful misbehavior. They may have a strong desire to go up to school personnel and tell them what they *really* think about their past programs.

As much as you may feel like saying "I told you so" to the school, this is a tactic that clearly should be avoided. Before you will be able to work together with school staff to develop the best educational plan for your child, you must develop a relationship based on mutual respect. This means you may have to forget many past wrongs so that you can look ahead to ways you can improve things for your child. Simply stated, what's past is past, and rarely does it do any good to continue to point out to the school that they were wrong and you were right.

A more constructive approach is to try to foster an improved climate in which to meet and discuss changes. As discussed earlier, it is wise to arrange for an inservice training program to help school personnel learn about Tourette syndrome and how it affects your child. Showing one or two videos from the TSA and sharing this book may also help.

Once the school personnel have a better understanding of Tourette syndrome, try asking them what they think would be some appropriate programming suggestions in light of their new knowledge. Afterwards, sort through this information and select the goals, objectives, and strategies that you feel are appropriate. Don't criticize any inappropriate ideas the school has, but focus on those that are useful. In other words, use positive reinforcement with school personnel for their worthwhile efforts. Next, contribute some of your own ideas of goals and techniques that would be helpful at school. By using this strategy, you can often see agreement in major areas of need where before it looked as though there was little common ground. This will also leave fewer points of disagreement to be resolved in developing your child's education program.

If your child is receiving special education services, both you and the school will, of course, have to follow the steps outlined in the

Individuals with Disabilities Education Act (IDEA). See Chapter 9 for a thorough explanation of this important federal education law. In this situation, it is especially vital that school personnel recognize that you have valuable ideas to contribute to the IEP. To ensure that school staff take your suggestions seriously, you may wish to bring one or two people along to the meeting. A friend, experienced parent, or professional advocate can make sure you cover everything you want to cover and provide invaluable emotional support.

Even if you deal with all school personnel in exactly the same way, you will probably find that some are more accepting and supportive of your child than others. If you look back through your child's academic history, you will usually find that things went better with some teachers than with others. Try to enlist the support and help of the teachers who have had particular success in working with your child. Ask them to be involved in educational planning for your child as long as it's feasible and as long as they have ideas to contribute.

Above all, keep the lines of communication open between you and your child's teachers. Encourage them to let you know when your child is doing well *and* not so well in school. Many parents like to keep in touch with teachers through regular meetings, email, phone calls, or a notebook in which they correspond about progress and problems. Try to anticipate problems that might result from a change of medication—and let teachers know ahead of time. You need to make sure the teachers understand that you are committed to helping them help your child, *and* to making the parent-professional partnership work.

Transfering the IEP From One Grade and Teacher to the Next

It's often very helpful to schedule a time to review the IEP with your child's teacher(s) before the new school year starts. This has several benefits. First, it assures you that the teacher has reviewed the IEP, and it provides you an opportunity to discuss your child's issues and accommodations with the teacher. Sometimes IEPs are not written clearly, and what was "understood" last year may not be apparent to this year's teacher(s). As your child advances in school, it may be useful to have each teacher sign off to confirm they have read the IEP and that they have no questions about the content. An older child with multiple teachers may find it helpful to carry an "IEP at a Glance," which outlines all of her classroom accommodations. That way, if she needs to self-advocate, she has a document on hand to back her up. (This can be especially useful with substitute teachers.)

∷ Conclusion

Tourette syndrome can be a challenging disorder for schools, parents, and children to deal with. But with sensitive and knowledgeable planning, most children with Tourette syndrome can make good progress in school. As a parent, you can do a great deal to ensure your child's continued progress: first, by making sure that your child's motivation to attend school and learn remain high; and second, by advising school personnel of special learning needs and strengths that they may not be aware of. By enlisting the support of enlightened educational and medical personnel, you *can* help your child learn the skills she needs to live up to her potential. No child deserves anything less.

∷ Parent Statements

This year our son is doing well at school, thanks to a combination of flexibility, routine, structure, and an understanding teacher.

❧

I think he gets on his classmates' nerves a lot. The teacher says his noise level (shrieks, shouts, and squeals) is loud, but she is easygoing about it.

❧

I always wondered why, after the diagnosis, the school wanted to change everything for my daughter. She was the same girl on Monday that she had been on Friday, we just had a name for what was going on.

❧

My daughter came home after the first week of middle school and announced that she was going to run for student body secretary. This involved getting up in front of 1100 students, tics and all, and making a speech. She said this was "sink or swim" time. She made her speech, first giving an intro on her tics and why she had them. She was elected student body secretary, and then reelected the next year!

❧

My son wasn't diagnosed with TS until the middle of fifth grade, but he had tics and behavior problems from the time he was three. His first grade teacher set the tone for his school career by promptly labeling him "Jumping John" at the beginning of the school year and staying on his case for the next eight months. I nominate her for the "Insensitivity Award" for that year!

❧❀❧

Because of her positive educational program and the care and concern of the staff, my daughter has gone from having very low self-esteem to being a success in school.

❧❀❧

Teachers have told me over the years that simple accommodations they made in the classroom for my daughter, like always writing the assignment on the board instead of calling it out to the students as they pile out of the classroom, ended up helping many other students also! Gee whiz!

❧❀❧

In middle school, a substitute teacher threatened to expel my daughter from class if she didn't stop her noises. She didn't believe that my daughter couldn't help it, despite the other students also trying to explain about TS. As the class got out of control, the substitute called for the principal to come to the classroom. The principal supported my daughter, commended the other students for supporting her, and explained TS to the substitute. Then we helped the school develop a simple program to alert all substitutes to "nontraditional" students they would be having in their classrooms.

❧❀❧

He's very accident prone because of his impulsivity. Luckily, the teacher is aware of our worries and doesn't just write us off as "overprotective parents." She noticed when Thomas skinned his tongue by licking a metal fence on a very cold day. Thomas has a very high pain tolerance, and the teachers need to be aware of that.

❧❀❧

The other kids call him "dummy" and "trouble maker."

❧❀❧

The sad truth is that children who present a challenge are sometimes seen as troublesome and disposable.

❧

My daughter's school is very good about working together with her to solve problem behavior. She feels validated and her sense of personal power and self-esteem is increasing.

❧

I see all the potential, the talent, the good, and the loveable. The school sees nothing positive about having to make basic, logical accommodations.

❧

I make a point of meeting with school personnel at the beginning of the year to vocalize my assumption that we are a team, working toward the same end—namely, helping my daughter succeed at school and become a life-long learner. I point out that this is the same goal they have for every other child. I make sure that every accommodation includes a description of my child's responsibility in that accommodation. During the course of the year, I also make sure I highlight the teacher's involvement in my daughter's successes.

❧

At the beginning of each new term of school, my daughter and I would meet with the new teachers to explain TS and her accommodations. Besides listing what the teachers needed to do, we also listed my daughter's responsibilities. For example, she took tests away from the classroom so the teacher had to be prepared for that. However, it was my daughter's responsibility to find a place ahead of time to take the test, perhaps in an office or another classroom during a teacher's prep time. This was good training for my daughter, helpful to the already burdened teachers, and demonstrated that we were all part of the team.

❧

Our kids have incredible coping skills to be able to go to school each day and be nonconformists in a mini-society that insists on conformity.

❧

My son spent so much time in the principal's office during the fourth grade that he lost a full grade level of reading skills. This was all hidden from me. I discovered the truth only when Joel began fifth grade.

❦

I've come into contact with many types of educational professionals, and I always appreciate it when I see a teacher or school psychologist who is committed to helping children with TS, and is willing to be flexible and creative in their approach.

❦

*The experts in the field of neurology and TS in particular let us know that there is still so much we don't know about Tourette syndrome. But some teachers and counselors come off like they know it all and have **the** answers.*

❦

Lorenzo told the teacher he was tired of being teased and beaten up every day at recess. The teacher said, "Go sit down." Then when Lorenzo decided he had no alternative but retaliation, the school acted shocked at his "inappropriate behavior."

❦

Waxing and waning of symptoms causes so much frustration at school. When tics are waning, teachers get fooled into thinking the TS is "better." Then when tics wax, teachers want to believe your child can control this—even after they've been told otherwise many times.

❦

Educators often don't read material that we provide on TS. Notes about her behavior continue to come home from school, even though we've explained her problems over and over.

❦

I've always tried to find at least one person in the school who is on my side.

❦

It's going real well in school. I'm very pleased with the cooperation we've received. The Early Education Special Services have been wonderful.

❦

Anthony was always class clown. He tried to camouflage his tics by doing things that were, if not acceptable, at least humorous.

❧

The first time anyone in school ever said anything good about my son was in fifth grade, right after his diagnosis of TS. His teacher said, "He's a neat kid. He's got a lot going for him!" That was the first time I felt that Michael had a chance to succeed.

❧

Because children with TS feel so out of control so much of the time, it's important to give them choices and "personal power." Let them have some input in their IEPs and their after-school time.

❧

Consequences for inappropriate behavior at school do not have to be punishment, detention, loss of recess or other privileges. Instead, parents and teachers must be creative. Try role playing, or reviewing the "incident" and making plans for the next time something similar happens.

❧

*When teachers don't want to make accommodations or adaptations for your child because it encourages him to be **dependent** on others, tell them this. True **in**dependence is self-confidence and the ability to be in control of your own life. Everyone needs help from others. Help is **inter**dependence, not dependence. Teachers' jobs depend on having students to help!*

❧

If teachers complain because your child is constantly losing control or needing to be restrained, examine the situation. What sets off these explosions? What attitudes, methods, or expectations are setting your child up for failure and frustration? The IEP obviously isn't working, so set up a new plan—devise other methods—until something does work!

❧

Elementary school was so supportive and safe for my child. But once he hit junior/senior high, it all changed. They were less willing to make any changes for my child and they didn't really read the IEP. My child had to go to a special high school program with kids with emotional problems and he was victimized all the time. It was a big mistake. Now I wish we had fought the district to provide his services in the home school building. He was victimized and bullied there too, but not as much.

❦

For years, I worried that other kids would make fun of my son's tics. Although he reported that some of his peers did make mild jokes, he regarded these as the sort of comments that people who trust one another can make. I know of one time when a kid made intentionally hurtful remarks and the school acted quickly to suspend him for a few days. I was really impressed by the level of support the school showed to my son in that regard.

❦

The best thing that ever happened to Kenny was to get involved in gymnastics in ninth grade. The coaches and other team members accepted him, included him, and encouraged him to be the best he could be and work as hard as he could. After working with these great people for a few months, he no longer wanted to hang around with the wild kids who had been the only ones in school to partially accept him, tics and all. He tried to straighten up and act in a way that would make his teammates proud. By the end of the school year, his "behavior" goals were taken off his IEP. By eleventh grade, he had lettered in gymnastics and received a sportsmanship award—not because of his exceptional athletic skills, but because of his enthusiasm, hard work, and helpful attitude toward the other team members. It was the proudest day of our life!

❦

While our son was in third grade, we realized that as the proverbial "square peg," he would probably not reach his potential in the "round hole" setting of public school. He spent the rest of his school career in small, challenging, and nurturing private schools, and is now at college, in a similar environment. It was definitely the best thing we've ever done for him, and we don't regret it for a moment, not withstanding the considerable expense.

❦

In fourth grade, before Joshua was diagnosed with TS but when his behavior was probably the most "inappropriate," he started taking piano lessons. He was always fooling around on the piano and trying to play simple tunes, so we figured he was musical. His teacher thought so too, but he hated to practice. It was just one more battle to fight, and we decided it wasn't worth it. Then in sixth grade, after his TS diagnosis, Joshua started playing trumpet in the school band. He drove the poor teacher crazy, but she loved and encouraged him and put up with his antics during practices, which he loved. He had to practice a certain amount of time each week, and we would scrupulously record his time, including every minute he spent hitting his mouth with the mouthpiece of his horn—one of his newest tics. Now that Joshua's a junior in high school, his tics have subsided a lot. He gets better at the trumpet every year, and is now competing in a state-wide music contest, playing solos on his trumpet. He's always playing the piano by ear in his spare time. His music teacher was right. He had "music in him," and in spite of the TS, it's still there and going strong!

9

LEGAL RIGHTS AND REMEDIES

Sonja D. Kerr

You are probably aware that there are laws to protect the rights of people with physical and mental disabilities. For example, there are laws requiring that public places be accessible to people in wheelchairs, and laws granting children with mental and physical disabilities the right to attend school. But you may not be aware that many important disability laws also apply to children with Tourette syndrome. Because TS is a neurological disorder, all the laws that apply to children with disabilities in general also apply to your child. Some of these laws guarantee your child the right to attend school and to participate in a work place. Others prohibit discrimination or grant your child financial and medical assistance, if he qualifies. Still other laws can complicate long-term planning for your child's future.

As a parent, you do not need to be an expert on these laws. But understanding what your child is entitled to can help you ensure that your child receives the education, training, and special services he needs. After all, some professionals have little or no experience in working with children with TS. At times *you* may have to tell *them* what your child needs and is entitled to under the law and be sure that they have up-to-date information about TS. You should also know enough about the law to be able to know what looks illegal and speak up for your child's rights if need be. Understanding how laws can sometimes work against families of children with disabilities can help you avoid pitfalls in estate planning.

To help you exercise your rights and fully protect your child, this chapter provides an overview of the purpose and contents of the most important federal laws, as well as information on how you can advocate for rights and services for your child. For information on state or local laws, you should contact your local Tourette Syndrome Association chapter or your state Protection and Advocacy office, as listed in the Resource Guide. Your local Bar Association should also be able to refer you to local lawyers who specialize in laws affecting people with disabilities. Remember, there is no substitute for consulting a knowledgeable lawyer. Although the information in this chapter is accurate and up to date, the author and publisher are not providing legal or other professional advice.

■■ Your Child's Right to an Education

Children with Tourette Syndrome have a right to an education. Some children with Tourette syndrome have little or no trouble learning in the regular classroom. Many others, however, run into academic

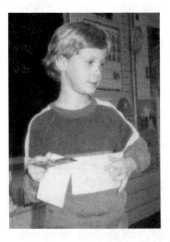

difficulties because of tics, learning disabilities, attention deficit disorders, or other symptoms. If your child has educational problems due to his TS or a related disorder, you need to learn about an important federal law: the Individuals with Disabilities Education Act (IDEA 2004).

IDEA is the basic federal law that protects your child's right to an education. The law was revised by the U.S. Congress in November of 2004 and there are important changes to the law that you should know about. Keep in mind that as this book is being written, we do not yet have the federal regulations that will also be revised as a result of IDEA 2004. (You may also hear this law referred to as the Individuals with Disabilities Education Improvement Act, "IDEIA," or as Public Law 94–142, which was the original version.) Be sure that you and anyone working with your child has the latest version of the law and the latest version of federal and state regulations.

IDEA 2004 is a sweeping and complex law that ensures every child with a disability will receive a "free appropriate public education designed to meet the child's unique needs." It does so by providing federal funds for the education of children with disabilities to every state whose special education programs meet federal standards. Currently, all states have accepted federal funding and must therefore provide a variety of approved educational services and rights to children with disabilities and their parents. States must have in place regulations and procedures to ensure full implementation of the federal law in that state. Check with your local state educational agency for information about such regulations and procedures. It is important to review state procedures, as they do vary, although a state law cannot be less protective than the federal law.

The sections below explore the major provisions of IDEA. As you read about what the law does and does not require schools to do, there are two important points to remember. These two points are: a child has the right to a meaningful education **and** his/her parents have a vital role in the development/planning of that education.

IDEA establishes the *minimum* requirements for special education programs. As the U.S. Supreme Court has ruled, states are required to provide your child a program that is reasonably calculated to allow him to gain "meaningful benefit." Think of "meaningful" or "appropriate" compared to what your child's unique needs require. This means a school does not have to provide "the best" program, but the educational program must be individually tailored to your child's unique needs and it must be reasonably calculated to result in educational benefit for your child.

Most importantly, you must be a part of developing your child's program of education. Parental participation is a key feature of this federal law. IDEA gives parents a vital role in their child's education. In fact, when Congress first enacted P.L. 94–142, it was largely in response to parents pressuring Washington for a say in their child's education. Through this law, Congress sought to correct the traditional imbalance of power between school personnel and parents. IDEA 2004 requires that children receive appropriate services and that parents be full participants at every step along the way in formulating their child's program of education. Parents are to be equal partners in the creation of a program of education for their child with TS. Parents must be notified if their child is being considered for special education, must be given the opportunity to help plan their child's educational program, must be notified of any changes in the program, and must be given a means of resolving disputes with the school system. What all this means is that there are many ways you can work with the school to create a more appropriate program for him or to insist through legal procedures that your child receive a more appropriate program.

■■ What IDEA 2004 Provides

The law requires that school districts determine if your child is eligible for special education and related services under IDEA 2004. Typically, this will mean that either you or your child's teacher may ask that your child be referred and evaluated. Parents must be given notice of the evaluation and consent to the evaluation.

■■ Coverage

IDEA defines a child with a disability as one who may have a variety of disabilities. Although Tourette syndrome is not one of these specific disability categories, your child may still qualify for services. Commonly, children with TS qualify as "other health impaired." Under the law, "other health impaired" means "having limited strength, vitality or alertness, including a heightened alertness to environmental stimuli, that results in limited alertness with respect to the educational environment, that... is due to chronic or acute health problems...and adversely affects a child's educational performance."

For the first time, IDEA 2004 specifically lists Tourette syndrome as an example of a condition that can cause other health impairment—under 34 C.F.R 300.8. [c] 9 (i). (AD/HD, too, is listed as an other health impairment.) If your child has learning disabilities in addition to TS, he may also qualify on the basis of having a specific learning disability (SLD). Some schools suggest that children with TS be classified as "emotionally behaviorally disturbed" (EBD). Because TS is neurologically (not emotionally) based, this practice is incorrect.

Children with TS can begin to receive services as soon as they are diagnosed. All states now serve children from age three, and many are beginning to serve them from birth. Children with TS may continue to receive services through age eighteen, or until age twenty-one, if the state where they live offers education services to students without disabilities who are older than eighteen.

Special Education and Related Services

If your child qualifies under IDEA, then the school district must provide him with special education and related services. Taken together, this means extra help beyond just going to school.

Special education is instruction individually tailored to meet your child's unique learning needs. For children with TS, it can include one-to-one tutoring, modified curriculum and grading, or special classes in weak areas. For children with milder forms of TS, it can even include such accommodations as overlooking poor penmanship caused by tics or giving extra time for tests or shorter assignments. Accommodations and modifications for testing are very important since most states have enacted state standards tests that children must pass to graduate from high school.

Related services are any services your child needs to benefit from his special education. Services can include occupational therapy, physical therapy, speech-language therapy, counseling, tutoring, personal aides, specially trained teachers, and transportation to and from school.

One of the most important services for children with TS is the development of a behavioral program. IDEA requires that a child receive specific assistance through behavioral programming if the child's behavior interferes with his own learning or the learning of others.

Least Restrictive Environment

IDEA requires that your child receive his education in the "least restrictive environment" in which he is able to learn. The least restrictive environment is the setting that allows him to have the maximum contact possible with children in regular education programs. For children with milder TS, the least restrictive environment is often a regular classroom within a regular neighborhood school. Although they may receive help from special aides or therapists or use special equipment such as tape recorders, they still spend 100 percent of their time in a regular classroom. Other children with TS may spend part of the day in a regular classroom with typical children and part of the day in a special classroom working on subjects they have trouble with because of learning disabilities or attention problems.

A few children with TS are unable to make appropriate academic progress within a regular school because the school district lacks the expertise to work with them. Often, these children have extremely severe physical tics that school personnel misinterpret as intentional misbehavior. In these very limited cases, the least restrictive environment might be a special education program located in a private or residential school for children with disabilities—at least until the school district acquires some expertise. Keep in mind that the least restrictive environment for your child depends on his *individual unique educational, including social skills,* needs and that the environment can change for your child from year to year. The best approach is to start with the assumption that a regular classroom is right for your child, and only look into more restrictive alternatives if he runs into academic or social difficulties.

Free Appropriate Public Education

Every decision about which services your child should receive and in what setting should be made in light of the requirement that he receive a "free appropriate education."

"Free" means exactly what it sounds like. Parents do not have to pay anything for their child's special education, no matter what special services he is found to need. The federal government and state governments provide additional funding to your school district if your child is eligible for services under IDEA. This includes costs for related services

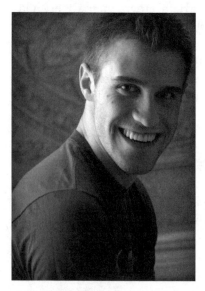

such as transportation and physical, occupational, or psychological therapy. Do not be afraid to ask for what you believe your child needs. The United States Supreme Court has held that a school district cannot deny your child what he needs because of cost.

"Appropriate" means what is educationally correct for your child's needs, so that he can learn and make reasonable progress in school. As mentioned earlier, it does not mean "best." It does not mean that your child's program must be designed to help him maximize his ability (unless your state law so provides). It does mean an educational program that is reasonably calculated to result in benefit, given your child's unique needs. You and your school's staff have to jointly decide what is "appropriate."

"Public" usually means a public school, and the standards of the public school. It can also, on occasion, mean a private school or private tutoring with tuition paid for by the public school. If the public school doesn't have an appropriate program for your child, but a private school does, the public school may have to pay the costs for your child to be educated in a private setting.

Remember, services must be free, appropriate, and the responsibility of the school district.

Identification and Evaluation

By now it should be clear that education programs cannot be appropriate unless they are tailor-made to take into account each child's educational strengths and needs. To make sure that schools have a clear picture of children's abilities and disabilities, the IDEA requires that states have procedures for identifying and evaluating children who would benefit from special education. Under the law, school districts are required to make an effort to identify all children with disabilities. But if your child has already been diagnosed with TS, you can take the first step and notify the school that your child may need special education. To set the process in motion, contact the school's special education department, explain your child's diagnosis, and request, in writing, that your child be given a special education assessment or evaluation.

In most cases, your child's evaluation should be completed within 60 school days. Your state law may also set a shorter specific timeline for completing an evaluation from the time it is requested by a parent.

The purpose of an evaluation is to determine your child's current level of educational performance and the areas that he needs assistance in. As Chapter 7 discusses, your child's need for special education may be evaluated in several ways. First, he may be given a variety of tests to assess his abilities in all developmental areas. In addition, he may be observed in the classroom and you may be interviewed about your child's strengths and needs. In fact, IDEA requires that multiple procedures be used to evaluate your child. That is, the school cannot rely solely on the results of tests, for example. In addition, you have the right to be notified of the type of tests to be given, and the tests must be administered by qualified personnel. Finally, the tests must not discriminate on the basis of your child's disability or racial or cultural background.

As a parent, it is important that you make sure the assessment paints an accurate and complete picture of your child. Otherwise, the program he receives may not be appropriate, given his needs. Offer your own information or questions about your child's abilities to the evaluator. And after the evaluation, request copies of all assessment data and other information in your child's records.

If you disagree with the evaluation completed by the school district, you have the right to ask the school district to pay for an independent education evaluation (IEE). For instance, you may not agree that your child reads at a particular level, is disruptive to others, or has no strong points. You will know if it "doesn't sound like" your child. When you make this request, indicate that if the school district is not willing to provide an IEE, that you may proceed to get an evaluation at your own expense and seek reimbursement later. After the school district receives your request for an Independent Educational Evaluation, it must either agree to pay for one or it must prove at a special hearing that its evaluation was correct. Because evaluations often cost much less than such hearings, school districts will often pay for independent evaluations in an effort to resolve disputes over assessments. Be sure to put your request(s) in writing, and keep a copy of the communication. While you wait for a response from your district, check with doctors, the TSA, or other parents for recommendations of an evaluator. Whether you pay for the evaluation or the school district pays, be sure to cooperate and provide the evaluation results in a timely fashion to the school district.

Individualized Education Program (IEP)

Once a child is determined to need special education, the school district must hold a meeting to discuss the assessment results and to develop an Individualized Education Program (IEP). The IEP is a written document which describes the education a child with disabilities will receive to meet his unique needs. It specifies:

1. your child's current abilities in academic, emotional, and other areas; any health problems; and any particular problems your child is having in school;
2. long-range goals to help your child learn or reducing the difficulties that prevent your child from performing bet-

ter (a long-range goal might be: "Dan, who reads at grade 4.0, will increase his reading ability to grade 4.5 by the end of the second semester, as measured by performance in reading 4.5 grade materials." These goals should include "progress markers"—stating the time and process by which the school will inform you of how your child is doing;

3. the types of special instruction, therapy, and other assistance your child will receive, as well as where he will receive these services;
4. the projected date services will begin and their expected duration;
5. how your child's progress will be measured;
6. the extent to which your child will be able to participate in the regular classroom, and any in-class modifications that will be used;
7. whether your child will be receiving services for longer than the traditional nine-month school year (as might be necessary if the lack of a consistent program causes your child to regress, take a long time to regain skills he had in the spring, or not become as self-sufficient as he could be with a longer year);
8. for children aged sixteen or older, the assistance and services that will be provided to help them make the transition to work or postsecondary education.

Your child's IEP will be developed at a meeting, or series of meetings, attended by a school administrator, your child's regular classroom teacher, other school staff who may have evaluated or worked with your child, you, and your child, if you deem it appropriate. You may also invite other family members, a friend, doctor, social worker, advocate, lawyer, or anyone else you feel comfortable bringing to the meeting.

At an IEP meeting, your child's needs in *all* areas should be discussed. Your role is to tell the school staff who your child is and what you think he needs. Some parents take a very active role in this process, while others are content to observe and ask questions. Do what feels comfortable to you. Think of it as painting a picture of who your child is now and a futuristic picture of who your child can be. What skills does he need in order to reach the futuristic picture?

All children with Tourette syndrome have differing needs. Share what those needs might be. For example, say: "My child can't follow directions" or "My child counts ceiling tiles" or "My child is impulsive and acts without thinking" or "My child swears at home, too." Then, make suggestions to help school staff deal constructively with problem behaviors. For instance, suggest: "Give my child an organizing notebook" or "If he is staring at the ceiling, remind him to look at his books" or "Tell the other kids that John doesn't mean to hit or swear."

Once your child's IEP has been designed, the school district must provide you with a copy of it, and you have a right to approve or disapprove it. If this is your child's first IEP, the school must have your written consent and must then begin providing services immediately. If this is a revision of an initial IEP, the school cannot legally change your child's program without notifying you. The school must inform you of any changes made and give you the opportunity to respond to the changes and accept or reject them. If you do formally object to the changes by requesting a special hearing, the school district must generally keep your child in the program he was in when you objected. This is referred to as the "stay put" provision of the IDEA. Hearings are described in more detail below.

There is one final point about IEPs it is important to remember. As your child's strengths and needs change, so should his IEP. Consequently, the IDEA requires that children's special education programs and their progress be reviewed at least once a year; many states encourage more frequent reviews. This ensures that your child will not be "stuck" in a program that is not meeting his needs. You have a right to be notified of all meetings about your child and to participate if you wish. If you do not want to attend a meeting, the school can have one without you, provided you were told about it. If you feel additional meetings are necessary, you can request them by writing to your child's teacher, the school principal, or special education director.

As a result of the passage of IDEA 2004, some states will be piloting a process for a "three year" IEP. These states can encourage parents to consent to writing an IEP for their child that will not need to be reviewed or changed for three years. Keep in mind that you have the right to participate or not participate in a three year IEP for your child. Your consent is required and the three years must be at a natural transition point (i.e., moving from elementary to middle school or middle school to high school.)

Notice of Procedural Safeguards

IDEA 2004, like its predecessors, requires that you be provided with information about how to obtain services for your child and your child's rights and protections under special education. All states must have in place a written explanation of these rights which are often called "Notice of Procedural Safeguards" (NOPS). Many states and school districts have a copy of this information on their websites. This information is very important, so be sure to read it. If you have any questions about the content, contact a local advocacy group, your state Protection and Advocacy office, your local school district, or your state department of education. The NOPS must, at a minimum, inform you of your right to object to any proposed program of education, how long you have to do so, and the process for objection. The NOPS must be in a language you can read and understand.

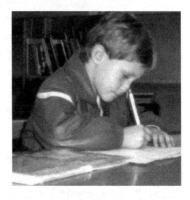

Behavioral Needs/Discipline/Manifestation Meetings

Children with TS often have behavioral difficulties. IDEA 2004 requires that IEP teams develop ways to address a child's behavior if the behavior interferes with the child's or others ability to learn in school. There are three keys to thinking about discipline. First, remember that your child must receive an education, even during times when the school may want to impose discipline. The rule is that services cannot cease for more than ten school days per year. Second, it is always best to proactively plan a behavioral program for your child. Finally, there are important exceptions to the usual rule that your child's program cannot be changed that happen in a disciplinary context so it is wise to consult with an advocate in those situations.

The first step to help your child is generally to conduct a functional behavior assessment (FBA). The purpose of an FBA is to identify what behavioral difficulties your child is having and how often and what purpose they serve (e.g., to escape from demands or to get attention). The next step is to create a behavioral intervention plan (BIP) that will help teachers and other staff work with your child to improve his behavior.

Many times, children with TS do not have appropriate behavioral planning, and, as a result, encounter regular school disciplinary approaches such as suspensions and expulsion. Remember, a child with TS can be suspended from school but not for longer than ten school days in one school year without being provided educational services.

If a school district intends to change the program of a child with TS because of behavioral problems, a meeting should be held known as a manifestation determination. A manifestation meeting is to decide if the child's misbehavior is a manifestation of his disability. If the misbehavior is a manifestation of the child's disability, the normal rule is that the child's program cannot be changed. There are three exceptions to this rule which allow a child to be removed to an interim alternative educational setting: 1) if the child brings a weapon to school, 2) has drugs at school, or 3) engages in behavior that inflicts serious bodily injury. This "removal" time is not to punish your child but to have your child in a safe place while his IEP team can determine how to adjust his program to avoid more problems. The removal period cannot last more than 45 school days.

In these disciplinary situations, you and your child have special appeal rights known as an "expedited" special hearing. If you are uncertain what to do, put in writing that you do not agree and want a hearing. Remember to read your NOPS if your child encounters disciplinary problems.

If your child is suspended for any reason, do not hesitate to contact a local advocacy group, an attorney, or your Protection and Advocacy Office. The rules are complicated and confusing and you will need assistance to do what is right for your child.

Resolution of Disputes

As mentioned earlier, one of the key provisions of IDEA 2004 is to encourage a team of people, including parents, to work together to plan a child's education program. Ideally, parents and school staff can openly discuss their concerns about a child's abilities and disabilities and jointly agree on the services and strategies that will best meet his special educational needs. Occasionally, however, disagreements arise. Examples of disputes are: 1) whether your child qualifies for special education services; 2) whether your child is too disruptive to be in a particular class; 3) whether your child needs occupational therapy or another specific related service.

The revised IDEA encourages parents and school districts to try various ways to solve disputes. There are four ways to solve disputes:

1. You may always request another IEP meeting.
2. You can request mediation.
3. You can file a complaint with your state education department.
4. A final option is that you can request a special hearing often called a "due process hearing."

There are three important changes in any use of the legal proceedings (due process hearings) available to parents of children with disabilities.

First, IDEA 2004 now gives parents and students generally only two years from the date on which you disagree with any aspect of your child's program to take formal legal action. Some states have even shorter periods of time. Read your NOPS to determine how long you have to bring a complaint to the district's attention if you are unhappy with your child's education.

Another important change has occurred by the Supreme Court decision in *Schaffer v. Weast* (2005). The Court examined who should have to "prove" that the school's program is not appropriate to a child with a disability. The Court decided that parents sometimes will have the burden to prove the inappropriateness of the program, unless the state has a different rule. Read your NOPS to find out the rule in your state.

A final change is that if parents inappropriately use legal proceedings, the IDEA now permits school districts to recover attorney fees from parents. That is, if parents are found to have improperly brought a due process hearing against the school district, they may have to reimburse the school district's legal fees. (This is in contrast to the earlier version of IDEA, which allowed parents to recover legal fees from the school district, but not vice versa.) This is an extremely unusual situation. Read your NOPS to learn more about this rule.

Informal Dispute Resolution

Many states give parents the opportunity to discuss disagreements with school staff in so-called *mediation* or resolution settings and these are encouraged by the IDEA 2004. The format of these meetings varies from state to state. Generally, a mediation session will be hosted by someone not directly involved in the dispute. Either you or the school can request such a meeting. If you request it, do so in writing. If you are wondering whether to participate in such a meeting, ask yourself four questions:

1. Will the meeting be moderated by an impartial third party?
2. Do you believe the disagreement can be resolved through honest discussion?
3. Are *both* you and the school interested in reaching a solution without resorting to more formal methods?
4. Is your participation truly voluntary?

If the answer to each of these four questions is "yes," then by all means meet with the school staff and try to reach a solution. But if the answer to some questions is "no," do not hesitate to investigate the more formal methods of resolution discussed below. Sometimes it is helpful to discuss with an attorney or lay advocate whether you should try these informal methods or proceed to more formal means. (A lay advocate is a parent, teacher, doctor, or other individual who has considerable knowledge about the IDEA or your child. Call your TSA for help finding one.) To find out whether your district or state has an informal dispute resolution process, contact your State Department of Education.

Formal Administrative Proceedings—Due Process Hearings

IDEA gives parents the right to formally appeal *any* decisions made by the school regarding their child's identification, evaluation, program, or placement. For example, you can challenge your school's refusal to qualify your child for services, or the types or amounts of therapy he is receiving, or the classroom setting he is in, or a behavioral plan that you do not believe is appropriate.

You can set the appeals process in motion by sending a letter to the school district's Special Education Director and in some states copying that to the state department of education. It is best to at least consult with an attorney or experienced advocate before requesting a special education due process hearing.

A request for a hearing must include at least: 1) your child's name, school of attendance, and residence; 2) the nature of the dispute or problem; and 3) what you see as a solution to the problem.

Send the request by some means that you can establish later. This can be certified mail, hand delivery, email (saved), or fax.

Once you request a hearing, the school district has the opportunity to request a resolution meeting. It is good to participate in such a meeting, because it will help you better understand from the school's perspective and there is always the possibility of resolution. The school district must either ask for clarification of your concerns within ten days or respond with its version of the dispute within fifteen days.

A school district can ask a special hearing officer to order you to be more clear on what your concerns are. Therefore, it is best to be clear in your initial request. Describe the problem as specifically as you can.

In general, the hearing must be held and completed within forty-five days of when the district or state department receives your request. The hearing will give you your first opportunity to present your case before someone who does not have any stake in the outcome. An "impartial hearing officer"—someone who has not had any direct dealings with your child and does not have any professional or personal interest in the school that might cloud his objectivity—will preside over the hearing. IDEA 2004 requires that hearing officers be knowledgeable in special education and in application of law to this type of proceeding, so many hearing officers will be attorneys. You may object to the hearing officer chosen if you do not believe that person is "impartial." Ultimately, the hearing officer will decide whether the school's or your arguments have more merit, so it is important that he or she be objective.

Both you and school district representatives must give the other a list of the people who will testify at the hearing, and copies of any evidence, including recommendations from any experts, five business days before the hearing. This is known as the "five day rule."

At the hearing, you can present information or "evidence" to prove that the school's decision will not give your child an appropriate education that meets his needs. Evidence may include your child's school records, independent evaluations, testimony from people such as the state TSA advocate who have special knowledge, and others. At a minimum, you should come prepared with relevant portions of your child's school history, information from his physician and other non-school care providers, a description of the school's proposed education program, and a description of the program that you feel would best meet your child's needs.

Besides presenting your own evidence, you generally have a right to review all the evidence to be presented by the school at least five days before the hearing. You can also require witnesses, including school staff, to attend and testify. You can question or cross-examine any witnesses the school district may bring. And you can ask an attorney or lay advocate to represent you at the hearing.

Remember that now, according to *Shaffer v. Weast*, where the burden of proof lies—which side must present the best information—varies from state to state. In some states, the burden is on the school district to prove that its program is appropriate. In others, the parents must prove that the school's program is inappropriate. Call your TSA to find out how it works in your state or review your NOPS on this point.

The hearing officer will hear both sides and must issue a decision, in writing, within forty-five days of your initial request for the hearing. If you ask for it, the school district must provide you with an electronic recording or transcript of the hearing. If the hearing officer rules against the school, he or she will order the school district to provide whatever you requested for your child.

If you prevail at the hearing, the school district must also pay your attorney's fees. This is a rather recent development, so be certain that any attorney with whom you consult is aware of the provision. You should also be aware that payment of attorney's fees might be limited or refused if you reject an offer of settlement from the school, proceed with a hearing, and then do not obtain a better result. In addition, the school district or state department of education must pay for all the other costs related to the hearing, whether or not you prevail. This includes the costs of the hearing officer, the court reporter, and copies of the electronic record or transcript. If teachers are called as witnesses, the school district must also pay for substitute teachers for them. Because of the possible expenses involved, many districts prefer to reach an agreement with parents without going to a hearing, unless the case is very important.

If the hearing officer rules against you, you have the right to appeal this decision. Until recently, appeals from the hearing officer were routinely heard by the State Educational Agency—the state department of education. Parents and advocates have challenged the appropriateness and fairness of permitting a state educational agency to review these decisions because that agency was not perceived as "impartial." As a result, most states are now moving to a system where the hearing officer's decision is final and appealable only to a court, or is reviewed by a truly impartial hearing review officer who is not a part of the state's educational agency. The impartial hearing review officer considers the evidence presented at the due process hearing and any additional evidence presented. Based on that evidence, the hearing review officer then issues an independent decision.

A hearing officer who finds that your child has been denied a free, appropriate education has broad authority to order relief. He or she can order a new evaluation, compensatory (make-up) services, or a new program, including private schooling. An IHO cannot order attorneys' fees in most states.

Although many parents have used due process hearings to obtain more appropriate programs for their child, it is best to think twice before embarking on a hearing. Going through a hearing can place significant emotional stresses on both your child and your family. You will have to meet with your lawyer. You may have to miss work. You will have to put your files in order and prepare what you plan to say. In some states, due process hearings are quite lengthy and very expensive, often involving attorneys for both sides. In other states, hearings are less complicated, and parents may be able to represent themselves, perhaps with the help of a lay advocate.

In deciding whether to ask for a due process hearing, it is important for you to find out what hearings are generally like in your state. Ask other parents, advocates, or attorneys about the average length and cost of hearings, how often hearings are requested, and whether they think you need an attorney. Consider whether you can afford to pay attorney's fees to your attorney if you lose. (You might also be able to find an attorney who will only charge you if you prevail and can recover attorney's fees.) Then weigh the importance of the issue being disputed against the emotional demands of making the request and proceeding through the hearing.

If you decide it is essential that your child receive a particular type of program or service which the school district has refused, do not be afraid to request a hearing. As mentioned above, when parents who know their rights request a hearing, schools may attempt to meet their demands rather than go to a hearing. If your dispute involves an issue that you and other parents frequently discuss, your child may need to be the "test case" to push the issue for all children. Generally, other parents and advocates are very supportive of parents going to a hearing. In fact, some parents have said they never felt so supported as they did before, during, and after their hearing.

Complaint Process

An alternative to a due process hearing is to file a written complaint with the state department of education. You do not have to have an attorney to file a complaint. The complaint should be provided in writing and you should be sure that your state department has received it and is actively investigating your complaint. In general, states must make a decision on complaints within 60 days of receiving it. The state must decide if your child has been denied a free, appropriate public education and if so, order an adequate remedy. Such remedies are similar to those you might obtain from a hearing—e.g., a new evaluation, compensatory education services, a new program. If you do not like the results, in some states you may appeal to court and in others you must first proceed through a due process hearing.

In general, you have up to one year and sometimes three years to file a complaint with the state department of education. Review your NOPS on this point.

Civil Court Action

If you are not satisfied with the results of a due process hearing or the appeal to a hearing review officer, or, in some states, a complaint, there are further steps you can take. You can take your appeal to a state or federal court by bringing a civil lawsuit against the school district. After reviewing the information from previous hearings and hearing additional evidence, the court must decide two questions. First, did the school district follow the procedures required under IDEA in making the decision about the child's educational program? Second, is the educational program proposed by the school district the appropriate placement for your child? If the court rules in your favor, the school district must comply with its order.

At this stage, parents generally employ an attorney, if they have not done so already. And once again, they may recover attorney's fees if the court decides in their favor. However, if your action is completely frivolous, then the court could, in a rare instance, order that you pay the school's legal costs.

Your attorney can further advise you of the specific appeal procedures from one court to the next. Basically, however, parents can appeal decisions of a court up to the highest court of the United States—the Supreme Court. Some parents have found it necessary to do so, and it is as a result of many of those cases that your child has the rights described in this chapter. However, this is very rare. Since the initial version of the IDEA, the Supreme Court has only heard a handful of cases.

■■ No Child Left Behind Act

One of the most significant changes to the IDEA 2004 is the requirement that children with disabilities have the right to "highly qualified teachers" pursuant to the No Child Left Behind Act. Because the NCLBA is new and the revision to IDEA 2004 is also new, it is not possible at this point to know exactly how the courts will interpret this provision of the IDEA. However, it is clear that parents can and should ask about their teacher's credentials and attempt to find out whether their child's special education teacher and related services personnel are "highly qualified teachers." Congress made this section of the IDEA 2004 effective immediately.

■■ Other Federal Antidiscrimination Laws

Rehabilitation Act of 1973

Section 504 of the Rehabilitation Act of 1973 protects the right of "an individual with handicaps" not to be discriminated against by agencies receiving federal funding, including school districts. A handicapped individual, under Section 504, is anyone having a physical or mental impairment that substantially interferes with "caring for one's self, performing manual tasks, walking, seeing, hearing, speaking, breathing, learning, and working." Someone with TS may fit this definition if his TS or associated conditions affect him in these ways. All public and private organizations receiving federal money must take action to accommodate people with disabilities so that they can "learn, work, and compete on a fair and equal basis." Agencies that don't accommodate people with disabilities can lose their federal funding.

Although Section 504 only covers discrimination in federally funded agencies, it can still be helpful to your child on a day-to-day basis. For example, if your child plays the violin well enough to belong to the orchestra at his public school, but the conductor wants to exclude him because he has loud vocal tics during concerts, you can charge the school with discrimination. Likewise, if a federally funded agency turns your child down for a summer job solely because of his TS behaviors, that is discrimination under Section 504. In addition, once your child reaches college age, he can receive accommodations and supports under Section 504 to help him succeed at college (e.g., extended time on tests, help with note-taking). (This is helpful because IDEA protections do not, in most states, cover students who have graduated from high school.) Because people with TS sometimes have trouble convincing agencies that they are covered under Section 504, be prepared to document that your child is disabled enough to be covered.

Keep in mind that children who attend private schools may be protected by Section 504 if the private school receives any federal funds. Such funds may be federal lunch funds, nursing funds, transportation, etc. Be sure to ask if the private school is subject to Section 504; do not assume it isn't.

The Americans with Disabilities Act

In 1990, Congress passed the Americans with Disabilities Act (ADA), which many people view as an extension of Section 504. The ADA is the latest, but very natural step in the evolution of federal civil rights laws

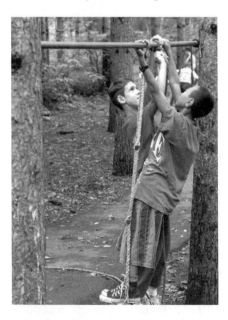

that protect people with disabilities. The ADA's purpose is simple—to eradicate discrimination in *all* aspects of life, not just in federally funded programs. It covers a large array of public and private sector activities. Under the ADA, discrimination on the basis of disability is prohibited in the following areas:

Employment. Under the ADA, a "qualified individual with a disability" is anyone who has a disability and can perform the essential functions of the job, with or without special accommodation. Basically, an employer cannot refuse to hire, train, or promote a "qualified individual" solely on the basis of Tourette syndrome or any other disability. Indeed, the employer is prohibited from asking whether a prospective employee has a disability. Furthermore, an employer is required to make modifications (accommodations) within the workplace that will enable an otherwise qualified person to perform the job. For example, if an employee with TS syndrome had difficulty with hand writing a project, use of a computer would be an accommodation. Under the ADA, workers with disabilities who feel they have been discriminated against can file a complaint with the Equal Employment Opportunity Commission (EEOC) or a state human rights office. If this agency is unable to resolve the dispute, the next step is to take the employer to court. During this stage, it is usually advisable to consult a lawyer with expertise in employment discrimination. Attorney fees can be recovered if the court finds in favor of the employee.

Consumer Services in Private Business. Any business that provides "public accommodations" is prohibited from discriminating against people with disabilities. That is, any facility that is open to the general public must also be open to individuals with disabilities, and under the same terms. For example, a restaurant could not seat someone with loud vocal tics in a remote corner of the room on the grounds that he might otherwise disturb other patrons. Or the managers of a movie theater or concert hall could not exclude a patron with Tourette syndrome because his tics might distract others. Unless it would impose an unreasonable cost, every store, health club, school, restaurant, hotel, motel, museum, laundry, doctor's office, dentist's office, and other business must allow people with disabilities to use their facilities on an equal footing with people without disabilities.

State and Local Government Services. Every service funded by state and local government must be accessible to people with disabilities. This includes voting. An important decision by the United States Supreme Court, Tennesee v. Lane (2004) has made it clear that even the courts of a state must fully accommodate individuals with disabilities. The key is to indicate what accommodation is necessary and make that request in writing.

Public Transportation. Under the ADA, all public transit must be accessible to people with disabilities. Buses, trains, subways, and other public conveyances must have some provision for transporting people with disabilities, and cannot refuse service on the basis of a patron's disability.

Telecommunication. Just like businesses in the private sector, telecommunications companies must make their services accessible to people with disabilities.

The exact scope and protection provided by the ADA will vary depending upon the situation at issue. It is best to consult an attorney if you believe there has been discrimination because your child has TS. You should do so *before* filing a complaint with any state human rights agency, EEOC, or the Office of Civil Rights. The ADA permits a person to bring a lawsuit if he feels he has been discriminated against. It also permits recovery of attorneys' fees if the suit is successful. To keep abreast of changes in interpretation of the ADA that may affect people with TS, periodically check with your local TSA or ARC.

▪▪ Government Benefits and Protection

In addition to protecting the rights of people with disabilities through the IDEA 2004 and other antidiscrimination laws, the federal government provides various programs and benefits for people with disabilities. Your child may qualify for some or all of these programs and services if he meets the eligibility requirements.

Developmental Disabilities Act of 1978

The Developmental Disabilities Assistance and Bill of Rights Act (DDA) offers a wide range of services to people with developmental disabilities. For purposes of the DDA, a developmental disability is one that occurs before age twenty-two and that limits a person's abilities to do certain activities necessary for self-sufficiency—walking, grooming, learning, earning money, and the like. Most people who are more severely affected by TS qualify for "DD" services, while people with milder symptoms do not. Different counties set different eligibility guidelines for these services. Your county Human Services agency can tell you how to find out whether your child qualifies.

If your child has severe symptoms, especially symptoms that cannot be controlled by medication, there are services available under the DDA which may be necessary to your family's survival. Services include:

1. Child development (early intervention)—the IDEA 2004 now requires that eligible children receive special education services from age three. But some states try to enhance the development and learning of children

with disabilities from birth on. These states typically offer early intervention services—occupational therapy, physical therapy, speech therapy, or other specialized help designed to help minimize problems that would otherwise affect the child's development. If your child received a diagnosis of TS before age three, he may qualify for these services.

2. Case management—When a child with disabilities needs the services of many educational and medical professionals, a case manager helps to arrange for these services and facilitates communication between parents and the professionals. A case manager may be an educational, medical, social work, or other professional who is dedicated to your child's protection and rehabilitation.

3. Provision of services such as assistance from in-home aides, behavior specialists, or respite care workers to help your child live as independently as possible within the community.

Protection and Advocacy Offices. The DDA also provides for the establishment of a Protection and Advocacy (P&A) office in each state. These P&A offices protect and advocate for the civil and legal rights of people with developmental disabilities. Many serve people with Tourette syndrome, depending upon the office's criteria. If you or your child encounter problems related to education, employment, housing, or other activities, the attorneys and advocates at your P&A agency should assist you at no cost. State P&A offices are listed in the Resource Guide at the back of the book.

Vocational Rehabilitation

Vocational Rehabilitation (VR) services are offered to all adults with disabilities in every state. Services are designed to help people with disabilities gain employment, and job training and placement assistance. VR services are supported by federal funding and are provided at no cost for those who cannot afford to pay.

If you think your child may need assistance in getting or keeping a job, begin inquiring about vocational programs when your child is still in high school so that you will have ample time to prepare for the transition from school to the workplace. The first step in obtaining services is to request a vocational needs assessment no later than age sixteen. If it is determined that your child has vocational needs, goals and objectives should be written into your child's IEP. To request services after high school, you will need to contact your state Department of Vocational Rehabilitation. Your child will be assigned a personal counselor and given an assessment, similar to that provided under IDEA. Once his needs are determined, an Individual Written Rehabilitation Plan (IWRP) will be developed, clearly setting forth the specific services to be provided. The types of services most commonly provided are vocational counseling and guidance in selecting the most appropriate career; medical examinations and other tests which help to determine job potential; instruction and training, books, equipment, and initial set-up materials for self-employment; placement; and follow-up services to make sure the adult with Tourette syndrome obtains employment and remains satisfactorily employed.

Even though your child may qualify for vocational rehabilitation services, it is important to realize that these services may not always be available. Often vocational rehabilitation offices have long waiting lists of people who are eligible for assistance, but the funding and personnel are simply not available to satisfy everyone's needs. Services are generally doled out to the people who are judged to have the severest problems first. This makes it doubly important for you to take advantage of any vocational assistance available through the school system before your child graduates, while he is still covered by IDEA.

Social Security Programs

Adults and children with TS can apply for and receive two types of Social Security before they are of retirement age. The benefits available are Supplemental Security Income (SSI) benefits, and Social Security Disability Income (SSDI). Both programs can provide additional income to qualified children with disabilities and their families. To qualify, your child must meet the strict requirements of the program and establish financial need. If your child is under eighteen or is living at home, need is based not only on your child's income, but also on the income and resources of you, the parents.

Supplemental Security Income (SSI)

Supplemental Security Income is designed to provide income for people who cannot work. It is available not only to people who have worked for a period of time and paid Social Security taxes during that time, but also to people who have never worked or have worked only for a limited period of time. Adults are eligible if they can demonstrate that they are unable to engage in "substantial gainful activity" because of a disability. Children who have disabilities similar to those that prevent an adult from working can also qualify. Both children and adults with disabilities must also meet the financial need requirement set by the Department of Social Security. Since the cutoff figure changes frequently, you should contact your local Social Security office to find out what the current income requirement is. They can also advise you as to how any assets in your child's name or earnings from a part-time job can reduce her benefits.

To apply for benefits for your child, contact your local Social Security Administration Office. Your first request will most likely be denied. Many people with TS are denied benefits because the agency may need more detailed information about the person's disability. Ask that your doctor explain in writing that your child's symptoms are chronic and will not disappear. Have the doctor detail all areas in which TS limits your child's abilities, including speech, reading, sight, hand and arm movements, and compulsive behaviors. Be persistent in your efforts.

Social Security Disability Insurance (SSDI)

Your child is eligible to receive Social Security Disability Insurance if one of his parents becomes disabled and is no longer able to work. The amount that parent and child receive is based on the number of years the parent worked before becoming disabled. A child who is disabled before the age of eighteen can also receive SSDI payments based on the amount of a retired or deceased parent's Social Security coverage. The process of applying for SSDI is the same as for SSI. Unlike SSI, however, applicants are not required to meet certain income qualifications.

Medicaid

Sometimes children with TS can qualify for Medicaid, a government-sponsored health insurance program. To be eligible, your child must qualify for SSI or have insufficient funds to pay for medical care. Usually, but not always, your child's medical needs will have to be pretty extensive for him to qualify. Medicaid can pay for medications, doctor visits, evaluations, and hospital stays. Call your local social services office to apply. Ask for a written explanation of what services are covered in your state.

■■ Planning for the Future

Tourette syndrome is a lifelong disability. But because TS symptoms may change in severity over the course of a lifetime, the needs of a person with TS are extremely difficult to predict. Most adults with TS are able to care for themselves, but some may need some assistance.

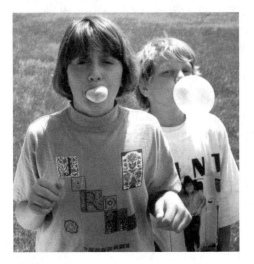

For example, when medication is not effective or produces severe side effects, adults with TS may not be able to care for themselves independently. Adults with learning disabilities may have difficulty getting a job that pays enough for them to fully support themselves. And adults with echolalia or coprolalia will most likely encounter obstacles to employment, housing, and other rights that nondisabled people take for granted. (Although such discrimination is definitely illegal under the ADA, people with TS need funds to fight it.)

If there is a chance that your child's Tourette syndrome will prevent him from caring for all his own needs as an adult, it is important that you plan now for his future well-being. You will, of course, also want to provide monetarily for your child in the event you die before he reaches adulthood. There are two key areas to consider. First, you will want to consider if your child needs a guardian or conservator. There are many different options in this area. Consult an attorney who practices guardianship/conservatorship law. Second, if you are planning to leave funds to your child, you need to determine how those funds will best be provided to ensure the best care for your child in the future.

Guardianship/Conservatorship. You will want to plan who will care for your child if you die or become unable to do so. Equally as important, however, will be to make a plan to assist your child if he will become an adult but will be unable to make all of his own decisions as an adult. In this case, you can consult an attorney about your state's options for guardianships and conservatorships. Many states have a variety of options and guardianships are not always as limiting today as they have been in the past. Most states appoint an attorney for your child to be certain that all of his rights are protected throughout the process. Because IDEA presumes that your child will have the ability to consent and/or agree to IEPs once he is 18 unless there is a guardianship or conservatorship in place, it is important to plan ahead. If you believe your child can advocate on his own, you can still be a part of the IEP process by having your child execute a power of attorney. Again, consult with an attorney or advocate in your area on this point.

Estate Planning

Many of the pitfalls associated with estate planning have to do with the concepts of financial need or cost-of-care liability. As explained above, many government benefits that may be available to your child are dependent upon financial need. If you would like your child to be eligible for these benefits after you are no longer around to look after him, this means you must take care that poor estate planning does not disqualify your child from receiving government assistance. Similarly, if you think your child might need services such as in-home care or health insurance provided by the state, you must keep cost-of-care liability in mind when planning your estate.

Cost-of-care liability is a provision that enables states to require a person with disabilities to use his own funds to pay for state services if he is able to do so. States can draw upon funds owned by the person with disabilities himself as well as funds in some types of trust funds. Some states can even require parents to pay for services for adult children with disabilities. This practice may sound fair in theory. But the catch is that the funds you or your child provide are seldom used to benefit your child directly.

The section below outlines some do's and don'ts of estate planning that can help you avoid the cost-of-care liability trap while ensuring that your child's needs will be adequately provided for. These strategies are provided primarily to help you evaluate the appropriateness of any estate plan you might have now or in the future. To develop an estate plan, it is of utmost importance that you seek professional legal counsel and advice from an attorney specializing in guardianship and estate planning for people with disabilities. Without assistance, all that you have worked for could be lost due to the high costs of care.

As mentioned above, most children with TS grow up to be self-supporting adults who are entirely capable of managing their own assets. If you are reasonably certain that your child will be able to manage on his own after your death, you can probably plan your estate much as any other family would. But if you think your child may need to rely on government benefits such as SSI, SSDI, or Medicaid once he reaches adulthood, or that he may need assistance from the state, estate planning becomes more complicated.

If you want to make sure that your child does not inherit money or property that would be subject to cost-of-care liability or jeopardize his eligibility for government benefits:

1. Be sure to leave a properly written will. If you die without a will, your estate will be distributed according to the laws of inheritance, and your child with TS and his siblings will likely share equally in your estate.

2. Don't rely on joint tenancy instead of a will. If both parents die simultaneously or if one spouse fails to execute a will after the other dies, the result can be the same as if you died without a will.

3. Don't leave property to your child with TS. Instead, leave it to siblings with the unwritten understanding that they will use it to help support their brother or sister with TS.

4. Don't create a support trust for your child with TS; the result is the same as leaving property to him.

5. Don't name your child with TS as a beneficiary in an insurance or retirement plan. Name a sibling or siblings as beneficiary instead, so they can use the funds on their sibling's behalf.

6. Don't establish a UGMA (Uniform Gifts to Minors) account for your child with TS, as these funds become his property once he reaches the age of eighteen.

7. Consider setting up a Special Needs Trust, or a discretionary or luxury trust for your child with TS. In some states, funds left to a child with disabilities through these kinds of trusts cannot be tapped by the state for cost-of-care liability. Consult a lawyer knowledgeable about estate planning for people with disabilities to find out if this is a viable option in your state.

Be sure to tell family members about these estate planning issues. If your child has relatives who may attempt to provide monetarily for his future in their own estate plans, it is essential that they know about all the pitfalls described above. Otherwise, they may leave property to your child via a will or support trust, only to have that property disqualify your child from receiving government benefits or fall into the hands of the state.

Last, but not least, remember that proper estate planning varies for each family, and every will needs to be tailored to individual needs. To develop an effective estate plan, you must let your attorney or estate planner know what the unique needs of your family are. You should be prepared to give your estate planner the following information:

1. nature and degree of your child's disability, including educational and IQ level;
2. functional capabilities and independence;
3. any special medical needs;
4. any work or earnings history;
5. any assets your child owns;
6. any current wills or trusts that exist;
7. current and anticipated educational and living arrangements; and
8. governmental assistance programs such as SSI or SSDI in which your child presently participates or could participate in the future.

Raising a child with Tourette syndrome can be financially and emotionally exhausting. Not only do you have a child with a disability, you have a child with a disability that most people have never heard of or do not understand. This means that it may sometimes be up to you to see that your child receives the special help and benefits he is entitled to and that all his rights are respected. But there are also many professionals who can help you know and exercise your rights. Remember, learn as much as you can about the laws and programs affecting your child, consult knowledgeable professionals, and then trust your own instincts as to what is best for your child.

Advocacy

There are probably many other rights and benefits besides those discussed in this chapter that you think your child should have. As our information about TS improves and as programs for persons with TS are created, it is important to advocate for the rights of persons with TS. The only way to make sure that new and improved laws get on the books is through advocacy. The only way to make sure that good laws get enforced is through advocacy. And the only way to make sure that people understand what your son or daughter needs is through advocacy.

To advocate simply means to plead another's cause. Advocacy can take many different forms. Informing teachers, doctors, and other professionals about the supports and services that your child needs is a form of advocacy. So, too, is educating strangers about appropriate ways to react to your child's TS behaviors. Writing or calling local or federal lawmakers to voice your support for legislation that would benefit your child is yet another form of advocacy. As the parent of a child with Tourette syndrome, you will likely feel compelled to get involved in at least one of these forms of advocacy sooner or later.

The Need for Advocacy

When your child was diagnosed with Tourette syndrome, you were thrust into a new world of parents who have children with special needs. You will find that there is much support and understanding from other parents who have children with disabilities. Other parents understand

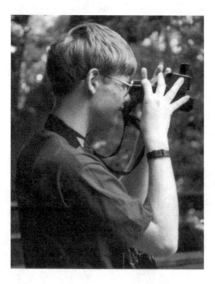

what you mean when you describe the frustrations and anger you have with the "system." But even though you will find much support and understanding from parents, you will also find that the system is not so understanding, and that it can be extremely difficult for you to get the services your child needs.

Because there are so many misunderstandings about TS, there is often a greater need for advocacy than for other disabilities. Your child has a disability that seems invisible to most people. The only visible signs of his disability may be behavioral difficulties such as motor tics, swearing, spitting, or aggressive behavior. These symptoms are *not* going to be recognized by most people as a form of disability. Most people who see these behaviors are going to incorrectly assume that you have a "bad" child or that you are a "bad" parent. Neighbors may not want their children to play with your child. Strangers may make rude comments to you. Because of these and many other gross misunderstandings about Tourette syndrome, your child will probably need someone to advocate for him on a *daily* basis.

Another important reason for advocacy on behalf of children with Tourette syndrome is to ensure that good employment, housing, and training programs exist in the future. Currently, there are precious few of these programs, and long waiting lists confront people who need them. Public officials do not spontaneously decide to establish programs that meet the needs of people with disabilities. They usually must be pushed, and sometimes pushed hard. This is done by advocates working in organizations like the TSA and by advocates working on their own. But unless people fight now and fight hard for services and programs in the future, there is a great risk they won't be there when your child might need them.

Children with TS need to have someone explain the symptoms of Tourette syndrome to their teachers, relatives, and others. Someone needs to explain to teachers what support services are needed in the educational system. Someone needs to explain to doctors what is and isn't working for your child. Someone needs to explain to insurance companies that your child needs medical coverage. This section on advocacy is designed to provide you with enough information about advocacy so that you can determine what is best for your child and what kind of advocacy *you feel most comfortable doing.*

As a parent, you must decide what type of advocacy you will provide for your child. Remember, your primary role in life is not as an advocate. *First and foremost, you are your child's mother or father. First and foremost, any child with disabilities is still a child.* It is essential to remember that being a good parent simply means doing your best.

You probably did not choose to be the parent of a child with Tourette syndrome. You certainly did not choose to be an advocate for the rest of your life. Advocacy is, in the words of many parents, "thrust upon you." Remember that you are a parent first, and then an advocate, *if you choose to be.* You must find your own style and determine what kind of advocate, *if any,* you will be for your child.

Many parents feel comfortable providing individual advocacy for their son or daughter. Others feel more comfortable in requesting the assistance of a professional advocate. You should choose the role you feel most comfortable with.

Gathering Information

The underlying purpose of advocacy is usually to convince someone to do something that they would not otherwise do for your child. For example, you might want to convince the school that your child needs a peer tutor. Or you might want to change your health insurance so it covers your child's Tourette syndrome. Whatever you want to accomplish, you need facts to back up your argument. You must be prepared to show why what you are asking for is in your child's best interests, as well as why your child will suffer if you don't get your way. Typically, the more information you learn about Tourette syndrome and how it affects your child, the more comfortable you will feel about telling others what your child needs. Here are some ideas on how to gather information:

1. **Read, read, read.** Request information from various sources on the Internet, including TSA, subscribe to their newsletter, consult the publications listed in the Reading List—read everything you can about TS. Many TS websites also host listserves for parents. For a complete list, see the Resource section of this book.

2. **Talk to other parents**—in the doctor's office, at school, in support groups. Find out what has and has not worked for their children. Find one parent you can regularly call. It is helpful to be able to get support and advice from someone who knows exactly what you are going through.

3. **Find out where the local advocacy agency is** in your area by calling your local TSA or ARC chapter. Get on their mailing list so you can receive information on advocacy workshops, new legal findings, community resources, and the advocacy efforts of others with an interest in TS.

4. **Watch your child.** Learn what does and doesn't work for him by observing him.

5. **Ask questions** of parents, professionals, and other *adults* who have Tourette syndrome.

6. **Gather more information** than you think you want or think you will read. If you don't read it now, just put it away and save it for later. It is better to have too much information available than not enough.

7. **Keep copies of all your child's medical and educational records,** and request written documentation of your child's needs from doctors and teachers.

Advocating in Your Child's School

As pointed out earlier in the chapter, federal law guarantees only that your child receive an "appropriate" education. It does not spell out what constitutes an appropriate education for any one child, but leaves that up to the school personnel and the parents to decide. Sometimes, teachers and parents agree on what services a child with TS should receive and where he should receive them. But more often, parents and school personnel have different ideas about what an appropriate education for a child with TS should be like. If disagreements arise, you do not have to let the school have its way; you can advocate.

Frequently, school personnel will disagree about how to handle your child's education simply because they know little or nothing about TS and how it affects your child's ability to learn. You may be able to bring them around to your way of thinking by educating them about TS. You can get literature written especially for teachers from the national TSA. Chapter 7 suggests some ways to explain TS to teachers and other school personnel.

If the professionals in your child's school are knowledgeable about TS, but still will not provide your child an education that you feel is appropriate, you may have your work cut out for you. You must find out *why* the school personnel don't want to do as you ask, and then try to counter their arguments. For example, are they refusing to provide your child with occupational therapy because of the cost involved? Then you need to gather documentation from professionals that your child's fine motor skills will continue to lag unless he receives OT. Are teachers refusing to give your child his tests orally because it takes too much of their time? Then you may need to work with them to figure out a time schedule that would be fair to your child and to them. (They can't refuse to test your child orally because of time constraints; oral testing is often necessary.)

Here are some pointers to keep in mind when advocating within the educational system:

1. Be familiar with your child's educational rights. That does *not* mean that you need to know all the laws, but before you go to an IEP or other meeting, call a local advocacy

agency and ask them for a brochure on the special education laws in your state, and reread this chapter.

2. Discuss potentially troublesome issues with teachers *before* they arise at a meeting. It is often easier to resolve issues informally before a meeting.

3. Make a list of concerns you have and give that to the school staff at a meeting. Walk through this list at the meeting asking for the school staff's input. Bring a notebook and take notes at meetings in case further court involvement or due process is necessary and you need to document what was said. You can also bring a tape recorder if that is easier.

4. Bring a friend or your spouse if that will make you more comfortable at the meeting.

5. Find an ally in the school system to act as a buffer between you and any angry, frustrated, or insensitive staff members. He or she may be able to provide you with inside information, calm down frustrated staff members, or assist you in indirect ways. For instance, he or she might help staff implement educational strategies in a positive way, help other staff members learn to trust and respect you, or direct you to "good people" within the system.

6. Keep a small note pad by your phone or in your briefcase at work. Whenever you discuss important issues with *any* school personnel, jot down the date and a few notes about the conversation, in case documentation becomes necessary.

7. Remember that everyone needs support, even professionals. Let your child's classroom teacher and other school personnel know that you appreciate the positive things they do. This will make it more likely that they will continue to go to bat for your child.

8. Compromise only on the small issues. Be persistent about your long-range goals, such as boosting your child's self-esteem through appropriate behavior management strategies or having an inservice on TS for school staff every year.

9. Determine what role you are comfortable with in the school system. You may decide to attend all meetings by

yourself, or you may want to bring a special education advocate to some. If you need to start a due process appeal, you may want a formal advocate or an attorney.

Advocating in the Medical System

In the educational arena, IDEA guarantees that parents have a say in decisions made about their child's schooling. Unfortunately, there are no equivalent laws requiring professionals to work with parents in making decisions about their child's medical care. Because of the nature of Tourette syndrome, however, there are many reasons a doctor *should* consult you when treating your child.

As Chapter 3 explains, the information you supply about your child's symptoms and responses to medications is invaluable in planning your child's treatment plan. Ordinarily, doctors have no problem requesting this information from parents, and parents have no problem providing it. But what happens if you would like to be more involved in your child's treatment plan? For example, what if you have read about a new medication that you think might help your child, but your doctor has never mentioned it? Or what if you think your child's medication causes too many side effects, but the doctor seems unwilling to consider a change? You can advocate for specific medical services just as you advocate for educational services. Here are some pointers to keep in mind:

1. Be informed. Read as much as you can about Tourette syndrome and the medications and treatments that have been successful. Always ask your doctor about anything you don't understand. Ask him or her to spell the names of medications and what the side effects of medications are.

2. Remember that there is much disagreement among physicians as to the treatment of TS. There is so much *new* information about TS that there is still much misunderstanding. Your doctor may not recommend a new treatment because he is waiting for more information about its risks and benefits, or then again he may not even be aware of the treatment. It doesn't hurt to ask what your doctor thinks.

3. If you want to discuss any aspect of your child's treatment with the doctor, try to schedule an appointment in the morning. Doctors are fresher then and less hurried. Be concise and prepared when you meet with the doctor.

It helps to come to the appointment with a written list of questions that you can check off as you ask them.

4. Ask for a second opinion if you are not satisfied with your doctor's answers.

5. Remember that you are the consumer. Switch doctors if you are not getting the help you are asking for. Ask other parents of children with TS or your local TSA for referrals to experts in the field.

Legislative and Class Advocacy

The previous sections have discussed ways that you, as a parent, can provide individual advocacy for your son or daughter. But there will also be times when the voice of one person is simply not enough. There will be times when laws need to be changed, and you may want to become part of a larger group to help change the system. Here again, as with individual advocacy, you must decide what you are comfortable with. There are many different ways to become involved in *class* advocacy—advocacy aimed at reforming the system as a whole. It may be as simple as voting for the right candidate or writing a short letter, or as complex as testifying before a legislative body or participating in a class action lawsuit.

It is extremely important to recognize the power that parents have as a large group, and to remember the changes in laws that parents have brought about. The special education laws that now *guarantee* your child's right to a free and appropriate education were a result of the efforts of organized parents. IDEA passed in large part because parents just like you were frustrated and angry that their children with disabilities were not being served by the educational system. They joined forces with other parents and *they changed the system.* It only takes one parent to start talking, and soon you have large numbers who do make a difference. *Never underestimate your power as a parent.*

Parents of children with Tourette syndrome should feel an urgency to band together. Because of widespread misunderstandings about the disability, many issues need the immediate attention of lawmakers. As a parent, you may already recognize many of these problems. For example, some professionals continue to disagree as to whether Tourette syndrome is a mental health issue or a developmental disability or a neurological disorder. Because of this, there is no guaranteed funding stream for service. Often Human Service and other agencies won't provide funding unless they can conveniently pigeonhole a disability. And insurance companies are able to get away with paying less than they should by claiming that TS is a mental illness. Furthermore, many professionals continue to give low priority to this disability because they mistakenly believe that the incidence of TS is low. As a result, medical researchers don't put enough time into looking for better treatments, and educators don't spend enough time looking for better ways to teach children with TS. To complicate matters, because of behaviors such as tics, spitting, and swearing, children with TS are not perceived by the general public as cute children. Therefore, many people, including legislators, would rather not think about the problem.

For parents of young children with Tourette syndrome, *now* is the time to organize with other parents. *Now* is the time to demand appropriate services and better funding so that adulthood will be easier for your child.

The first step is to locate the local and national advocacy groups already in existence. The national Tourette Syndrome Association needs your support. There may also be a local or state TS group in your area; contact the TSA or visit their website to determine if there is. If there are no local groups, you may need to gather the strength and just start one. If you do, you will be amazed by the number of people who will come out of the woodwork to join. Parents of children with TS have a desperate need to network and find others.

Reaching the Lawmakers

As a member of an advocacy group, you will be in the best position to change the system through legislative reforms and court decisions. You will also find it easier to keep abreast of any legislative issues that may affect your child. This is important because—as with individual advocacy—the key to successful legislative advocacy is to be informed and know the issues.

One of the best ways for your local TS group to find out about pertinent legislation is to have your group's name added to the mailing list of larger advocacy groups that watch the state and national legislative changes. Examples of these groups are listed in the Resource Guide at the back of the book, and include Children and Adults with Attention Deficit/Hyperactivity Disorder (CHADD) and the ARC. Most organizations of this nature develop "Action Alerts" in response to proposed legislation. These alerts will inform your group of actions that individual members should take to help get a desirable bill passed, or an undesirable bill defeated. They may, for instance, recommend that you write letters to legislators or sign petitions. These larger advocacy groups can also provide you with information sheets that describe a proposed bill and how it may affect your child.

Once you know the formal name of a bill or proposed law and how it will affect your child, the next step is to contact your legislator. There are many ways you can do this, but the simplest, most effective ways are to simply call or write your legislator.

Calling Your Legislator

Parents are often reluctant to call their legislator, fearing that their opinions couldn't possibly matter and that their phone calls would be an unwelcome intrusion. But nothing could be further from the truth. Legislators must vote on hundreds of issues each year and they simply do not have the time or the expertise to learn about each issue on which they are voting. If a bill is proposed that will affect your child, chances are very likely that your legislator knows *nothing* about TS and will need information before voting. Because your child has TS, you are an expert compared to most people. Many legislators will base a vote on as little as one or two phone calls if that is all the information they have. One phone call can make a difference.

To call your legislator, first jot down a few notes about the major points you want to make. Then when you actually talk to someone, you will know exactly what you want to say. (Don't forget to mention that you are a constituent and you do vote!) Often if a bill is coming up for a vote, a secretary or aide will answer the legislator's phone and just tally the yes and no calls. Legislators really do count these calls and listen to their constituents' opinions. So make that call and urge other parents you know to do the same thing.

Writing Your Legislator

Letters and emails are also an extremely effective way of getting your legislator's ear. Writing is an especially good method if you have a number of facts to convey that you think might help sway your legislator's vote. Here are some guidelines to help you put your opinion in writing:

1. Keep your letter or email short and concise.
2. Start with a pleasant introduction, being sure to identify yourself as a parent of a child with Tourette syndrome.

3. Focus on the issues and how they affect you and your child personally.

4. Always refer to the proposed legislation by the proper bill number and title.

5. Conclude with your request or recommendation for a vote and thank the legislator for his or her time.

6. If your group organizes a letter-writing party, don't send form letters. Personalize your letters.

7. When bills pass that will help your child, write your legislators and thank them if they voted for it.

Recharging Your Batteries

Earlier chapters have emphasized how important emotional support is to coping with a wide range of issues—from adjusting to the initial diagnosis to managing your child's daily care. Support is also important when you are advocating, whether individually or in a group. You are dealing with such emotionally charged issues on such a regular basis that you need the opportunity to share what you are going through with others.

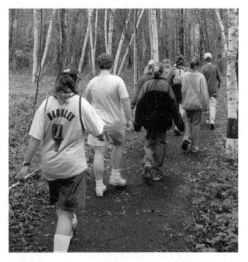

Becoming a member of an advocacy group, as suggested above, is an excellent way to find support. You can get comfort and practical advice from other parents who have experienced *the very same issues* you are facing. If you are married or have a partner, not only can you share some of the emotional burden, but also the advocacy work. You can take turns attending meetings, if possible, and also divide the advocacy work so that each of you winds up with the role you feel most comfortable with. For example, one of you may want to become the expert on medical issues related to TS, and the other may want to become the educational expert. Or, one of you may prefer to gather all the information you need to support your argument, while the other attends meetings and presents your case.

Whatever you do, don't let the need for advocacy rule your life. Recognize that it is okay to feel tired and worn out. Don't become a martyr parent. Recognize your limits and periodically refuel yourself. Even if you think you only have five extra minutes a day, don't forget about your own needs. Remember to play, sleep, love, laugh, work, and just take time for yourself. Taking a break is especially important if you are a single parent and must handle all the advocating on your own. Try to space apart educational meetings and medical appointments. If you can schedule two meetings in two weeks, rather than two meetings in one week, it may be an easier schedule for you to live with.

Finally, to keep your motivation high, periodically take stock of your accomplishments. Write down the things you have accomplished for your child. Have you helped your child's teacher *really understand* that he can't control his tics? Have you helped the doctor find a combination of medications that improves your child's tics? Have you helped to raise money for a candidate who is sensitive to the needs of children with disabilities? Make a habit of focusing on your successes, not your failures. And above all, believe in yourself.

∷ Conclusion

There are many ways you can advocate for your son or daughter. And when you do, you are not only advocating for your child, but for all the children who will eventually be born with Tourette syndrome. Every minor, positive change that you are able to make in the system will affect thousands of other people in the future. As a parent, you are incredibly powerful and you can make a difference.

Margaret Mead said it best: "Never doubt that a small group of thoughtful committed citizens can change the world; indeed, it's the only thing that ever does."

∷ Parent Statements

Don't go to an IEP meeting unless you know your child's legal rights. Don't expect the school to let you know what they are. I learned everything the hard way until I met other parents of kids with TS. They are the people with real helpful information.

❧❀❧

I am treated as a respected and equal member of my child's IEP team. This makes me feel "listened to" and helps me put my trust in the professionals who have such an important role in Holly's life.

·ᡓᢤᢖ·

The most frustrating aspect of having a child with Tourette syndrome is dealing with the schools. They resist programming for Dan's special needs (including learning disabilities), and instead just drop him into the most handy EBD [emotional-behavioral disorder] slot they have available.

·ᡓᢤᢖ·

I learned quickly that public schools are not prepared for the child with "special needs" or anyone who doesn't fit into the "round peg in round hole" school system. They need help to make a way for the "square peg." I think the changes help all the children to learn to accept differences and to think more creatively.

·ᡓᢤᢖ·

Once parents learn about the laws and their child's rights, they're in a much better position to negotiate with the school.

·ᡓᢤᢖ·

When I first got involved in legislative advocacy, I was amazed at the impact each individual can have on the system if he is committed to a cause.

·ᡓᢤᢖ·

Get everything in writing and make copies!

·ᡓᢤᢖ·

I've needed to learn advocacy for my child just like the parents of a kid with a hearing impairment need to learn sign language and the parents of a kid with cystic fibrosis need to learn pummeling. It's never accomplished once and for all; it never ends.

·ᡓᢤᢖ·

Long before I realized that I had rights (and that Kenny had rights), the only time I got any action from the school was when I said, "Well, I guess I'll just have to keep him home then." Now I know the reason that threat got results was because if I kept Kenny home from school, we would end up in court. That's the last place schools want to end up.

❦

Being involved in advocacy helps reduce the feelings of powerlessness encountered when you have a child with TS. In two short years, I have made great strides in educating people in my child's world about Tourette syndrome.

❦

Often the attorney can get the school to pay her fees. The first time the school procrastinates in meeting your child's needs, find an attorney who knows special education law. Every bad day at school chips away at your child's self-esteem and potential.

❦

Something that has been hard for me to accept is that an "appropriate" education does not necessarily mean "best" education. The schools are only required to go so far.

❦

I have been my child's advocate for four years now, and my son is now beginning to take over and learn to advocate for himself. Through this experience, he will learn so much about people, negotiations, and feeling personal power.

❦

When we showed the school the law that they had to provide services, they wrote a nice IEP, but it was never enforced.

❦

*I'd say that if the school punishes your child for his symptoms **after** you've explained to them that he can't help it, get an attorney.*

❦

One thing the laws can't legislate is understanding and tolerance. I worry about this sometimes when I think about what kinds of problems my son could run into on the job.

❦

I'm tired of parent advocacy groups always saying "the parent is the best advocate." When you spend twenty-four hours a day coping with your child with TS and the rest of your family, where do you get the energy necessary to become an advocate?

❦

I wish someone had told us when our child was diagnosed that we would have to become pseudo-lawyers just to have our child's legal rights upheld.

❦

I have been very fortunate. I have not had to take our school district to a due process hearing. The right people have been in place to advocate for his special needs.

❦

Because there was no one else to advocate for my child, I fell into the role of his advocate. I have learned a lot, just by believing in my child's rights and by taking a risk to be assertive.

❦

I learned much from advocating for my child at school. In my case diplomacy worked better than anger. Even though I was angry that the school didn't see the problems and come up with their own common sense strategies, I kept my anger to myself and tried to work as a team with the school professionals. They did try to help my son.

❦

I find that a good teacher or school psychologist makes all the difference in the school year. Some teachers are better with flexible planning than others. Finding that match is crucial. I found one person in the system to be my advocate and help me find the right teacher for my child.

❦

If you have the time, volunteer in the school district in areas that help lots of kids, not just yours. I've been on boards that work on equity issues, harassment, and discipline policy, curriculum adoption, even changing boundaries. I connect with lots of people in the district and have learned the politics, as well as where to go to get something done.

LIVING WITH TOURETTE SYNDROME: "I AM NOT MY TICS!"

William V. Rubin, M.A.

∷ My History

I have lived with Tourette syndrome for approximately fifty-five years. Since the age of about six I have had a variety of head and facial tics (blinking, head shaking, nose and mouth movements); other body tics (leg and foot movements, stomach contractions, hand tightening, and arm and shoulder movements); vocalizations (sniffing, barking, grunting, and throat clearing); and rituals (checking that the coffee pot is unplugged,

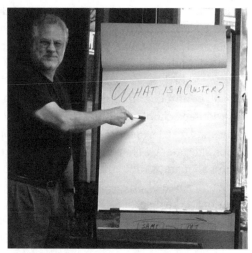

William V. Rubin

pushing my bed up to the wall until it feels right, feeling that I have to be places on time).

When I began having these symptoms as a child, nobody knew much about TS. I was very lucky, though, and generally had no problems in school or out in public. I was almost never teased or ridiculed by classmates, or reprimanded by teachers, parents, or other adults. Still, I often felt isolated, even in a room filled with my friends. I couldn't understand why I had to have strange "habits" and be so different from the other kids.

Once I reached adolescence, my parents became less accepting. My father wanted to know why I kept "making these noises to disturb everybody?" I could control them for periods of time, so why did I have to make sounds at all? It must have been just to "get them," he decided. My father and I battled for several years over my tics. Luckily, my parents finally realized that no matter what, I could not control the symptoms, and the confrontations ended.

After high school, I attended Brandeis University, and graduated with a bachelor's degree with honors in psychology. I next enrolled in graduate school at the University of Nebraska on a National Institute of Mental Health Fellowship in Clinical Psychology. I had completed most of my courses for the Ph.D., and was completing an internship in Child Clinical Psychology, when one of the psychologists there agreed to help me try to eliminate my tics and noises. We thought this would be good for my professional career. We attempted several behavioral approaches, including aversive electric shock, before one of the psychiatric residents suggested that I try a powerful antipsychotic medication called Haldol. This drug is used to treat severe psychiatric disorders; however, it had begun to be used, in small doses, to treat tics. I started taking Haldol and it "miraculously" reduced my symptoms by about 75 percent. Shortly afterwards, however, I decided to drop out of school as a result of unrecognized side effects of the medication. I later returned to graduate school in Industrial Psychology at Case Western Reserve University, in Cleveland, Ohio, but again dropped out because of medication side effects. These included short-term memory loss, depression, doubts about my skills, and difficulty understanding complex materials. Although some of my professors may have suspected TS, no one ever mentioned the disorder.

I was finally diagnosed as having Tourette syndrome at the age of thirty-five. This occurred following a vacation to Connecticut where I met the TSA state coordinator. She gave my first wife information about TS, which she shared with me on our trip home. At about the same time, my parents saw a television show in which neurologists described this unusual syndrome. They mentioned to me what they had seen, and several months later I went to the pediatric neurology department at the Cleveland Clinic for my formal diagnosis.

People frequently ask how I felt after being diagnosed. Although I firmly believe that knowing that you have TS is very important, it still takes time getting used to. For me, knowing that I had TS was a double-edged sword. On the positive side, I finally knew why I had to make the strange sounds and movements. On the negative side, however, I had to acknowledge that there was something "wrong" with me. Accepting the reality of a disabling condition doesn't mean giving up, but it does mean coming to grips with something that, for me, will probably never go away. It took me about six months to begin to accept these realities.

As a parent, you too will need to come to grips with the realities—and unknowns—of Tourette syndrome. While new research suggests that some of the symptoms of TS may decrease over time, more research needs to be done to understand how many people see their symptoms improve and in what ways. This is why parents must begin, as quickly as possible, to help their children understand TS and to help them work through the feelings they will have.

Once I began to accept the fact of my TS, I became active in the Tourette Syndrome Association of Ohio, serving as its Vice President for four years and its first Director of Training, Research, and Development. Between 1985 and 1993, I helped the Tourette Syndrome Association of Minnesota operate its Family Learning Camp. It was the first camp for children with TS and their families in this country. While I was no longer affiliated with the local TSA, I continued, until the mid-90s, to provide consultation and workshops on TS in schools, mental health facilities, correctional facilities, and even homeless shelters.

Over the past ten years, my growing business has left me with less time to dedicate to issues related to Tourette syndrome. Synthesis, Inc., the company I founded in 1987, continues to be both rewarding and challenging. We conduct mental health service system research and consult with local human service agencies. We have become recognized leaders in the development of a clinical service planning and quality improvement technology called Cluster-Based Planning and Outcomes Management (Rubin & Panzano, 2002) which is used to manage and evaluate mental health and substance abuse services. We have also been designated a Coordinating Center of Excellence by the Ohio Department of Mental Health. My personal life has not always run smoothly. My first marriage ended after thirty-one years. However, I have remarried and, in that process, found new happiness, gained a business partner, and inherited three grown children who have given me exciting new experiences and the opportunity to learn a new role as "an additional parental presence."

While it wasn't the primary problem, my Tourette syndrome did play a role in the matters that strained my first marriage, and the issues and transitions were not easy. Counseling from a psychologist really helped me through it, and in the process, I came to a greater understanding of the symptoms of my TS and their relationship to who I am. I also began to think of my journey through life in terms of a "recovery" process. Boston University researcher William Anthony, one of the leaders in the psychiatric rehabilitation movement, describes recovery as "a deeply personal, unique process of changing one's attitudes, values, feelings, and goals… a way of living a satisfying, hopeful, and contributing life, even with the limitations caused by illness." Recovery is not an end product, but a journey.

Since my childhood, major strides have been made in understanding Tourette syndrome and in educating the community about it. However, the condition continues to be misdiagnosed, inappropriately treated, and misunderstood by health care professionals, educators, employers, parents, and the general public. It is little wonder that children, their parents, and adults with TS are themselves often misinformed. Many must face the world with only a poor sense of who they are and what they are capable of accomplishing. Without proper diagnosis, treatment, basic information, and supports, children with TS have a hard time acquiring the coping strategies they need. This can lead them to feel that they cannot take charge of their own lives and make choices for themselves.

Over the years, I have been very lucky in the way my family and society have reacted (or in fact, not reacted) to my symptoms. While I certainly have been, and continue to be, affected by my disorder, I have not suffered the great ridicule and isolation that some with TS experience. In writing this chapter, I have tried to pinpoint what it is about my experiences that has enabled me to live a productive life with Tourette syndrome. I have also drawn upon the conversations and experiences I have had over the years with many children and adults with TS. I hope my recollections and perspectives will help children with Tourette syndrome and their families better understand the condition and begin to engage in a recovery process of their own—one that will allow them to overcome the negative impact of TS while accepting its continued presence.

∷ Understanding Tourette Syndrome

What Does It Feel Like to Live with TS?

When I think about this question, I identify two separate types of feelings. These are: 1) how I feel physically before, during, and after having symptoms; and 2) how I feel emotionally about what I do.

Physically, I am aware of almost every tic or sound that I make. This awareness is in the form of a feeling of tension in a specific body location. It also feels as if something "is going to happen." That is, it feels as if I am going to blink or shake my head forward. Although I am aware of these events, my mind does not constantly focus on them. In computer terms, the awareness "runs in the background." It's only when tics are really interfering with my activities or when I am trying to suppress them that the awareness becomes heightened. For example, when I used to play competitive volleyball and was very tired, I would have ankle, leg, and hip tics that would slow down my movements and interfere with my jumping. Sometimes I became so conscious of these tics that I would have to force myself to concentrate on the rest of the game.

From my observations over the years, I believe that children are less aware of some of their symptoms. In other cases, they may say they are not aware of them because they have absolutely no explanation for why they do such strange things. As a result, they may "lie about," or deny, having done something (for example, poking at a classmate as he walks by). Some children even purposely become disruptive or act as class clowns to cover up for their inability to control their behavior. (Sometimes it's more acceptable to be a "problem child" than a "crazy child.") Even though my parents noticed my tics at about the time I started school, I really don't remember being very aware of them until I reached junior high school. I can remember that all the way through high school I "lied" to people about my symptoms, calling them "habits" when I really had no idea what was going on. In any event, we all know when we are having bad days—when our tics are more pronounced and can wear us out physically and mentally.

Once I have the tic (or other symptom), there is a release of tension. It's not that it feels so good *while* I'm expressing the symptom, but that the tension is gone *after* I've expressed it. I have only mild compulsive symptoms, but I can still recognize that tension will be relieved, for instance, after I *check* to make sure the stove burners are turned off, even though I'm standing right across the kitchen and can see them. This is why it's so difficult for us when we are asked not to perform the behaviors that are part of our obsessive-compulsive symptoms. It usually takes specific

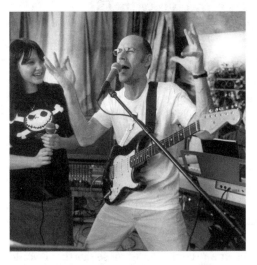

behavioral approaches and/or medications to help reduce our need to act on these feelings.

Motor tics, vocalizations, and other behaviors can also have specific physical effects on your body. Fatigue and pain come from both the repetition and the severity of symptoms. My neck muscles, for example, are always tight and stiff. For many years, I had a head-shaking tic that was made worse by wearing dress shirts with ties or anything up around my neck. Sometimes I would shake my head and sniff so many times that I would give myself a headache and severe neck pains. About twenty-five years ago I stopped wearing ties or the types of shirts that increase these tics, but they still occur at a lesser level.

Over time, severe tics can even result in temporary or permanent physical damage. For example, the neck tics described above, coupled with years of competitive sports, have resulted in my having microfractures and compressions in the vertebrae in my neck. In addition, more than twenty years ago, when changing medications from Haldol to clonidine, my symptoms got very severe for about two months. This is called a *rebound effect,* and can occur after long-term use of some medications. I made such loud noises that my larynx was damaged. Years later, I still have difficulty carrying a tune.

When I do training workshops for parents or professionals, I always have them experience how it feels physically to have tics. If you want to get a sense of what it's like, just stand in front of a mirror and blink by squeezing your eyes shut about fifty times. As difficult as the physical discomfort can be to deal with, I think the most damaging part of Tourette syndrome is its emotional impact. What does it feel like emotionally to have tics or compulsions, or to make noises? It's frightening, frustrating, terribly embarrassing, and very saddening. It can make you feel about as small as you can possibly feel. We have grown up (or are growing up) doing things that we can't seem to control. They don't make sense and we don't know why we do them. Even when we have a diagnosis and intellectually know that we have a neurotransmitter imbalance, we live every day knowing that we will always stand out. No matter where we go, some people will be looking at us, wondering, and some even laughing.

While public service announcements, newspaper articles, and educational efforts at the national level have increased awareness of Tourette syndrome, you still never know exactly how people will respond to your symptoms. The feedback can be violent (being hit, ridiculed, shunned, or kicked out of class) or very subtle (a raised eyebrow, a snicker, a waiter being distracted while taking your order). When others respond negatively, I get angry at them for their stupidity and cruelty. And then I hate myself for being so different that it makes me their target. As a result of many years of negative responses from those around us, I think most of us with TS live with an ongoing sense that we are being watched. This awareness produces a constant level of stress. Even though my symptoms would be considered moderate and generally not socially unacceptable, I routinely encounter the more benign responses mentioned above. If you want to experience some of the emotional feelings that your child may be having, ask a good friend to stand right in front of you and watch while you blink, or grimace, or shake your head for about a minute. When you are through, talk with them about how you felt; ask them also how they felt, and what it was like looking at you.

Years ago, I wondered whether there were ways to reduce this stress of being watched in specific situations. On several occasions, I tried a little experiment while sitting in airport waiting areas. I closed my eyes and pretended to sleep so that I would get no visual feedback from other passengers. In fact, this strategy did make me more comfortable. I didn't really care if they were looking, or wondering, or laughing. It was like a demonstration of the old expression, "what you don't know can't hurt you." I have used this technique now for many years in waiting rooms and other situations where everyone is expected to be quiet and still. I do it for myself—not for the others in the room. In many ways, I think we have to be able to emotionally close our eyes for periods of time so we can get on with our lives.

What Does It Feel Like to Know Your Tics Bother Other People?

I am sometimes asked how it feels to know that tics, vocalizations, or other behaviors that I have annoy other people. First, it is important to recognize that your symptoms may not always be as annoying as you believe. When I think back to my childhood, I realize that one of the things that enabled me to live with TS was the fact that, in the beginning, my parents were virtually the only ones who said anything about my tics and noises. No teachers or classmates asked me to stop making noises, twitching, or shaking my head. This was extremely unusual. But my experience has shown me that there are several factors that greatly affect others' ability to ignore my symptoms of TS: 1) their general attitude of acceptance, 2) their getting to know me over time, and 3) my openness about my TS.

In work settings, after initially being very aware of my tics, most of my co-workers hardly notice them unless I am having a period of very severe symptoms. In fact, co-workers and close friends are so at ease with my symptoms that they have even remarked to me about funny movements (tics) or sounds that other people may have. Recently, the chief financial officer of my company told me that when she first interviewed for a position with Synthesis fifteen years ago, she wasn't sure how she could work with someone with my symptoms. However, this changed the moment in the interview when I mentioned, in a matter-of-fact way, that I had TS and it caused the tics and noises she was seeing. My ability to provide an explanation eliminated her need to care about my symptoms.

Although there are obviously some symptoms that are not easily tolerated, I believe many people can adapt to many symptoms. Indeed, it is critical for parents, siblings, friends, teachers, employers, co-workers, and others to learn to ignore symptoms. Since stress exacerbates the symptoms of TS, knowing that people are listening or watching for your tics only makes them worse. Trying to suppress your tics does the same. When I think of the Family Camps I helped run in Minnesota, I realize just how much you can accomplish when most of the people around you accept or ignore most of your symptoms (including coprolalia).

The other side of this issue, though, is that at times (and over time) some symptoms *are* annoying to others. In the past when I would go to symphony concerts, I would try to suppress my tics, and still worry about annoying other patrons who expect quiet during the performance. It is even more distressing to me that some of my tics and noises have interfered with my wife's sleep, because my tics start almost immediately when I awaken (even in the middle of the night). Worse still is when I put my arm around the woman I love and bark in her ear.

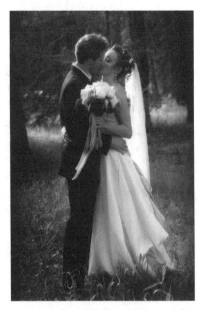

There will always be some symptoms that challenge your relationship with your spouse, family, and friends. Sometimes you can laugh about them, sometimes you cry, and sometimes you get angry. Without apologizing for the symptoms, I think people with TS must accept responsibility for trying to reduce the effect of their symptoms on those they care about. I don't mean we need to feel responsible for the symptoms, but only that we recognize the impact the symptoms can have on others and try to reduce that impact.

What About Suppressing the Symptoms?

Many people with TS can suppress symptoms for varying lengths of time. How successfully they can do so usually depends on the severity of their disorder, the symptom, and the specific situation. For example, I can usually suppress symptoms better when I go to a movie than when I go to watch a football or basketball game. My love of sports and the excitement of the game make my tics and noises worse. At the same time, with everybody else shouting and jumping around at the game, who cares?

On the other hand, suppressing tics at a movie or concert takes much more energy for me to be both quiet and still. Withholding symptoms is like repeatedly trying to hold your breath for as long as you can, then catching a quick breath, and then holding your breath again. At the end of a two-hour movie or a concert, not only am I physically tired, *but my tics come out even more intensively on the way home.*

Trying to suppress tics and other symptoms also requires that you focus part of your mind on that effort. If you try holding your breath over and over, you will find that after a while you start thinking about your chest or mouth or head. You must split your concentration between what is going on around you and the portion of your body (or mind, if you have obsessive thoughts) that you are trying to control. Having to divide your attention like this can certainly affect your ability to study or perform other complex tasks. That's why I believe we must expect the symptoms to occur and learn to adapt to them. From my experience, expecting a child to suppress tics in school will tell her she is "not OK." It will wear her down physically, make it more difficult for her to concentrate on the material to be studied, and mean she will have more tics when she gets out of school.

I don't know any parents who haven't felt guilty for having *expected* their children to stop having tics, and I think most of us with TS have felt at some time or another that we should be able to stop. But for a number of reasons, *expecting* individuals with TS to suppress symptoms is both unrealistic and harmful. As described above, holding back symptoms takes considerable physical and mental energy. This adds to the difficulty the person may already have in learning, taking care of her day-to-day needs, or interacting with others. I have emphasized the word "expecting" because those of us with TS will try to suppress our own symptoms anyway. We are just like anybody else. We don't want to look funny, disturb others, or be ridiculed or thrown out of movies or school. We want our parents, friends, and spouses to love us, so we don't want to do things that irritate them. But when I feel that somebody expects me to suppress my tics, I feel they are really saying that I'm not OK with them. This heightens the already difficult emotions (e.g., anger or shame) I have toward my tics. Likewise, when people with TS themselves feel that they ought to suppress all their symptoms so as not to bother others, we are saying to ourselves that we are not OK with ourselves.

I Am Not My TS—But My Tourette Syndrome Is a Part of Me

As I indicated earlier, I believe it is important to recognize that many symptoms of Tourette syndrome make little sense to those of us who have them or to others—especially when viewed in the context of the rest of our lives. Having to shake my head violently when I'm driving doesn't make any sense. Or what sense does it make for an eleven-year-old girl to yell obscenities in church every week? I sincerely believe that the more we can learn to view our TS symptoms as "add-ons" to who we really are, the better we will be able to get on with our lives.

▪▪ How Can We Get On With Our Lives?

I think one of the most important factors in being able to live with TS is developing the strength from within to go out and take on the world. Over the years, I have met some remarkable people with serious symptoms of TS or other disabling conditions who go out day after day and live their lives. For example, I had an employee with cerebral palsy who used enormous physical energy just to go from his office to the rest room. Another friend with TS had to allow himself at least two hours to dress each morning because of his compulsions. A young woman I knew attended college while experiencing very severe full-body tics and coprolalia.

When children are confronted with the reality of Tourette syndrome, their strength from within must first come from the support of others. As we are growing up, we all develop a sense of how well we can master our environment. The child who grows up with loved ones who support her but don't coddle her learns that "I am OK. I may not always succeed, but I can still go on with my life."

I really can't say enough about how much my family and friends have contributed to my own feelings about myself. Their love and support never wavered, even in the face of my mystifying behaviors. *They looked right past my tics to the person I really was becoming, and responded to that person.* That even included punishing that evolving person when he did something wrong. My parents never seemed to let my symptoms come between them, and until their deaths, they were both there for me. My brother and our friends never let my symptoms get in the way, either. They never even mentioned the movements and noises I made. Although I believe that people with TS, their parents, siblings, spouses, and friends must be able to talk comfortably about TS, I don't feel it needs to become a regular topic of conversation. To allow it to do so only focuses attention and effort away from the rest of our lives.

Today, growing up seems very different for most of the children with Tourette syndrome I have met. Much more emphasis is placed on appearance, and "fitting in" seems even more important. However, once teenagers with TS begin to feel more comfortable with who they are, they become more eager and able to make friends. They may have fewer friends than other children do, but they start doing and experiencing the same things that other teens do. They play sports or play in the band; they have girlfriends and boyfriends; they like (and are liked by) some of their teachers, and don't like (and are not liked by) others; they want to learn to drive; they don't always do what adults want them to do, and so forth.

In order to learn to live with Tourette syndrome, I think we must all learn to live—period. That is, we must try to focus on things we would do if we did not have TS, and figure out ways to accomplish those things. During the years I helped to run the Family Camp in Minnesota, we would videotape many activities. When I 'd review the tapes, I would see members of twenty-five to thirty families running around, doing arts and crafts, eating, swimming, playing volleyball, and generally having a good time—just like any other families. I even saw some kids fighting, pushing, or teasing, just like other kids.

I'm not trying to minimize the problems that some symptoms can cause, but I *am* trying to emphasize that we can become so focused on those symptoms that we forget that we are very much like other families or individuals. Families talk about not being able to go out and do things together. Adults with TS complain that their options are limited. Many families have the same problems that we do. For example, if we can figure out how *any* three children and their parents can take a two-week vacation together in their minivan without killing each other, surely we can figure out how to do it when one of the children has TS. Or maybe we learn that a one-week vacation is better for our family.

There is, of course, no way to totally ignore the many additional problems TS creates for us. But the more we can try to "live our lives as others do," the better we will be able to handle the special burdens placed on us by the symptoms of TS.

■■ Coping and "Recovery" Strategies

Dr. Patricia Deegan, a psychologist who herself is in recovery from a psychiatric disability, writes "Recovery does not refer to an end product or result. It does not mean that my friend and I were 'cured.' In fact, our recovery is marked by an ever-deepening acceptance of our limitations. But now, rather that being an occasion for despair, we find that our personal limitations are the ground from which spring our own unique possibilities. This is the paradox of recovery, i.e., that in accepting what we cannot do or be, we begin to discover who we can be and what we can do."

Part of "learning to live as others do" means developing coping and recovery strategies. Although many people develop them, people with TS must learn how to handle more unusual and difficult situations than others need to do. We must learn to live with a body that we do not totally control, and a mind that sometimes won't pay attention or won't let us stop thinking about some things.

Learning to cope is important because the world doesn't really change very quickly. That is, attitudes toward people with TS and other disabling conditions change slowly, so we must learn to live in a society that—while not specifically *against* us—is certainly not actively *for* us. That is why parents must help their kids by being patient and supportive as they try out different approaches to coping.

Parents can help their children learn to cope in several important ways. The key is that your child must see you as an ally in her journey through childhood and adolescence. You show your child that you're on her side when you acknowledge her feelings, her struggles, and her desire to figure things out. Keep in mind, also, that your child's understanding of situations will be limited by her age and developmental level.

Another way parents can help their children learn to cope is by acting as good role models when dealing with uncomfortable situations. For example, if a store manager is concerned about your child touching boxes on the store shelves, you may quietly but quickly approach the manager and explain that this is one of your child's tics or compulsive behaviors. You can also calmly assure the manager that if anything is broken, it will be paid for, but that damage is unlikely. More importantly, parents can be very effective in helping their child figure out ways to head off problems before they occur.

Coping is not always about dealing with unpleasant situations. In most cases, it's about working out ways to do the things we want to do. For example, what ideas can you and your child brainstorm for dealing with times when she wants to go out somewhere, but she is ticcing a lot?

Finally, it's important to remember that developing coping and recovery strategies is a personal process. There is no one correct way. Eventually your child must become responsible for what she does, and for the consequences. As your child is learning and growing, you as parents must share in the celebration of her successes and be supportive when her efforts are unsuccessful.

I certainly don't claim to have all the answers about how to live with Tourette syndrome, but I feel very strongly that each of us must develop our own coping mechanisms that will enable us to deal with other people and situations. We must each "discover who we can be and what we can do," so we can live successful lives. There's no way to describe how to cope with every different situation people with TS may face. But, I'd like to discuss at least a few of strategies that I've found make my life easier and, I hope, more productive.

First, it's important to understand that the goal of my coping strategies is to live my life as normally as possible. Most of my strategies involve how I try to cope with:

1. Being out in public;
2. Interacting with people who don't know me well (students, employees, new clients, acquaintances);
3. Relating to people very close to me;
4. Accomplishing specific tasks (work, school assignments, sports, etc.).

My coping strategies for each of these situations are rooted in non-confrontation and in presenting an image of competence.

Being Out in Public

If I'm out in public and become aware that others are staring or making comments about me, I generally ignore them and go on as if nothing were wrong. I usually don't try to confront people unless they directly interfere with what I'm doing. Rather, I try to demonstrate my competence. This is because many times people feel my symptoms might indicate that I am unstable. For example, if I'm in a department store and a clerk notices my tics, I don't walk away or confront her by asking what she is staring at. Instead, I ask the clerk about something I'm interested in purchasing. Or, if I'm ready to buy something, I do it with my charge card. This says to the clerk that while I may do some funny things, I am competent enough to be able to buy something, and I earn enough to have a charge card at the store. If I'm out of town on business and in a restaurant, I will pay with a business credit card and give the waiter/waitress a good tip. In these ways I am saying, "I'm not so different from your customers. (Maybe I'm even a *better* customer)."

A child could use the same tactics. For example, since many adults expect inappropriate behavior from children, a child could ask a question *politely* about an item in the store, pick up something off the floor that another customer has dropped, purchase the item she came for, or just slowly leave the store.

I've also found that speaking to others first is a way of putting them at ease about my various symptoms. It's also more difficult to laugh at, be afraid of, or make fun of someone after you've just had a brief but pleasant conversation with her about the basketball game last night,

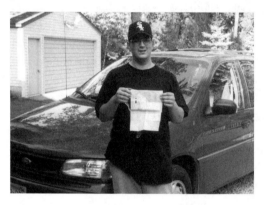

the math exam yesterday, the bad cafeteria food, or even just the weather. (Parents can do this also, if they see someone who appears to be upset by the child's symptoms).

Sometimes when people are really unpleasant, it's difficult to just ignore them or disarm them by having a chat. I know teenagers who have had to fight their way off the schoolyard each day until the other children finally stopped teasing them. I know other adults whose symptoms are much more serious than mine who must sometimes respond to others' comments, threats, or insults. Sometimes they do this by walking up to their tormentors and informing them about TS (before ducking); sometimes they just walk away; and sometimes they have had to fight—verbally or physically. There is no simple rule about how to cope with people who continue to ridicule or threaten you. It is very important, though, for children with TS to tell their parents and/or teachers when they are being confronted or harassed. They must work together to develop strategies to resolve the issue, but harassment and bullying should not be accepted.

In general, I don't believe that people with TS should avoid going places or doing things just because their symptoms might disturb or annoy others. When I choose to avoid situations, it is for only one of two reasons:

1. *I* am likely to be uncomfortable in the situation or with the way people may respond, or

2. My symptoms are *so severe or disruptive* that it's not fair to others for me to be there.

Places I would not generally visit for the first reason include bars where I know the patrons' response to my tics might make me uncomfortable. I also generally avoid going out to dinner or to evening movies when I am very tired after a long week at the office, because crowds make my symptoms worse, and trying to control them would make *me* very uncomfortable.

Places that should be avoided for the second reason depend on the symptoms an individual has that might be considered very inappropriate for a particular situation. For example, if someone has a compulsion to break drinking glasses or dinnerware, going to a fine restaurant would only cause her trouble. Or if one's coprolalia could not be controlled, going to the theater or a school play might be too disruptive for actors and audience members. On the other hand, I know of children with coprolalia who have attended church regularly because the members of the congregation know and accept their symptoms. You just have to use your judgment in deciding how disruptive is *too* disruptive. There are no hard and fast rules for determining whether or not a situation should be avoided. However, my rule would be, when in doubt, go.

Dealing with Acquaintances at Work, School, and in the Community

As I indicated earlier, I had an easier (but not easy) time than most children growing up with Tourette syndrome. That is, I was almost never teased, ridiculed, isolated, or rejected by my playmates, classmates, or teachers. I think this was partly due to luck, partly to the times, and partly to the way my family and I coped with the strange behaviors I was exhibiting. Not knowing that I had TS, and finally accepting that, no matter what, it didn't seem as if I could stop the symptoms, my family and I went back to trying to live our lives.

One of the most valuable things my family did, I believe, was to model for others how I should be treated. That is, my family made it clear that they saw me as a valued and "OK" child, and this helped others to see me the same way. Even if others weren't sure about me, my family established the expectations for others' behavior toward me. For example, when I was a child, we used to go regularly to a dinner buffet at an older hotel near our house. While hotel staff and other patrons must certainly have noticed my symptoms, nothing was ever said to me. If anything was ever said to my parents, I don't know. However, I do know that we ate at this restaurant for many years, and I was always treated with courtesy and friendliness.

In establishing expectations, what family members and friends *don't* do is often as important as what they do. For example, if my brother had laughed at me or teased me or told our playmates that I was weird, I could have easily been more isolated. Instead, he was one of my best friends. If my aunt had told my parents that they could come for dinner only if I would try to be quiet and still, I would have become even more self-conscious about being in social settings. If my first wife had asked me to try to stop the twitching when we were out on a date, I most certainly would never have married her, or even felt comfortable dating. Although I definitely recognize that in all of these examples, members of my family may sometimes have been annoyed or embarrassed, or have thought I was odd, they seldom, if ever, let me know.

The expectations my family set for themselves and others—coupled with their consistent emotional support—played a critical role in teaching me how to cope with classmates, roommates, teammates, employers, co-workers, clients, and employees. And today, I follow my family's lead and try not to let my Tourette syndrome be the focus of any relationship. For example, I've often been asked what you should say about your TS in a job interview. Clearly, federal law prohibits potential employers from asking about disabling conditions except in specific situations. In my case, the chances are always good that the employer will witness some of my symptoms during the interview. In contrast to someone in a wheelchair, a person with TS can have symptoms that appear much more bizarre. We may be mistaken for emotionally unstable, nervous, or high on drugs. Consequently, for me, it is important to mention TS in an interview. I wouldn't, however, do this the moment I walked in. When I've interviewed for jobs, I have tried to work it into the interview at an appropriate place that made me look good. For example, if I were applying for an entry-level position and I was asked about my organizational skills, I might describe my volunteer work with the Tourette Syndrome Association, scheduling appearances at health fairs. I would then take the opportunity to mention what TS is and that I have it. Again, my whole focus would be on demonstrating competence, understanding, and acceptance of my TS, and being open about it.

Of course, when in the interview you talk about your TS depends upon the severity of your symptoms and how well you can control them

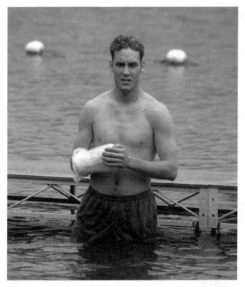

in the interview. I didn't get every job I applied for using this approach, but many times over I found that these strategies were successful in disarming and reassuring others.

Children and their parents can use basically the same approach when trying out for a youth baseball league, applying for ballet school, and the like. That is, they can concentrate on demonstrating and talking about their skills and interests, and then work in a mention of TS—perhaps by talking about medication or that their eyes are OK and that the blinking is caused by Tourette syndrome.

In the long run, the best strategy is to demonstrate the relationship and interaction you expect from others. When I interview new staff people for my company, I only mention my TS if the subject comes up naturally. In some cases I have told them about my TS during the interview process and in other cases, only after I've hired them. Whenever I do tell them, I want it to be part of a normal interaction. Once again, I try to reinforce the notion that "I am not my TS."

Relating to People Very Close to You

Family members, spouses, girlfriends, boyfriends, and others who are close to us should be the easiest for us to get along with. Yet sometimes I think they're the hardest. This is because they're the people we care most about, the people who care most about us, the people we want to please the most, and the people (aside from ourselves) whose lives are most seriously affected by our conditions.

I believe that coping involves beginning to share, with those close to us, how we feel about our symptoms. Sharing our feelings about TS is like sharing feelings about other very important aspects of our lives. Our ability to share and the way we do it depends not only on how old we are, but on the relationships we have with the important people in our lives. This means, for example, that children of different ages will understand information about TS differently, express their feelings differently, and relate to their parents differently. There is almost no way for an elementary school student to come to grips with the concept of a "neurobehavioral disorder." She must first be assured that she won't die from it, that others can't catch it, that her parents know it is frightening for her, and that her parents will try to protect her from doing anything *too* strange or crazy-seeming.

For many of the children with TS I have met, their symptoms have become so much a focus of their family's life that I think it's important not to talk *so* much about the disorder at first and *not to push them* to share their feelings. Rather, parents, siblings, and other relatives need to demonstrate that they understand how difficult it must be to live with TS and acknowledge that the child has legitimate feelings about what is happening to her. For example, your child should not always have to tell you how hurt she was by a problem that developed in school because she could not "keep her hands to herself." All you might need to do is put your hand on your child's shoulder and say, "I know you're trying really hard, and it's frustrating when the other students can't seem to understand that you can't stop doing certain things." Over time, this acknowledgement of a child's feelings will help her learn to share them more directly with parents and others.

Coping also involves beginning to understand how our symptoms affect others. It involves understanding that parents, siblings, and spouses are human too . . . that they occasionally need their "space" and distance from us . . . that they sometimes get tired of having to deal with our symptoms (at home or in public) . . . that they get beaten down by schools, human service systems, employers, and neighbors as they try to help us learn to cope. Understanding and working through these situations is very painful but essential.

Naturally, people who live together have some conflicts. Yet it's very difficult for those of us with TS when these conflicts are caused by things we can't control. This makes us worry that we'll lose those we love because of something we can't change. For example, some children with TS have compulsions to repeat or question what others say—over and over again, *ad infinitum*. Parents, siblings, and others can become quite frustrated with this repetition, even when they know it is part of the TS. Thus, coping must start with openness and sharing. If the caring is there, and families are willing to work hard together, the coping will follow.

Accomplishing Tasks

Developing coping strategies to accomplish work, school, or other projects means beginning to take control of our lives. Although we cannot totally control our symptoms, we *can* take steps to help reduce their impact on our lives. We can use our minds to figure out how best to get things accomplished. Because my Tourette syndrome was undiagnosed for many years, many of my coping strategies just seemed to develop naturally. For example, we all know that fatigue makes TS symptoms increase. I have always been an early riser, so in college I found myself doing most of my studying in the morning and early afternoon. Whenever possible, I also scheduled classes during the morning. Even after a late night of partying on the weekend, I would get up at 7 a.m. to study while my dorm mates slept. I tended to visit the library at off hours when there were fewer people to disturb, because trying to withhold my tics made reading and concentrating very difficult.

After college, I continued to adjust my schedule to my tics. For instance, when I began reviewing research for the Ohio Department of Mental Health, I would get to work at 7 a.m. I seldom reviewed a grant after 2 p.m. because I knew my tics would be worse and disrupt my ability to concentrate on the technical material.

Another coping strategy that I stumbled upon before I knew I had TS was to participate regularly in sports and physical exercise. I discovered that my ability to cope with my TS, as well as the many stresses of everyday life, was enhanced by taking part in these activities. One reason is that being quiet and still is extremely difficult for people with TS, but that symptoms seem to be reduced when the body is in motion. I have found that when I participate in sports in which there is more continuous activity (racquetball, volleyball, weight training, swimming), I have fewer tics than when I play sports in which there is more time between activities (for example, softball, baseball, golf).

Physical activities help with coping in other ways, too. First, sports and other physical activities such as dance and karate can give children with TS an opportunity to succeed through hard work. This does not mean that every child must be a star, but that they can see progress and a temporary reduction of symptoms. (It is important to remember that when fatigue sets in after the activity, the symptoms will likely be worse for a time.) In addition, team sports and other physical activities offer opportunities for children and their families to be with other children and families. This gives parents a chance to model how others should view and treat their child. Parents can also explain TS to others (when needed), have fun with their children, or just cheer them on. Finally, exercise and sports are good for anyone's overall health.

Of course, developing coping strategies for getting things accomplished involves more than managing our tics and other symptoms. It also requires that each of us look carefully at how our symptoms affect our ability to do essential tasks, and then try to make the adjustments needed to accomplish our goals. It is equally important to develop the ability to make legitimate demands on others to accept us and make accommodations that enable us to succeed. For example, an employee with TS and her boss might mutually adjust a work schedule to enable the employee to work a shift when her symptoms would be less disruptive. Or even more important, the employee might share information about TS with coworkers while supervisors and management model an attitude of acceptance. This is the balancing act of accepting responsibility for the fact that we have TS while refusing to apologize for it, or be limited or defined by it.

When we are children, this responsibility falls on our parents, but as we become teenagers, we must empower ourselves and learn to play a much larger role in this process. This role becomes especially important if your child needs an individualized education program (IEP) at school.

In my experience, developing a successful IEP rests on getting a clear picture of the child's tics, noises, and behaviors, understanding how they are affecting her school performance or behavior, and figuring out what specifically will help her. The more input the child herself can give about these issues, the better. For example, suppose that a student is not getting her homework assignments completed. Is it because attention problems are causing her to miss the assignments? Are arm and head tics preventing her from writing down the assignment fast enough? Are vocal tics preventing her from hearing the assignment? Have medication side effects caused short-term memory loss, or has fatigue made her tics get so severe that she can't complete her homework at night? Has she become so alienated by her teachers' lack of understanding that she is refusing to do schoolwork at all? Is she such a good student that the class bully steals her homework every day and threatens a beating if she tells? Any of these may be the problem. We must, however, understand what is really going on before we can devise a strategy to resolve the situation.

Because of the fluctuating nature of Tourette syndrome, we must also recognize that what works one time might not work as well another time. My tics and other symptoms can be somewhat reduced for a while, and then they get worse for no apparent reason. This is known as "waxing and waning." Fatigue can also trigger some of my more disruptive symptoms. For example, after several long days at the office followed by late nights of sports and limited sleep, I used to get mouth and stomach movements that made eating very difficult. Some of my leg and head movements also affected my sports activities, and back when I played volleyball it used to be very frustrating to be playing well one week and not nearly as well the next. These are times when those of us with TS must keep doing most of the things we normally do, but be willing to accept a somewhat lower level of performance. These are times when we have to remember that *nobody* performs at their highest level all the time, and that people who don't have TS also perform inconsistently, although for some different reasons.

As individuals and families coping with TS, we must really try to understand the condition. We must seek out accurate information. We must ask questions. And we must learn to trust and use our own observations and judgment about our symptoms.

Keeping Your Perspective

Finally, I think one of the most important ways to cope with Tourette syndrome is to cultivate a sense of humor about it. Being able to laugh about TS with loved ones can really help.

All of us can think of humorous stories about our symptoms and others' reactions to them. For example, in the past, when I came home from work, I would purposely make some noise like singing, whistling, or calling to my first wife to make sure she knew it was me and not a burglar. Every once in a while she would teasingly remind me that she always knows where I am in the house. After all, what kind of burglar comes into a house grunting, sniffing, and clearing his throat?

Or how about the time long ago when my niece was three years old and first started to notice that Uncle Bill made some funny noises and faces? She wasn't sure what I was doing, so she stared at me. My brother and sister-in-law tried to explain TS to her and told her not to stare. So for the rest of the weekend, she very pointedly avoided even *looking* at me.

Over the years I have had several opportunities to meet with groups of young adults with TS. One of the funniest experiences of my life occurred during such a meeting at the TSA National Conference in 1989. Twenty competent, bright, motivated individuals, including professionals, managers, students, and administrators, all with motor tics and vocalizations, were gathered in a small meeting room. Suddenly, several individuals with coprolalia began responding to each others' statements. Others in the group goaded them on. Raucous laughter filled the room. We spent a very productive two days identifying issues for adults with TS, but most importantly, shared many good, long-needed laughs.

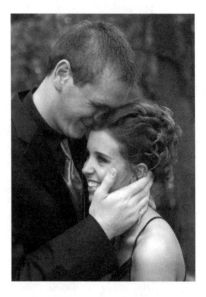

If people with Tourette syndrome and our families can occasionally laugh at our symptoms, we can definitely see ourselves as distinct from our TS. This successful separation allows us to get a better sense of who we are and allows for an eventual re-integration and incorporation of the symptoms of Tourette syndrome into our lives. I believe this step can help us begin to take control of those portions of our lives over which we have control and learn to better cope with those portions over which we have little or no control. That TS affects our lives every day is inescapable. That having to live with it and adapt to it helps shape the person we become, is also undeniable. Living with TS is not easy living, but we have much more to offer the world than our sounds, tics, compulsions, and other strange behaviors. WE ARE NOT OUR TICS, but Tourette syndrome is part of our lives.

∷ References

Anthony, W.A. (1993). Recovery from mental illness: The guiding vision of the mental health service system in the 1990s. *Psychosocial Rehabilitation Journal, 16(4)*, 11-23.

Rubin, W. V. & Panzano, P. C. (2002). Identifying meaningful subgroups of adults with severe mental illness. *Psychiatric Services, 53*, 452-457.

Deegan, P.E., (1988). Recovery: The Lived Experience of Rehabilitation. *Psychosocial Rehabilitation Journal, 11(4)*, 11-19.

❌ Personal Statements

Accomplishing my goals and living my life has been complex and at times difficult. I have had to come up with ways of accomplishing my goals that other people don't have to worry about. My college textbooks must be put on computer discs, I use note takers and record lectures, and it will take me six years to finish my degree. However, my disabilities have also led me to be more determined, confident, and open-minded. Whenever someone tells me I can't do something, I become interested in finding out a way that I can do it.

❧

Life can be frustrating at times. Writing is tough and books are hard to read because I tear paper easily. Also, sometimes I hit and drop electronics, which makes having a cell phone, computer, camera, etc. difficult. Even with the difficult times, when I look at my life overall, and what has happened to me, I can't complain about having TS. I am very proud to be a person with Tourette syndrome and would not want my life to be any other way.

❧

I know that my family doesn't see me as any different from someone who doesn't have TS; they see me as a normal person like everyone else because that is what I am.

❧

The way my sister deals with my TS now is different from how she dealt with it when I was first diagnosed fourteen years ago. My sister was eight when I was diagnosed and she had a difficult time getting use to my disability. It was really hard for her when we were in public because people would look at me and laugh at what was going on. Now, when I look back at those times, I realize that that is how any child that age would react to people staring at them or the people they are with.

❧

Once in a while, I meet someone who is rude to me or makes fun of me because of my TS. When this happens, I just ignore it or I will be silly and say something to make that person feel silly about their being rude to me. If someone is rude to me, I am not rude back, otherwise I am just

like them, and they will be less likely to listen and learn from what I have
to say to them.

❧

My friends treat my TS like my family does: it is natural to them. To me,
my disability is no big deal. When other people, my friends, and others
in my community see that it is no big deal to me, then it becomes no big
deal to them. Also, I am very open about my TS, and this makes people
a lot more comfortable around me because I am willing to talk about
and answer questions.

❧

My grandmother told me that making noises wasn't something a good
girl did and that I was disappointing her. That really upset me, so I used
to leave when I needed to tic because I wanted her approval. Even to
this day, I feel uncomfortable having tics in front of her.

❧

I didn't even know I had TS until I was eleven. Life was really hard before
my tics were diagnosed. The kids at school would tease me. They decided
to torment me because they didn't know about my problem. When I was
diagnosed the school nurse talked to them and then they understood.

❧

As far back as first grade, I can recall knowing I was different from other
kids, but not being able to place my finger on what it was. The other
children used to tease me then, but even so, I really don't think I knew
exactly what was different.

❧

Sometime during the third grade, the blinking started. I remember blinking so hard that my eyes would water like a dam had burst. But even
though I continued to blink and have other minor tics, I don't remember
it bothering me socially. Socially, I was accepted, and although I was a
fairly hyper child, I didn't cause problems for my teachers.

❧

I was about seven when I had the first vocal tic I can clearly recall. It was
a guttural, grunt-like noise. My parents tried to make me stop because

they thought I did it to annoy them. When they did, I used to think, "But I really need to do this now; I can't stop." That thought scared me because I believed I should be able to control it.

❧

I have met a lot of friends at a camp for kids with TS that I go to one week out of the year. Camp is a place for your family to learn about TS and a place for kids to have fun.

❧

I started dating in about ninth grade. Outside of the normal nervousness that teenagers have about first dates, I had no worries about my tics, for two reasons. First, my tics weren't that severe. The second reason was the sense of humor that I was either born with or brought up with or both. The ability to laugh at myself, and not take myself too seriously, helped me deal with my tics.

❧

I'm tough because I don't let things get to me. I'm hardworking. Once I get started on something, I keep going. I'm alert and observant. I see everything that's going on.

GLOSSARY

Absence (petit mal) seizure—Type of seizure characterized by brief loss of consciousness, usually for not more than ten seconds.

Adaptive behavior—The ability to adjust to new environments, tasks, objects, and people, and to apply new skills to those new situations.

Acetylcholine—A chemical in neurons that carries information across the synaptic cleft, the space between two nerve cells.

AD/HD. *See* **Attention-deficit/hyperactivity disorder.**

Advocacy—Supporting or promoting a cause. Speaking out.

Advocacy groups—Organizations that work to protect the rights and opportunities of people with disabilities and their families.

Affect—An emotion.

Affective disorder—A mental disorder involving the emotions; includes depression and bipolar disorder (manic depression).

Afferent cell—the nerve cell carrying the message away from the synapse to the next cell.

Akathisia—A feeling of inner restlessness that is relieved by moving about. A common side effect of neuroleptic medication.

Alpha-Adrenergic Agonists—Drugs that bond to alpha-adrenergic receptors in nerve cells; originally used to control blood pressure but now sometimes prescribed to control tics.

Anafranil—*See* **Clomipramine.**

Anticonvulsant—A drug used to control seizures. Even though all seizures are not convulsions, this term is commonly used.

Asperger's disorder (Asperger syndrome)—A type of autism spectrum disorder. Children with AS have difficulties with social skills and unusual preoccupations or interests; communication skills develop at a normal rate, although subtle differences in speech (overly grown-up vocabulary, differences in intonation patterns) may be present.

Applied behavior analysis—A method of teaching designed to change behavior in a precisely measurable and accountable manner. Also called **behavior modification.**

Assessment—Process to determine a child's strengths and weaknesses. Includes testing and observations performed by a team of professionals and parents. Usually used to determine special education needs. Term is used interchangeably with **evaluation.**

Associated behaviors—The spectrum of behaviors often seen in association with Tourette syndrome; includes OCD, AD/HD, impulsivity, and aggression.

Attention—The ability to concentrate on a task.

Attention deficit disorder (ADD)—Sometime used interchangeably with **attention-deficit/hyperativity disorder**, but primarily refers to the "inattentive" type of AD/HD.

Attention-deficit/hyperactivity disorder (AD/HD)—A condition beginning early in life that is characterized by inattention, hyperactivity, and/or impulsive behavior.

Attention span—The amount of time one is able to concentrate on a task. Also called **attending** in special education jargon.

Auditory—Relating to the ability to hear.

Auto Immune Reaction—Illnesses that occur when the body tissues are attacked by its own immune system. Patients with these diseases have unusual antibodies in their blood that target their own body tissues.

Babbling—The sound a baby makes when he combines a vowel and consonant and repeats them over and over again (e.g., ba-ba-ba, ga-ga-ga).

Basal ganglia—Part of the brain that some researchers believe could be the location of abnormalities which cause tics.

Behavioral dysinhibition—The inability to control inappropriate behavior because of neurological impairment.

Beneficiary—The person indicated in a trust or insurance policy to receive any payments that become due.

Biofeedback therapy—Use of biofeedback machine to teach oneself relaxation of muscles.

Bipolar disorder—The current term for manic-depression, a disorder involving extreme ups and downs in mood.

Blood level—The amount of medication in someone's blood; determined by taking a blood sample.

Bradycardia—Very slow heart rate.

Brainstem—Portion of the brain between the cerebellum and spinal cord.

Bruxism—Grinding of teeth repeatedly.

Busipirone—A drug used as an adjunct to tic medications, often used to treat anxiety or OCD in people with TS.

Case manager—The person responsible for coordinating services and information from members of interdisciplinary team.

CAT scan (CT scan)—Computerized axial tomography. A test involving X-raying the brain to find any possible malformations.

Catapres—*See* **Clonidine.**

Cause-and-effect—The concept that actions create reactions.

Central nervous system—The brain and spinal cord. The part of the nervous system primarily involved in voluntary movement and thought processes.

Cerebellum—Part of the brain that helps coordinate muscle activity and control balance.

Cerebrum—The largest part of the brain, located in the upper part of the head. Believed to control intellectual functions such as thinking, remembering, learning.

Childhood schizophrenia—A major psychiatric disorder, probably with multiple causes. Symptoms include disturbances in form and content of thought, perception, emotions, sense of self, volition, relationship to the external world, and psychomotor behavior. Childhood schizophrenia is very rare.

Chorea—Abrupt, quick, jerky movements of the head, neck, arms, or legs.

Chromosomes—Microscopic, rod-shaped bodies in cells which contain genetic material.

Chronic—Long-lasting.

Chronic tic disorder—A tic disorder involving the presence of motor or vocal tics—but not both—for over one year.

Clomipramine—An antidepressant medication used in Tourette syndrome to treat symptoms of OCD.

Clonidine—A high blood pressure medication used in treatment of TS. It can be helpful in controlling tics and AD/HD symptoms.

Cognition—The ability to know and understand the environment.

Cognitive Behavior Therapy—psychotherapy which focuses on changing thought patterns that are negative or irrational. CBT is based on the idea that thoughts determine feelings and behaviors. Changing these thinking patterns can change behavior and feelings.

Cognitive dulling—A common side effect of neuroleptic drugs; involves short-term memory loss and slowed thinking.

Comorbid condition—Medical term meaning a medical condition that occurs along with another medical condition, although one condition does not directly cause the other.

Compensatory skill—A skill used in place of another skill that an individual is unable to perform. For instance, a compensatory skill for someone who is unable to handwrite legibly might be typing.

Compulsion—The feeling of being compelled or forced to do a behavior, even though the person experiencing the compulsion does not want to do it. For example, evening things up, washing hands, cleaning.

Congenital—relating to a condition that exists at birth.

Consciousness—The state of awareness.

Convulsion—Involuntary contractions of the muscles. A seizure.

Cost-of-care liability—The right of a state providing care to a person with disabilities to charge for the care and to collect from that person's assets.

Cytogeneticist—A doctor or professional who studies chromosomes and genes and their effect on heredity.

Depression—Disorder producing depressed mood, appetite changes, sleep changes, and sometimes suicidal thinking. Can have a neuro-chemical basis and can often be treated with medication.

Desipramine—A tricyclic antidepressant used in the treatment of AD/HD associated with TS.

Development—The process of growth and learning during which a child acquires skills and abilities.

Developmental disability—A disability or impairment originating before the age of eighteen that is expected to continue indefinitely and that constitutes a substantial disability.

Developmental milestone—A developmental goal such as sitting or using two-word phrases that functions as a measurement of developmental progress over time.

Developmentally delayed—Having development that is slower than normal.

Diabetes—*See* Type two diabetes mellitus.

Diagnostic and Statistical Manual of Mental Disorders (DSM IV-TR)—A manual published by the American Psychiatric Association (APA) which describes all of the diagnostic criteria and the systematic descriptions of various mental disorders.

Discretionary trust—A trust in which the trustee (the person responsible for governing the trust) has the authority to use or not use the trust funds for any purpose, as long as funds are expended only for the beneficiary.

Dispute resolution procedures—The procedure established by law and regulation for the fair resolution of disputes regarding a child's special education.

Dopamine—One of the neurotransmitters (brain chemicals) involved in motor and vocal tics, as well as in AD/HD.

Drug vacation—Time off from taking any medication, usually in summer months.

DSM IV-TR—*See* Diagnostic and Statistical Manual of Mental Disorders.

Due process hearing—Part of the procedures established to protect the rights of parents and children with disabilities during disputes under IDEA.

These are hearings before an impartial person to review the identification, evaluation, placement, and services a child is receiving under IDEA.

Dysarthria—Impaired articulation due to problems in muscle control.

Dysinhibition of aggression—Inability to control aggressive behavior, as a result of neurological impairment.

Dyskinesia—A general term for involuntary movements.

Dyslexia—One type of learning disability that affects reading ability.

Dyspraxia—Difficulty planning movements or putting them into sequence.

Early development—Development during the first three years of life.

Early intervention—The specialized way of interacting with infants to minimize the effects of conditions that can delay early development. May be provided by infant educators, occupational therapists, speech therapists, physical therapists, as well as by parents.

Echolalia—A parrot-like repetition of phrases or words just heard (immediate echolalia), or heard hours, days, weeks, or even months ago (delayed echolalia).

EEG—*See* Electroencephalogram.

Efferent Cell—A nerve cell carrying the message toward the synapse.

EKG—*See* Electrocardiogram

Electrocardiogram—A recording of the electrical activity of the heart on a moving strip of paper. It detects and records the electrical potential of the heart during contraction.

Electroencephalogram (EEG)—The machine and test used to determine levels of electrical discharge from nerve cells.

Emotional lability—Instability of expression of emotions. For example, having a "short fuse" and being quick to anger. Common in people with TS.

Enzyme—A secretion from cells that changes chemicals in other body substances.

Epilepsy—A recurrent condition caused by abnormal electrical discharges in the brain that causes seizures.

Estate planning—Formal, written arrangements for handling the possessions and assets of people after they have died.

Etiology—The study of the cause of disease.

Evaluation—*See* Assessment.

Executive Function—A group of cognitive skills that enable a person to consciously manage his learning and behavior—for example, to set goals and stay on task until they are achieved; to continue to pay attention in class even when bored; and to avoid making past mistakes again.

Expressive language—The ability to use gestures, words, and written symbols to communicate.

Extinction—A procedure in which reinforcement of a previously reinforced behavior is withheld.

Extrapyramidal effects—Side effects of neuroleptic medications. Examples are bradykinesia, akathisia, and dystonia.

FDA—The Federal Drug Administration; the U.S. agency responsible for ensuring the safety of medications, foods, medical devices, and cosmetics.

Febrile seizures—Seizures that are associated with fever.

Fight or Flight Response—Natural response to fearful situation where the body reacts by increased heart rate, flood of adrenalin, widening of pupils, preparing the body to fight or run away.

Fine motor—Relating to the use of the small muscles of the body, such as those in the hands, feet, fingers, and toes.

Fluoxetine—An antidepressant used in TS to treat OCD and depression.

Fluphenazine—A neuroleptic drug used in treating TS. It is a dopamine blocker and may help reduce tics.

Focal motor seizure—Type of seizure that causes jerking of a few muscle groups without an initial loss of consciousness.

Generalization—Transferring a skill taught in one place, or with one person, to other places and people. For example, being able to use "please" and "thank you" appropriately in any situation or setting.

Genes—Material within the chromosomes that determines specific traits, such as hair and eye color and stature.

Genetic—Pertaining to a trait determined by the genes; inherited.

Glutamate—A central nervous system neurotransmitter that is affected by some of the medications used in TS and associated disorders. It is an excitatory neuromuscular transmitter.

Grand mal seizure—*See* Tonic clonic seizure.

Gross motor—Relating to the use of the large muscles of the body.

Haldol—*See* Haloperidol.

Half life—The time it takes a drug to decrease in potency in the blood by fifty percent.

Haloperidol—A neuroleptic medication used in treating the tics of TS.

Hyperactivity—A specific nervous-system-based difficulty which makes it hard for a person to control muscle (motor) behavior.

IDEA (The Individuals with Disabilities Education Act)—A federal law that guarantees qualified students with disabilities in the U.S. the right to a free appropriate public education. Formerly known as the Education for All Handicapped Children Act (Public Law 94–142).

IDEIA (The Individuals with Disabilities Education *Improvement* Act)—Sometimes referred to as IDEA 2004 or Public Law 108-446. Refers to the 2004 reauthorization (with changes) of IDEA.

Identification—The determination that a child should be evaluated as a possible candidate for special education services.

IEP—Individualized Education Program. The written plan that describes what services the local education agency has promised to provide your child under IDEA.

IFSP—Individualized Family Service Plan. The written document that describes what services a child will receive through his early intervention program.

Imitation—The ability to observe the actions of others and to copy them in one's own actions. Also known as **modeling**.

Impulsive—Lacking impulse control; prone to "acting without thinking."

Inclusion—The practice of placing children with disabilities in the same classrooms and schools as children without special needs, to the maximum extent possible, while still allowing them to make progress on their individualized learning goals.

Inhibition—The ability to inhibit or stop messages sent by the brain to other parts of the body.

Input—Information that a person receives through any of the senses (vision, hearing, touch, feeling, smell) that helps that person develop new skills.

Insistence on sameness—A tendency to become upset when familiar routines are changed.

Interdisciplinary team—A team of professionals who evaluate your child and then develop a comprehensive summary report of his or her strengths and needs.

Interpretive—The sessions during which parents and teachers review and discuss the results of a child's evaluation.

Intracranial—Within the skull.

Intractable—Difficult to control, treat, or cure.

Involuntary movements—Uncontrolled movements, such as tics.

I.Q. (Intelligence Quotient)—A measure of cognitive ability based on specifically designed standardized tests.

Language—The expression and understanding of human communication.

Learning disability—A disorder that results in a child having greater than expected difficulty learning in one or more specific areas (reading, math, spelling, etc.) given his or her overall level of intelligence.

Least restrictive environment—The requirement under IDEA that children receiving special education must be made a part of a regular school to the fullest extent possible. Included in the law as a way of ending the traditional practice of isolating children with disabilities.

Limbic system—Seen as the "emotional center" of the brain. Studied in TS research.

Lithium—Medication used to treat bipolar disorder, which is sometimes an associated condition with TS.

Local Education Agency (LEA)—The agency responsible for providing educational services on the local (city, county, and school district) level.

Long QT syndrome—an inherited heart condition that can result in abnormally rapid heart rate, resulting in fainting or even death if the heart does not regain its natural rhythm.

Luxury trust—A trust that describes the kind of allowable expenses in a way that excludes the cost of care in state-funded programs in order to avoid cost-of-care liability.

Magnetic Resonance Imaging (MRI)—A type of computerized brain scan.

Mainstreaming—The practice of involving children with disabilities in regular school and preschool environments. Now usually called inclusion.

Marijuana—an illegal drug made from the dried stems, leaves, and flowers of the cannabis plant; most commonly rolled into cigarettes to smoke.

Medicaid—A joint state and federal program in the U.S. that offers medical assistance to people with low incomes.

Medicare—A federal medical insurance program for the elderly and disabled.

Mental retardation—Below average cognitive abilities in association with below average "adaptive functioning" (i.e., ability to get along in the real world). Children with mental retardation learn more slowly than other children, but have a very wide range of abilities, just as other children do.

Metabolic Disorder—a disease caused by abnormal metabolic processes (usually the inability of the body to break down a substance, resulting in the dangerous accumulation of that substance).

Metabolism—The chemical and physical changes in human cells that provide energy.

Methylphenidate—A stimulant drug often prescribed for AD/HD; can sometimes cause increase in tics of TS. Common brand names include Ritalin, Concerta, Metadate.

Modeling—*See* **Imitation**.

Motor—Relating to the ability to move oneself.

Motor patterns—The ways in which the body and limbs work to make sequenced movements.

Motor planning—The ability to think through and carry out a physical task.

MRI—*See* Magnetic Resonance Imaging.

Multidisciplinary team—*See* Interdisciplinary team.

Neurobiological disorder—Brain disorders caused by a disorder of the neurological system of the brain; examples include Tourette syndrome, OCD, and Asperger syndrome.

Neuroleptic—An antipsychotic medication. Used in small doses, some neuroleptics are effective in treating the tics of Tourette syndrome.

Neurological impairment—Dysfunction of neurological functions in the brain.

Neurologist—A physician specializing in medical problems associated with the brain and spinal cord.

Neuromotor—Involving both the nerves and muscles.

Neurons—Nerve cells in the brain.

Neuropsychiatric disorder—A behavioral disorder which is influenced by both environmental and internal neurological factors.

Neurotoxin—A toxin (poison) that acts specifically on nerve cells (neurons). These toxins can be exogenous (from the environment) or endogenous (from inside the body).

Neurotransmitter—The chemical substance between nerve cells in the brain which allows the transmission of impulses (messages) from one nerve to another. There are many different types of neurotransmitters, including copamine, norepinephrine, and serotonin.

Norepinephrine—One of the brain's neurotransmitters involved in formation and function of dopamine and serotonin. Also known as noradrenalin.

Norpramine—*See* Desipramine.

Obsessions—Recurrent disturbing thoughts that will not go away. In OCD, compulsions may be performed in an attempt to deal with the obsession.

Obsessive compulsive (OC)—Having symptoms of obsessional thinking and/or compulsive behavior. A child with Tourette syndrome may sometimes experience OC thoughts or behaviors, which may or may not be severe enough to qualify for the diagnosis of obsessive-compulsive disorder.

Obsessive-compulsive disorder (OCD)—A neuropsychiatric disorder involving obsessive thinking and compulsive behavior which severely interferes with life functions.

Occupational therapist (OT)—A therapist who specializes in improving the development of fine motor and adaptive skills. May also be qualified to work on sensory integration problems.

OCD—*See* Obsessive-compulsive disorder.

OHI—*See* Other health impaired.

Oral motor—Relating to the movement of muscles in and around the mouth.

Oral tactile defensiveness—An over-sensitivity to touch around the mouth.

Orap—*See* Pimozide.

Other health impaired—A disability category used in IDEA and defined as: "having limited strength, vitality, or alertness, including a heightened alertness to environmental stimuli, that results in limited alertness with respect to the educational environment...." Tourette syndrome and AD/HD fall under the OHI category in federal law.

Parallel play—One or more people playing alongside, but not together, with one another.

Parent-professional partnership—The teaming of parents and teachers (or doctors, nurses, or other professionals) to work together to facilitate the development of babies and children with special needs.

Partial seizure—Type of seizure in which the abnormal discharge takes place in one specific part of the brain. A focal or local seizure.

Perseveration—Repetitive movement or speech that is thought to be created by the person's own inner preoccupations.

PET scan—*See* Position Emission Tomography.

Pharmacotherapy—The use of medications in treating a disorder.

Phenotype—The observable characteristics of an individual that are caused by a particular disorder, gene, etc. That is, two children may both have TS, but their phenotype (traits attributable to the disorder) may differ widely, depending on genetic and environmental factors.

Physical therapist (PT)—A therapist who works with motor skills, helping a child acquire or reacquire gross motor skills such as sitting up, walking, or riding a bicycle.

Pimozide—A neuroleptic drug used to help reduce tics of TS.

Placement—The selection of the educational program for a child who needs special education programs.

Polypharmacy—Use of more than one medication in treating a condition; common in TS.

Position Emission Tomography (PET scan)—Test that identifies metabolic activity.

Pragmatic Speech Therapy—Type of speech therapy for children who have Pragmatic Speech Disorder (difficulties with the practical, social use of language), which is seen in children with autism spectrum disorders such as Asperger syndrome.

Prognosis—A prediction about the likely course of a disease or condition in an individual.

Prolixin—*See* Fluphenazine.

Prompt—Input that encourages a child to perform a movement or activity. *See* Cue.

Proprioception—the body's sense of position and movement; it enables us to know where our body parts are in space without looking at them.

Prozac—*See* Fluoxetine.

Pseudoephedrine—Over-the-counter medication commonly used for colds, flu, and allergy symptoms. Can exacerbate tics of TS. Sold under brand name Sudafed.

Psychomotor (complex partial) seizures—Seizures that cause decreased alertness and changes in behavior.

Psychosis—a psychiatric disorder that causes delusions or hallucinations and interferes with the ability to participate in daily life; for example, schizophrenia.

Psychotropic drug— Any drug that affects the mind.

Punishment—An undesirable consequence that is applied following a behavior to reduce the probability of that behavior occurring again.

Receptive language—The ability to understand spoken and written communication as well as gestures.

Rehearsal—Practicing a desired behavior with a child in preparation for him to do it on his own.

Reinforcement—Providing a pleasant consequence (positive reinforcement) or removing an unpleasant consequence (negative reinforcement) after a behavior in order to increase or maintain that behavior.

Related services—Services that enable a child to benefit from special education. Related services include speech, occupational, and physical therapies, counseling, and psychological services, as well as transportation.

Remission—A complete absence of symptoms for a period of months to years. Sometimes occurs in TS.

Respite care—Skilled adult- or childcare and supervision that can be provided in your home or the home of a care provider. Respite care may be available for several hours per week or for overnight stays.

Ritalin—*See* Methylphenidate.

School phobia—Fear or avoidance of school attendance. Seen often in children with TS, it can be a side effect of neuroleptic medications, or a result of harassment or ridicule at school.

Screening test—A test given to groups of children to sort out those who need further evaluation.

SEA—The State Education Agency.

Sedation—Sleepiness; common side effect of some TS medications.

Seizure—Involuntary movement or changes in consciousness or behavior brought on by abnormal electrical discharges in nerve cells in the brain.

Selective Serotonin Reuptake Inhibitors (SSRIs)—Medications that slow down the process in which nerve cells in the brain take serotonin back up into the cell, which keeps more serotonin in the synapse of the cells. This makes more serotonin available to send messages to the next cell. SSRIs, which include Prozac, Paxil, Celexa, and Zoloft, are often used in the treatment of OCD, depression, and anxiety.

Self-help—Relating to the ability to take care of one's self, through such skills as eating, dressing, bathing, and cleaning.

Self-injurious behaviors (SIB)—Behaviors that result in self-inflicted injuries—for example, biting, head banging, picking scabs, cutting self.

Sensory ability—The ability to process sensations, such as touch, sound, light, smell, and movement.

Sensory impairments—Problems handling information relayed to the brain from the senses.

Sensory integration therapy—Treatment aimed at improving the way the brain processes and organizes sensations.

Sensory seizures—Seizures that produce dizziness or disturbances in vision, hearing, taste, smell, or other senses.

Sensory tics—Tics that produce disturbances in vision, hearing, taste, smell, or other senses.

Serotonin—One of the brain's neurotransmitters; abnormalities in serotonin are believed to play a role in depression and OCD.

Serum blood levels—The level of medications in the blood. Used to monitor drug therapy in the control of seizures or other conditions.

Side effects—Secondary, unwanted effects of using a medication.

Sight word approach—A method of reading in which the child says what he sees rather than sounding out words.

Single Photon Emission Computed Tomography—Device which measures brain function through blood flow and glucose metabolism.

Social ability—The ability to function in groups and to interact with people.

Special education—Specialized instruction based on an evaluation of the strengths and needs of a child with disabilities, and precisely matched to the child's educational needs and learning style.

Special needs—Needs generated by a person's disability.

SPECT—*See* Single Photon Emission Computed Tomography.

Speech/language pathologist (SLP)—A therapist who works to improve speech and language skills, as well as to improve oral motor abilities.

SQ3R—Study, Question, Read, Recite, Review; a educational method designed to help students learn and remember material.

SSDI (Social Security Disability Insurance)—Federal benefits available to workers who become disabled. In addition, children and adolescents who become disabled before the age of twenty-two may collect SSDI under a parent's account, if the parent is retired, disabled, or deceased.

SSI (Supplemental Security Income)—A Social Security Benefit available for low-income people who are disabled, blind, or aged. Based on need, not on past earnings.

Steady state—This term describes the drug level in the blood once it has reached a therapeutic level. Daily doses of medication maintain this level.

Stereotypies—-Constant repetition of certain meaningless gestures or movements, as in certain forms of autism spectrum disorders.

Stimulant—A psychotropic drug such as Ritalin and Dexedrine often used to treat AD/HD in children. It acts on dopamine in the brain.

Stimulus—A physical object or environmental event that *may* have an effect upon the behavior of a person. Some stimuli are internal (earache pain), while others are external (a smile from a loved one).

Strattera—A nonstimulant medication (atomoxetine) used to treat AD/HD. In contrast to stimulants, Strattera acts on (increases) norepinephrine in the brain, rather than dopamine.

Support trust—A trust that requires that funds be expended to pay for the beneficiary's expenses of living, including housing, food, and transportation.

Symptomatic—Having a cause that is identified.

Synapse—The microscopic space between two nerve cells in the brain; signals travel from one cell to another by releasing chemicals (neurotransmitters) that cross the synapse and cause an electrical charge in the next cell.

Tactile—Relating to touch.

Tactile defensiveness—Abnormal sensitivity to touch.

Tardive dyskinesia—Involuntary movements of the mouth, tongue, and lips, trunk and limbs that can rarely occur as a side effect of some medications. Some medications prescribed for Tourette syndrome can contribute to the development of this condition.

Therapeutic blood level—For any given individual, each drug has a level at which it is most effective. The therapeutic blood level refers to the amount of a medication within the blood that provides the most effective results.

Therapist—A trained professional who works to overcome the effects of developmental problems.

Tic—An involuntary movement (motor tic) or involuntary vocalization (vocal tic).

Titrate—To increase the dose of medication slowly over time until the optimum level is achieved.

TMJ (Tempromandibular Joint Disorders)—A group of muscle and joint disorders that cause pain and dysfunction in the jaw joint and muscles that control jaw movement. Common symptoms are pain in the chewing muscles or jaw joint, jaw muscle stiffness, limited movement or locking of the jaw, painful clicking, and popping or grating in the jaw joint when opening or closing the mouth.

Tourette syndrome—A chronic, physical disorder of the brain which causes both motor tics and vocal tics, and begins before the age of twenty-one.

Tricyclic antidepressant—Antidepressants such as desipramine and imipramine, sometimes used in treatment of obsessive-compulsive disorder.

Type two diabetes mellitus—-Diabetes is a disease in which the pancreas fails to produce insulin or the body cannot use insulin the body does produce, resulting in abnormally high levels of glucose (sugar) in the blood. Type two diabetes is most often acquired in adulthood, but has been increasingly diagnosed in children. It is most often caused by obesity, but may also be caused by certain drugs, pregnancy, etc.

Uniform Gifts to Minors Act (UGMA)—A law that governs gifts to minors in the United States. Under the UGMA, gifts become the property of the minor at age eighteen or twenty-one.

Vestibular—Pertaining to the sensory system located in the inner ear that allows a person to maintain balance and enjoyably participate in movement such as swinging and roughhousing.

Visual motor—Pertaining to the combined use of visual and motor skills, such as when putting a puzzle piece into a puzzle or catching a ball.

Vocational training—Training for a job. Learning skills to perform in the workplace.

Waxing and waning—A naturally occurring rising and falling of severity and frequency of tics.

READING LIST

:: Tourette Syndrome

Publications for Adults

Bruun, Ruth Dowling and Bruun, Bertel. **A Mind of Its Own: Tourette's Syndrome: A Story and a Guide.** New York: Oxford, 1994.

Cohen, Brad and Wysocky, Lisa. **Front of the Class: How Tourette Syndrome Made Me the Teacher I Never Had.** Acton, MA: Vanderwyk & Burnham, 2005.

Seligman, Adam Ward and Hilkevich, John S., eds. **Don't Think about Monkeys. Extraordinary Stories Written by People with Tourette Syndrome.** Duarte, CA: Hope Press, 1992.

Shimberg, Elaine Fantle. **Living With Tourette Syndrome.** New York: Fireside, 1995.

Van Bloss, Nick. **Busy Body: My Life with Tourette's Syndrome.** London: Vision Publishing, 2006.

Walkup, John T., Mink, Jonathan W., and Hollenbeck, Peter J. **Tourette Syndrome: Advances in Neurology.** Philadelphia: Lippincott & Wilkins, 2006.

Wilensky, Amy. **Passing for Normal: A Memoir of Compulsion.** New York: Broadway, 2000.

Publications for Children

Buehrens, Adam. **Adam and the Magic Marble.** Duarte, CA: Hope Press, 1990.

Buehrens, Adam. **Hi, I'm Adam: A Child's Story of Tourette Syndrome.** Duarte, CA: Hope Press, 1990.

Byalick, Marcia. **Quit it!** New York: Yearling, 2004.

Corman, C.B. *Simon and the Barking Dog; Simon's Special Sneeze Test; Simon Spells Tourette Syndrome.* Bayside, NY: Tourette Syndrome Association, n.d.

Niner, Holly L. and Treatner, Meryl. **I Can't Stop! : A Story About Tourette Syndrome.** Morton Grove, IL: Albert Whitman & Company, 2005.

Tourette Syndrome Association. **I Have Tourette's But It Doesn't Have Me.** [DVD]. Available from: TSA, 42-40 Bell Blvd., Bayside, NY 11371. www.tsa-usa.org.

Tourette Syndrome Association. *That Darn Tic.* [Newsletter]. Available from: TSA, 42-40 Bell Blvd., Bayside, NY 11371. www.tsa-usa.org.

▪▪ Associated Disorders

Publications for Adults

Attwood, Tony. **Asperger's Syndrome: A Guide for Parents and Professionals.** London: Jessica Kingsley Publishers, 1998.

Ayres, A. Jean. **Sensory Integration and the Child: Understanding Hidden Sensory Challenges.** Los Angeles: Western Psychological Services, 2005.

Bashe, Patricia Romanowsk, Kirby, Barbara L., Baron-Cohen, Simon, and Attwood, Tony. (2005) **The OASIS Guide to Asperger Syndrome: Completely Revised and Updated: Advice, Support, Insight and Inspiration.** New York: Crown, 2005.

Baer, Lee. **Imp of the Mind: Exploring the Silent Epidemic of Obsessive Bad Thoughts.** New York: Plume, 2002.

Barkley, Russell A. **Taking Charge of ADHD. The Complete Authoritative Guide for Parents (Revised Edition).** New York: The Guilford Press, 2000.

Bruey, Carolyn Thorwarth. **Demystifying Autism Spectrum Disorders: A Guide to Diagnosis for Parents and Professionals.** Bethesda, MD: Woodbine House, 2004.

Dendy, Chris A. Zeigler. **Teenagers with ADD: A Parent's Guide.** 2nd edition. Bethesda, MD: Woodbine House, 2006.

Foa, Edna and Wilson, Reid. **Stop Obsessing.** Bantam Books, New York, 2001.

Greene, Ross W. **The Explosive Child: A New Approach for Understanding and Parenting Easily Frustrated, Chronically Inflexible Children.** New York: Harper Collins, 2001.

Kranowitz, Carol Stock. **The Out-of-Sync Child Has Fun, Activities for Kids with Sensory Integration Dysfunction.** New York: Berkley, 2003.

Kranowitz, Carol Stock. **The Out-of-Sync Child, Recognizing and Coping with Sensory Integration Dysfunction.** New York: Skylight Press, 1998.

Lynn, George T. **Survival Strategies for Parenting Your ADD Child with Obsessions, Compulsions, Depression, Explosive Behavior and Rage.** Nevada City, CA: Underwood Books, 1996.

Kutscher, L. Martin, Attwood, Tony, and Wolff, Robert R. **Kids in the Syndrome Mix of ADHD, LD, Asperger's, Tourette's, Bipolar, And More!: The One Stop Guide for Parents, Teachers and Other Professionals.** London: Jessica Kingsley Publishers, 2005. Levine, Mel. **A Mind at a Time.** New York: Simon and Schuster, 2003.

Manassis, Katharina and Levac, Anne-Marie. **Helping Your Teenager Beat Depression: A Problem-Solving Approach for Families.** Bethesda, MD: Woodbine House, 2004

Myles, Brenda Smith and Southwick, Jack. **Asperger Syndrome and Difficult Moments: Practical Solutions for Tantrums, Rages, and Meltdowns.** Revised ed. Shawnee Mission, KS: Autism Asperger Publishing Company, 2005.

Ottinger, Becky and Engh, Fred C. **Tictionary: A Reference Guide to the World of Tourette Syndrome, Asperger Syndrome, Attention Deficit Hyperactivity Disorder and Obsessive-Compulsive Disorder for Parents and Professionals.** Shawnee Mission, KS: Autism Asperger Publishing Company, 2003.

Rapaport, Judith. **The Boy Who Couldn't Stop Washing: The Experience and Treatment of Obsessive Compulsive Disorder.** New York: Plume Books, 1990.

Smith, Corinne and Strick, Lisa. **Learning Disabilities: A to Z: A Parent's Complete Guide to Learning Disabilities from Preschool to Adulthood.** New York: Free Press, 1999.

Vail, Priscilla. L. **Smart Kids with School Problems: Things to Know and Ways to Help.** New York: Plume, 1989.

Wagner, Aureen Pinto. **What to Do When Your Child Has Obsessive-Compulsive Disorder: Strategies and Solutions.** Lighthouse Point, FL: Lighthouse Press, 2002.

Whitney, Rondalyn Varney. **Bridging the Gap: Raising a Child with Nonverbal Learning Disorder.** New York: Berkley, 2002.

Publications for Children

Dendy, Chris Zeigler and Zeigler, Alex. **A Bird's-Eye View of ADD and AD/HD: Advice from Young Survivors.** Cedar Bluff, AL: Cherish the Children, 2003.

Fisher, Gary, Cummings, Rhoda, and Urbanovic, Jackie. **The Survival Guide for Kids with LD (Learning Differences).** 2nd ed. Minneapolis: Free Spirit, 2002.

Harrar, George. **Not as Crazy as I Seem.** Boston: Houghton Mifflin, 2003.

Hesser, Terry Spencer. **Kissing Doorknobs.** New York: Laurel Leaf, 1999.

Jackson, Luke and Attwood, Tony. **Freaks, Geeks and Asperger Syndrome: A User Guide to Adolescence.** (2002) Paperback. Jessica Kingsley Publishers.

Kranowitz, Carol Stock. **The Goodenoughs Get in Sync.** Las Vegas: Sensory Resources, 2004.

Levine, Melvin. **All Kinds of Minds: A Young Student's Book about Learning Abilities and Learning Disorders.** Educator's Publishing Service, 1992.

Levine, Melvin. **Keeping a Head in School: A Student's Book about Learning Abilities and Learning Disorders.** Educator's Publishing Service, 1990.

Moss, Deborah. **Shelley, the Hyperactive Turtle.** 2nd ed. Bethesda, MD: Woodbine House, 2006.

Walker, Beth. **A Girl's Guide to AD/HD: Don't Lose This Book!** Bethesda, MD: Woodbine House, 2004

Quinn, Patricia O. and Stern, Judith. **Putting on the Brakes: Young People's Guide to Attention Deficit Hyperactivity Disorder.** Washington, DC: Magination Press, 2001.

Wagner, Aureen Pinto. Up and Down the Worry Hill: **A Children's Book about Obsessive-Compulsive Disorder and Its Treatment.** Lighthouse Point, FL: Lighthouse Press, 2004.

:: Education

Dornbush, Marilyn and Pruitt, Sheryl K. **Teaching the Tiger: A Handbook for Individuals Involved in the Education of Students with Attention Deficit Disorders, Tourette Syndrome, or Obsessive-Compulsive Disorder.** Duarte, CA: Hope Press, 1995.

Dendy, Chris Zeigler. **Teaching Teenagers with ADD and ADHD: A Quick Reference Guide for Teachers and Parents.** Bethesda, MD: Woodbine House, 2000.

Tanquay, Pamela B. and Thompson, Sue. **Nonverbal Learning Disabilities at School: Educating Students with NLD, Asperger Syndrome and Related Conditions.** London: Jessica Kingsley Publishers, 2002.

Understanding Tourette Syndrome: A Handbook for Educators. Toronto: The Tourette Syndrome Foundation of Canada, 2001.

Strichart, Stephen and Mangrum, Charles. **Teaching Learning Strategies and Study Skills to Students with Learning Disabilities, Attention Deficit Disorders, and or Special Needs.** 3rd ed. Boston: Allyn and Bacon, 2001.

Wright, Peter and Wright, Pamela. **From Emotions to Advocacy: The Special Education Survival Guide.** Harbor House Law Press, 2006.

:: Family Life

Baskin, Amy and Fawcett, Heather. **More Than a Mom: Living a Full and Balanced Life When Your Child Has Special Needs.** Bethesda, MD: Woodbine House, 2006.

Marshak, Laura and Prezant, Fran. **Married with (Special Needs) Children: A Couple's Guide to Keeping Connected.** Bethesda, MD: Woodbine House, 2006.

McHugh, Mary. **Special Siblings: Growing Up with Someone with a Disability.** Baltimore: Paul H. Brookes, 2002.

Meyer, Don. **The Sibling Slam Book: What It's *Really* Like to Have a Brother or Sister with Special Needs.** Bethesda, MD: Woodbine House, 2005.

Meyer, Don. **Views from Our Shoes: Growing Up with a Brother or Sister with Special Needs.** Bethesda, MD: Woodbine House, 1997.

Satter, Ellyn. **How to Get Your Child to Eat … But Not Too Much.** Boulder, CO: Bull Publishing, 1987.

∷ Medical Issues

Schwartz, Jeffrey M. and Begley, Sharon. **The Mind and The Brain: Neuroplasticity and the Power of Mental Force.** New York: Regan Books, 2003.

Roberts, Elizabeth J. **Should You Medicate Your Child's Mind? A Child Psychiatrist Makes Sense of Whether to Give Kids Psychiatric Medication.** New York: Marlowe and Co., 2006.

Wilens, Timothy. **Straight Talk about Psychiatric Medications for Kids.** Revised ed. New York: Guilford Press, 2004.

RESOURCE GUIDE

The organizations, companies, and other resources listed below offer a variety of services that can be helpful to families of children with Tourette Syndrome and associated disorders living in North America. For further information about any of these organizations, call, write, or visit their web page, where you will find a plethora of great resources, articles, books, and services.

There are thousands of resources now online. Since there are too many resources on the Internet to even begin to list, I suggest you google search your topic and you will see how much help there is in cyberspace.

This resource guide is just a beginning in a quest for information on TS and associated disorders. We did not include specific scientific articles because there are so many and they change so fast. The national Tourette Syndrome Association publishes an annual research update, which is an excellent way to keep up-to-date.

In addition, there are some long-established, reputable websites that provide free, up-to-date research information and are worth visiting:

- **PubMed** (a service of the U.S. National Library of Medicine) at www.pubmed.gov—This website enables you to search medical journals and read the "abstracts" of most articles. These are short summaries of the articles. Sometimes you receive the full article. You can go to the website and search for Tourette, Obsessive Compulsive Disorder, Attention Deficit Disorder, Sensory integration—whatever specific topic you are looking for.
- **Google Scholar** at www.scholar.google.com—This is another good online search engine that searches through scholarly papers on many different topics.
- **Education Resources Information Center (ERIC)** at www.eric.ed.gov—This website, associated with the U.S. Department of Education, enables you to search over a million articles on education topics, and, in many cases, retrieve the full text of the original article.

When using one of these websites to search, you can set the search engine to limit what years of material is searched. It is important to look at the date on any research article, as there is often outdated information in older studies.

■■ Organizations & Websites

All Kinds of Minds Website
www.allkindsofminds.org
> Website with information on learning differences and links to many other online resources on learning disabilities, AD/HD, and other learning differences.

American Association of University Centers on Disabilities (AUCD)
1010 Wayne Av, Ste. 920
Silver Spring, MD 20910
301-588-8252
www.aucd.org
> Services and programs for children with disabilities are available through many universities. The national office above can help you locate the university affiliated program closest to you.

American Occupational Therapy Association
4720 Montgomery Lane
P.O. Box 31220
Bethesda, MD 20824-1220
301-652-2682; 301-652-7711 (fax)
www.aota.org
> The AOTA is a professional organization for occupational therapists. The organization distributes publications, and can refer you to an OT in your area.

American Physical Therapy Association
1111 N. Fairfax St.
Alexandria, VA 22314
703-684-2782; 800-999-2782
www.apta.org
> This professional organization for physical therapists offers publications of interest to parents and educators, education, advocacy, and research.

American Speech-Language-Hearing Association
10801 Rockville Pike
Rockville, MD 20852
800-638-8255; 301-897-0157 (TDD)
www.asha.org
> ASHA can provide information on speech and language therapy and audiologists in your area. It also distributes brochures on speech and hearing disorders.

The Arc of the US
1010 Wayne Av, Ste. 650
Silver Spring, MD 20910
301-565-3842
www.thearc.org/welcome.html
> Formerly known as the Association for Retarded Citizens, this is an organization for people with disabilities and their families. It has a publications catalog with publications on many aspects of developmental delays, and also supports a large network of local chapters.

Autism Society of America
7910 Woodmont Ave., Ste. 300
Bethesda, MD 20814
800-328-8476; 301-657-0881
www.autism-society.org
    The oldest membership organization for families of people with autism in the United States, the ASA is a good starting point for gathering information if you suspect that your child might have Asperger syndrome or another autism spectrum disorder.

CH.A.D.D. (Children and Adults with Attention Deficit Disorders)
8181 Professional Place, Ste. 150
Landover, MD 20785
800-233-4050; 301-306-7090 (fax)
www.chadd.org
    CHADD is a membership organization for families and individuals with attention deficit disorders which provides support and education for families, advocates for the rights of individuals with ADD, supports research, and offers a variety of publications. Website has local contacts.

Children's Defense Fund
25 E St. NW
Washington, DC 20001
800-CDF-1200; 202-628-8787
www.childrensdefense.org
    CDF is a legal organization that works to expand the rights of children, including children with disabilities. It can provide information on topics such as insurance and childcare.

Consortium for Appropriate Dispute Resolution in Special Education (CADRE)
P.O. Box 51360
Eugene, OR 97405-0906
541-686-5060; 541-686-5063 (fax)
www.directionservice.org/cadre
    CADRE provides technical assistance to state departments of education on the implementation of mediation requirements under IDEA. CADRE also supports parents, educators, and administrators by proposing options that will facilitate resolution for issues of conflict in special education programs. Offers pertinent articles and lists state contacts for CADRE projects.

Council for Exceptional Children
1110 North Glebe Rd, Ste. 300
Arlington, VA 22201
888-232-7733; 703-264-9446 (TDD)
www.cec.sped.org
    This is a membership organization for educators interested in the needs of children who have disabilities or are gifted. Their publication catalog offers a number of materials on education-related topics. Website has information on Canadian CEC.

The Dana Foundation & The Dana Alliance for Brain Initiative
745 Fifth Ave., Ste 900
New York, NY 10151
212-233-4040
www.dana.org
　　The Dana Foundation is committed to advancing education about current brain research findings and immunology. The website has fun educational games and great articles on the brain. Dana Press offers free newsletters on Brain research in a variety of areas of interest. There is also a European branch.

Jim Eisenreich Foundation for Children with Tourette Syndrome
P.O. Box 953
Blue Springs, MO 64013
800-442-8624
www.tourettes.org
　　This foundation, founded by the author of this book's foreword and his wife, strives to "build avenues of success for every child with TS through programs and services which address the needs of families, educators, peers, and medical professionals." The website offers free resources guides for principals, teachers, counselors, and support staff, as well as an extensive list of helpful publications for children with TS of all ages. The foundation also hosts stadium visits with Jim Eisenreich and children with TS at local baseball stadiums.

Epilepsy Canada
1470 Peel St., Ste. 745
Montreal, Quebec H3A 1T1
Canada
514-845-7855
Website: www.epilepsy.ca/eng/mainSet.html
　　Dedicated to improving the quality of life for people with epilepsy and their families, Epilepsy Canada offers a variety of informational brochures and publishes a newsletter.

Epilepsy Foundation of America
4351 Garden City Dr.
Landover, MD 20785
800-EFA-I000; 301-577-2684 (fax)
www.efa.org
　　The EFA works for the prevention and cure of seizure disorders and promotes independence and optimal quality of life for people with epilepsy. It has a lengthy publication catalog, provides information and referral, supports local parent and family networks, and advocates on behalf of individuals with epilepsy.

Families USA – The Voice for Health Care Consumers
1201 New York Ave NW, Ste. 1100
Washington, DC 20005
202-628-3030
202-347-2417 (fax)
Website: familiesusa.org/index.html
　　This national nonprofit, nonpartisan organization provides information and resources related to healthcare public policy and tracks the progress of legislation affecting managed care and Medicaid. Lists links to pertinent web sites and has publications, which can be mailed or downloaded on computer, regarding health insurance, especially Medicaid, and prescription medications. Lists relevant information state by state.

Family Village
www.familyvillage.wisc.edu
This website describes itself as "a global village of disability-related resources." It includes full text articles on specific disabilities, education issues, legal issues, recreation, and more, as well as opportunities to connect with others and extensive links to information, products, and resources.

Family Voices, Inc.
National Office
2340 Alamo SE, Ste. 102
Albuquerque, NM 87106
505-872-4774; 888-835-5669
www.familyvoices.org
A grassroots clearinghouse for information and education concerning health care of children with special health needs. Offers a newsletter, fact sheet, list of publications, and an advocacy handbook.

Henry Occupational Therapy Services, Inc.
500 N Estrella Pkwy, Ste B2-454
Goodyear, AZ 85338
623-882-8812
www.ateachabout.com
Henry Occupational Therapy Services provides training and products to professionals on sensory integration. Their mission is to promote understanding and awareness of issues related to sensory processing, sensory integration, and the sensory systems. Their website has information, links, and books on the subject of sensory integration.

International Dyslexia Association
8600 LaSalle Rd.
Chester Bldg., Ste. 382
Baltimore, MD 21286-2044
410-296-0232; 410-321-5069 (fax)
www.interdys.org
Formerly known as the Orton Dyslexia Society, this nonprofit organization supports research into dyslexia, publishes periodicals and books, and provides information and referral services through its local branches. Great website!

Internet Mental Health Website
www.mentalhealth.com
Website with information on OCD, ADHD, depression, TS, etc. There are links to more articles on these and related issues.

Learning Disabilities Association of America
4156 Library Rd.
Pittsburgh, PA 15234
412-341-1515
www.ldanatl.org
The LDA has over 500 local affiliates dedicated to supporting individuals with learning disabilities. The national office offers a wide range of publications, and can provide information on educational programs, laws, and advocacy.

Learning Disabilities Association of Canada
323 Chapel St.
Ottawa, Ontario K1N 7Z2
Canada
613-238-5721; 613-245-5391 (fax)
www.ldac-taac.ca
This nonprofit organization advocates for, and offers information about people with LD in Canada.

Learning Disabilities Online
www.ldonline.org
Website with information on learning disabilities, ADHD, etc. There are many useful articles, resources, and links.

National Alliance on Mental Illness
Colonial Place Three
2107 Wilson Blvd, Ste. 300
Arlington, VA 22201-3042
703-524-7600; 703-524-9094 (fax)
888-999-6264
www.nami.org
NAMI is the U.S.'s largest grassroots mental health organization dedicated to improving the lives of people with mental illness and their families. Their website has information on advocacy, programs, resources, and it lists all state contacts for child/adolescent network locations. There are links to many other good sites.

National Association of Cognitive-Behavioral Therapists
P.O. Box 2195
Weirton, WV 26062
800-853-1135; 304-723-3982
www.nacbt.org
From the website of this professional association, you can search for a mental health professional in your area who is a certified cognitive-behavioral therapist.

National Association of Private Schools for Exceptional Children
1522 K Street NW, Ste. 1032
Washington, DC 20005
202-408-3338; 202-408-3340 (fax)
www.napsec.org
This professional association publishes a newsletter and a directory of private schools for children with special needs.

National Association of Protection & Advocacy Systems (NAPAS)
900 Second Street, NE, Ste. 211
Washington, DC 20002
202-408-9514; 202-408-9520 (fax)
www.protectionandadvocacy.com
NAPAS can refer you to your local protection and advocacy office for help with IDEA disputes, discrimination complaints, etc. Interesting information on a variety of issues on the website.

National Attention Deficit Disorder Association (ADDA)
P.O. Box 543
Pottstown, PA 19464
484-945-2101
www.add.org/index.html
    ADDA is an organization focused on the needs of adults and young adults with AD/HD and their families. This organization offers relevant articles, answers to frequently asked questions, means to contact AD/HD professionals, and information regarding support groups, conferences, books, and other resources.

National Center for Learning Disabilities
381 Park Ave So, Ste. 1401
New York, NY 10016
212-545-7510; 212-545-9665
888-575-7373
www.ncld.org
    This parent-professional organization dedicated to working for the success of individuals with learning disabilities of all ages has a great website on learning disabilities organized by age group with resources, publications, advocacy, and online experts.

National Council on Disability
1331 F Street NW, Ste. 850
Washington, DC 20004
202-272-2004; 202-272-2022 (fax)
www.ncd.gov
    The NCD is an independent federal policy agency that makes recommendations to the president and congress on disability policy and represents all people with disabilities, regardless of severity, age, or cultural background. Website has links to other major federal agencies concerned with disabilities, resources including means to contact your state senators and representatives, a guide to disability rights laws, information regarding IEPs and IFSPs, etc.

National Council on Independent Living
1710 Rhode Island Ave. NW, 5th Floor
Washington, DC 20036
202-207-0334; 703-525-3409 (fax)
www.ncil.org
    A source of information on affordable and accessible housing for people with disabilities.

National Disability Rights Network
900 2nd St., Ste. 211
Washington, DC 20002
202-408-9514
www.napas.org
    NAPAS can refer you to your local protection and advocacy office for help with IDEA disputes, discrimination complaints, etc.

National Dissemination Center for Children with Disabilities (NICHCY)
P.O. Box 1492
Washington, DC 20013
800-695-0285; 202-884-8200 (voice/TDD)
www.nichcy.org
    This clearinghouse specializes in providing information on educational programs and other issues important to families of children with disabilities. Many publications can be download free from the web site, or ordered for a nominal fee in hard copy. Especially useful are NICHCY's "State Sheets," which list a variety of support and other organizations in each state.

National Health Information Center
Office of Disease Prevention and Health Promotion
U.S. Dept. of Health and Human Services
Office of the Secretary
1101 Wootton Pkwy, Ste. LL100
Rockville, MD 20852
240-453-8280
www.health.gov/nhic
    The NHIC was established to help both professionals and the general public locate health information. Offers an information and referral system and a database of organizations and government offices with health information that can be searched online.

National Organization on Disability (NOD)
910 Sixteenth Street, NW, Ste. 600
Washington, DC 20006
202-293-5960; 202-293-7999 (fax)
www.nod.org
    NOD is a national disability network organization concerned with all disabilities, all age groups, and all disability issues. Provides a fact sheet on ADA, as well as answers to frequently asked questions regarding disability and accessibility.

National Rehabilitation Information Center (NARIC)
4200 Forbes Blvd., Ste. 202
Lanham, MD 20706
800-346-2742; 301-587-1967 (fax)
www.naric.com/naric/index.html
    The staff of NARIC collects and disseminates the results of federally funded research projects related to disability and rehabilitation.

Nonverbal Learning Disabilities Association (NLDA)
2446 Albany Ave.
West Hartford, CT 06117
860-570-0217; 860-570-0218 (fax)
www.nlda.org
    Children with NLD tend to have good verbal abilities, but difficulties with nonverbal tasks, such as visual-spatial skills, math, and organization. NLD is common in children with Asperger syndrome. The NLDA, a membership organization, offers an online forum, informational articles, and conferences.

Obsessive Compulsive Foundation
676 State Street
New Haven, CT 06511
203-401-2070; 203-401-2076 (fax)
www.ocfoundation.org

OCF is a national organization composed of people with OCD and related disorders, their families, professionals, and other concerned individuals. This is the first source for information on OCD, with local and state contacts at the website.

Office of the Americans with Disabilities Act
Civil Rights Division
U.S. Dept. of Justice
950 Pennsylvania Ave. NW
Washington, DC 20530
800-514-0301; 800-514-0383 (TDD)
www.usdoj.gov/crt/ada/adahom1.htm

This is the federal agency charged with distributing information and answering questions from the public about the Americans with Disabilities Act. Information can be obtained on the website or sent by fax or U.S. mail.

Office of Special Education and Rehabilitative Services (OSERS)
U.S. Department of Education
400 Maryland Ave. SW
Washington, DC 20202
800-872-5327
www.ed.gov/offices/OSERS

This federal organization offers information on civil rights, federal benefits, medical services, education, and support organizations. It publishes OSERS News in Print, a newsletter regarding federal activities affecting people with disabilities, and Pocket Guide to Federal Help for Individuals with Disabilities, a summary of services and benefits available to individuals who qualify.

Online Asperger Syndrome Information and Support (O.A.S.I.S.)
www.udel.edu/bkirby/asperger

Website by parents of children with Asperger syndrome. This website has a lot of information and support for families, teachers, and other professionals who work with children with AS. There is information on social skills, school issues, adult issues, support groups, etc. There is a very comprehensive bookstore with books on many topics of interest to families with TS with or without Aspergers.

Parents Advocacy Coalition for Educational Rights (PACER)
8161 Normandale Blvd.
Minneapolis, MN 55437-1044
952-838-9000; 800-537-2237
952-838-0199 (fax)
www.pacer.org OR www.fape.org

An organization founded by parents to help other parents locate the support and resources they need in raising children and young adults with disabilities. Offers a catalog of publications, a computer resource center, relevant articles, and a summary of services available to individuals who qualify.

School Psychology Resources Online

www.schoolpsychology.net

Online resources for psychologists, parents, and educators. Website has information on TS and many related disorders with book lists and educational articles that can be downloaded and taken to school. There are articles on many possible issues such as sensory integration, bullying, depression, anxiety disorders, etc.

Senate Document Room

Hart Building B-04
Washington, DC 20510
202-224-7701 (fax)
www.senate.gov/legislative/common/generic/doc_room.htm

You can obtain a copy of any federal bill or law, including IDEA or the ADA, by contacting this office or going to website.

Sensory Integration International

P.O. Box 5339
Torrance, CA 90510-5339
310-787-8805; 310-787-8047 (fax)
www.sensoryint.com

The Ayres Clinic is a nonprofit organization committed to increasing knowledge about sensory integration disorders. They promote education about how sensory processing affects every area of a person's life. Their website offers articles, publications, workshops, research, and training for people with SI disorders, professionals, and families.

Social Security Administration

Office of Public Inquiries
6401 Security Boulevard
Room 4-C-5 Annex
Baltimore, MD 21235-6401
800-777-1213
www.ssa.gov

A government program offering economic protection to retirees and people with disabilities, as well as their survivors. Website offers online application for SSI and Medicare, downloadable forms and many pertinent publications, and an explanation of Social Security statements.

TASH

29 W. Susquehanna Ave., Ste. 210
Baltimore, MD 21204
410-828-8274
www.tash.org

TASH is an international advocacy organization that works for the inclusion of people with disabilities in every aspect of life. It publishes a journal and a newsletter.

Tourette Foundation of Canada

#206, 194 Jarvis Street
Toronto, Ontario M5B 2B7
800-361-3120; 416-861-8398
416-861-2472 (fax)

National TS Foundation of Canada should be the first stop for families with TS who live in Canada. This organization has state chapters, which you can find at their website.

The website lists upcoming conferences and information on TS and associated disorders and includes a Kid's Korner, bulletin board, and links to many other resources.

Tourette Syndrome Association
42-40 Bell Boulevard
Bayside, NY 11361
718-224-2999; 718-279-9596 (fax)
www.tsa-usa.org
 TSA National is a must-have resource for families with TS. Committed to finding the cause and cure for TS and controlling the effects of TS, the TSA can link families with many resources in education, medical knowledge, counseling, research, science, advocacy, and fund raising. The website has state and local contact information and many helpful links.

Tourette Syndrome Online
www.tourette-syndrome.com
 Great website with every kind of article on TS and associated disorders, links to other resources, chat and email chat, pen pals, and a TS store with lots of books. Hosted by the father of a boy with Tourette syndrome.

Tourette Syndrome Plus
www.tourettesyndrome.net
 This is my very favorite website on TS and associated issues. It is the most comprehensive as far as current articles for families covering TS and associated disorders. These articles are very easy to read, or to download and take to teachers, family members, or other professionals. There are book lists and other links to help families with TS. This website is run by Leslie Packer, Ph.D., who is a parent of two children with TS. She is also a psychologist and an activist in making life better for people with TS and their families.

U.S. Department of Education
Clearinghouse on Disability Information
400 Maryland Ave., SW
Washington, DC 20202
800-USA-LEARN; 202-205-8245
202-401-0689 (fax)
www.ed.gov/index/html OR http://ericec.org
 The mission of the US Department of Education is to ensure equal access to education and to promote educational excellence for all Americans. Its website provides information regarding initiatives, grant opportunities, research, statistics, and publications. ERIC, the clearinghouse on disability information, gathers and disseminates professional literature, information, and resources on the education and development of individuals of all ages who have disabilities and/or who are gifted.

:: Products

Autism Asperger Publishing Company
P.O. Box 23173
Shawnee Mission, KS 66283-0173
877-277-8254; 913-897-1004
www.asperger.net
 This company publishes books for parents and professionals on autism, Asperger syndrome, and other pervasive developmental disorders.

Hope Press
P. O. Box 188
Duarte, CA 91009-0188
800-321-4039; 626-358-3520
www.hopepress.com
    This publishing company specializes in books on TS, AD/HD, oppositional defiant disorder, and similar conditions.

Mend Solutions
www.mend.net
    Website by Dr Carl Hansen, one of our chapter authors. This website has information and products to help people live a healthy life and reach their full potential. It has practical information written in simple language to help people with TS improve their health and manage symptoms.

Online Clinic
www.online-clinic.com
    Website by one of our chapter authors, Dr Larry Burd. This website has links to booklets written by Dr Larry Burd on TS, OCD, ADHD, and learning disorders.

Sensory Comfort
P.O. Box 6589
Portsmouth, NH 03802-6589
www.sensorycomfort.com
888-436-2622
    This company sells products designed to "help make the world a friendlier place for those with sensory processing differences."

Sensory Resources, LLC
2500 Chandler Ave., Ste. 3
Las Vegas, NV 89120-4064
888-357-5867; 702-433-0404
702-891-8899 (fax)
www.sensoryresources.com
    Resources for raising children with sensory motor, developmental, and social/emotional challenges. The company sells books, videos, and tapes on sensory-related problems; website includes helpful links to other resources and information on upcoming workshops on SI.

Southpaw Enterprises
P.O. Box 1047
Dayton, OH 45401
800-228-1698; 937-252-7676
www.southpawenterprises.com
    A company that specializes in products, equipment, and resources for children with sensory integration and developmental challenges.

Therapy Works, Inc.
4901 Butte Place, NW
Albuquerque, NM 87120
877-897-3478; 505-899-4071 (fax)
www.alertprogram.com
    This company markets "The Alert Program"—a program to teach parents and children to regulate their nervous systems through learning strategies, awareness ,and skills to help make the nervous system respond in ways that help us live successful lives. For children with TS, who have nervous system disorders, this program may be very interesting and helpful.

CONTRIBUTORS

Dr. Larry Burd is a professor in the Department of Pediatrics at the University of North Dakota School of Medicine. He is also affiliated with the Child Evaluation and Treatment Program (CETP) at the Rehabilitation Hospital in Grand Forks, ND. Over the past twenty-one years, Dr. Burd has evaluated and developed intervention programs for several thousand children with developmental disorders. He has published more than 100 professional papers on topics dealing with development and behavior in children and adolescents, as well as written three handbooks for parents and teachers on Tourette syndrome, attention-deficit/hyperactivity disorder, and obsessive-compulsive disorder.

Dr. Patricia Furer is a Clinical Psychologist with the Anxiety Disorders Program at St. Boniface General Hospital in Winnepeg, Manitoba, and an Associate Professor in the Department of Clinical Health Psychology at the University of Manitoba.

Dr. Carl R. Hansen, Jr., is a graduate of the University of Minnesota Medical School and was a Child Psychiatry Fellow at the Yale University Child Study Center, 1982 through 1984, where he was honored with the Berger Research and Merck fellowships. Dr. Hansen is the President and Executive Director of MEND (Developmental Neurobiology and Ecology, Inc.), which is a solution-oriented research and development company. In his private medical practice at the Hansen Neuropsychiatric Clinic, Dr. Hansen specializes in the diagnosis and treatment of neurobiological and developmental disorders. He is an authority on neurobiological conditions such as Tourette syndrome, obsessive-compulsive disorder, and attention deficit disorders, and has published a number of scientific papers, abstracts, letters, and chapters in the area of toxicology, neurobiology, and psychiatry.

Robin Jewers is a Senior Occupational Therapist for Rehabilitation Services at St. Boniface General Hospital in Winnipeg, Manitoba, and performs clinical duties for the Tourette Syndrome Service.

Marilynn Kaplan is the parent of a young adult son who experienced severe Tourette Syndrome and associated neuro-biological difficulties during his school years. She is a past-president of Minnesota TSA and served on the board of directors of National TSA, PACER (Parent Advocacy for Educational Rights), and the Governor's Ombudsman's Committee on Mental Health and Retardation for Minnesota. She founded the Tourette Traveling Troupe to educate the public about TS. She has received several local and national honors for her volunteer work on behalf of children. Marilynn holds a Master's Degree in Special Education and is employed as a special education teacher.

Dr. Jacob Kerbeshian is a board certified child and adolescent psychiatrist who holds the rank of Clinical Professor of Neuroscience at the University of North Dakota School of Medicine and Health Sciences. He practices at the Altru Health System in Grand Forks, ND.

Sonja D. Kerr received a J.D. from the Indiana University School of Law in Indianapolis and an M.S. from Purdue University in Counseling Psychology. She is presently an attorney with Alaska Legal Services and also maintains a small private practice in special education and related projects. Prior to her employment with ALS, she was Supervising Attorney with the Disability Law Center of Alaska, where she practiced in the areas of special education, the Americans with Disabilities Act, and mental health law. In addition, she was in private practice in Minnesota and other Midwestern states for fifteen years exclusively in the area of special education, and represented many children with disabilities, including Tourette Syndrome. Ms. Kerr is past chair of the Counsel of Parent Attorneys and Advocates (COPAA), has served on the advisory board for TSA Minnesota, and has been active in a variety of disability organizations.

Tracy Marsh is the mother of two adult children, one of whom has Tourette syndrome. She holds a B.S. in social work and has experience in adolescent counseling. She is a past president of TSA Minnesota, past director of MN TSA Family Learning Camp, and has worked as a parent advocate and educator. She was also the editor of the first edition of *Children with Tourette Syndrome* (Woodbine House, 1992).

Rosanne Papadopoulos is an Occupational Therapist in private practice in Winnipeg, Manitoba.

John Piacentini, Ph.D., is Professor-in-Residence and Director of the Child OCD, Anxiety, and Tic Disorder Program at the UCLA Semel Institute for Neuroscience and Human Behavior and Chair of the Tourette Syndrome Association Behavioral Sciences Consortium.

William Rubin is the founder and president of Synthesis, Inc., a mental health research and consulting company in Columbus, Ohio. He received his bachelor's degree with honors in psychology from Brandeis University and earned a master's degree in psychology from the University of Nebraska. Although his tics began as a child, Bill was not diagnosed with Tourette syndrome until age thirty-five, after which he became active in the Tourette Syndrome Association of Ohio. He served as an officer for several years and its first Director of Training, Research, and Development. He also helped the Tourette syndrome Association of Minnesota to start the first U.S. camp for children with TS and their families.

Dr. Gary Shady is a Clinical Psychologist with the Child and Adolescent Program, St. Boniface General Hospital, Winnipeg, Manitoba. He is also Consultant to the Tourette Syndrome Service and Associate Professor in the Department of Clinical Health Psychology, University of Manitoba.

Dr. Rox Wand is a Consultant Psychiatrist at Simon Fraser Youth Day Treatment Program, Coquitlam, B.C.

INDEX

ABOUT THE EDITOR

Tracy Lynne Marsh is editor of the previous edition of *CHILDREN WITH TOURETTE SYNDROME*. She is a past president of the Minnesota chapter of the Tourette Syndrome Association, and has done in-service training for schools and community groups. She has a degree in social work from the University of Minnesota. The mother of two, including a son with Tourette syndrome now in his twenties, Marsh lives with her family in Lakeville, Minnesota.